ADVANCED PRACTICE NURSING IN THE COMMUNITY

CARL O. HELVIE R.N., Dr.P.H.

Professor of Nursing, Old Dominion University,
Norfolk, Virginia

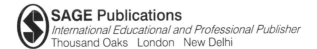
SAGE Publications
International Educational and Professional Publisher
Thousand Oaks   London   New Delhi

For information:

 SAGE Publications, Inc.
2455 Teller Road
Thousand Oaks, California 91320
E-mail: order@sagepub.com

SAGE Publications Ltd.
6 Bonhill Street
London EC2A 4PU
United Kingdom

SAGE Publications India Pvt. Ltd.
M-32 Market
Greater Kailash I
New Delhi 110 048 India

Printed in the United States of America

Library of Congress Cataloging-in-Publication Data

Main entry under title:

Advanced practice nursing in the community / edited by Carl O. Helvie.
    p. cm.
  Includes bibliographical references and index.
  ISBN 0-7619-0034-9 (cloth: acid-free paper).—ISBN
0-7619-0035-7 (pbk.: acid-free paper)
   1. Community health nursing. 2. Public health. I. Helvie, Carl O.
RT98.A37 1997
610.73′43—dc21   97-4752

This book is printed on acid-free paper.

99 00 01 02 03 10 9 8 7 6 5 4 3

Acquiring Editor:	Dan Ruth
Editorial Assistant:	Jessica L. Crawford
Production Editor:	Sanford Robinson
Production Assistant:	Denise Santoyo
Copy Editor:	Linda Gray
Typesetter/Designer:	Rebecca Evans
Indexer:	Julie Sherman Grayson
Cover Designer:	Ravi Balasuriya

This book is dedicated to Wilfried Kunstmann, Dortmund, Germany, colleague, friend, teacher, thinker, and questioner, and to those students who also questioned and helped me clarify my thoughts.

Brief Outline

Contents

PART III Community Assessment

Acknowledgments

I am grateful to many individuals who offered assistance in the preparation of this text. To acknowledge them all would be impossible within the limits of this section and the memory of the author. Thus, I apologize for any oversights, which are unintentional.

First, I acknowledge my graduate students in community health nursing who offered comments and stimulating questions over the past years as I taught the course on which this book is based. I am grateful to each of you. I am especially grateful to Chris Elnitsky, currently a doctoral student, and to James Hosack, a White House nurse, who stimulated me to refine the energy theory.

Next, I thank each of the contributors for the case studies and for the chapter on rural nursing. Their experience in applying the concepts in practice has added greatly to the book. In addition, their promptness in submitting the materials facilitated the meeting of deadlines.

I thank each of the reviewers of the original proposal for their comments and confidence in me and the reviewers of the completed manuscript for their valuable comments for refining the manuscript. These have strengthened the book. I thank my chair of nursing, Dr. Brenda S. Nichols, who reviewed and commented on the proposal and who approved a semester's leave from my teaching position for writing the book. Thanks also go to Dean Lindsay Rettie and Vice President for Academic Affairs JoAnn Gora, who also had confidence in me and who approved my leave for writing. I also thank my colleague, Dr. Laurel Garzon, who provided continued support and encouragement.

I also thank members of the leadership group of community health nursing of the American Public Health Association for their encouragement. I am especially grateful to Dr. Caroline White, past chair, Community Health Nursing Section of APHA who provided support and continued encouragement.

Last but not least, I acknowledge Christine S. Smedley, previous sponsoring editor, Sage Publications, for her confidence in offering a contract for the book. I also recognize Mr. Daniel Ruth, my current editor at Sage, for his support and help in obtaining reviews of the manuscript, providing contracts to contributors, and providing other assistance that facilitated the production process and enhanced the quality of the book.

Preface

This book is written for beginning graduate students in community health nursing or for nurses who need a community or aggregate focus in practice. It is the result of needing to use large numbers of articles for teaching graduate students in community health nursing over several years because a text that focused on multiple aspects of the community, aggregates, or both was not available. The text is different from other community health nursing texts and the author's previous community health nursing texts because it has a narrow and in-depth focus on the community and aggregates rather than covering the total field of community health nursing.

Part I presents a book overview and a review of community health nursing concepts. The review covers timely concepts such as generalist versus specialist, community-based and population-focused nursing, and community health nursing or public health nursing, roles, and models. This review is useful for the nurse who has not studied or practiced community health nursing recently.

Part II discusses a theoretical framework for the book. The theory selected to view the community or aggregate is the Helvie energy theory, a systems theory developed around the concept of energy. Models for using this theory in practice are included.

Part III explores community assessment. Chapters 3, 4, and 5 in this section discuss the influence of economic, environmental, and sociocultural forces on the health of the community. Concepts and models related to these topics are presented. Special social and cultural aggregates, such as the homeless and migrant populations and African American, Native American, Asian American, and Latino American populations, are included. In addition, two case studies by community health nursing leaders in practice using the concepts presented for economic and environmental forces influencing health and nursing are presented. Chapters 6 and 7 present concepts and models for community assessment and community analysis. These concepts are applied to a fictitious community, and a nursing leader applies the concepts of community assessment to an actual community.

Part IV covers community planning and interventions. Chapter 8 discusses the planning of community interventions and includes the planning process, concepts of community organization, community change, multilevel models of planning interventions, and other related concepts and models. Chapter 9 explores the planning for diffusion of programs and the maintenance of program changes initiated in the community. A case study by a nursing leader who used diffusion theory in the community to maximize the effects of a program is included. Chapter 10 looks at the first two community- or aggregate-focused interventions and includes concepts and models related to using mass media and the political process to introduce change into a community. Case studies by nursing leaders for these two interventions are included. Chapter 11 presents empowerment, coalition building, and involving professionals and the lay community as community interventions. Models and concepts appropriate to these overall concepts and three case studies by nursing leaders are presented. Chapter 12 discusses concepts of nursing centers, mass immunization clinics, community partnerships, and school nursing as aggregate interventions. A case study by a nursing leader who has developed and implemented a nursing center is included. Chapter 13 discusses the application of these interventions in a rural setting.

Part V introduces community evaluation and presents concepts of outcome variables for measuring community change, components of evaluation, study outcome variables, and other appropriate concepts.

It is the desire of the author that the book will assist the nursing student or practitioner to view the community as the focus of practice. This should be the domain of community health nursing.

PART I

OVERVIEW

CHAPTER 1

INTRODUCTION

OBJECTIVES

1. Contrast official definitions of community health nursing.

2. Differentiate between different views of public health nursing and community health nursing.

3. Summarize a usable philosophy of community health nursing.

4. Discuss multiple roles of community health nurses.

5. Relate community health nursing to the objectives of *Healthy People 2000* and the World Health Organization's goal for the year 2000.

6. Use an epidemiological preventive model in community health nursing.

BOOK OVERVIEW

This text is for the graduate student in community health nursing who is studying the community as the focus of care or the practitioner who needs to strengthen concepts related to community-focused care. Part I, containing this chapter, offers an overview of the book's organization and a brief review of major concepts in community health nursing. The review should be useful to nurses who have not worked in or studied community health nursing recently. Part II, containing Chapter 2, provides a theoretical framework for the book based on the energy theory developed by Helvie (1991, 1995). This theory uses a systems approach that revolves around the concept of energy.

Part III presents concepts needed in community assessment. Chapters 3, 4, and 5 evaluate selected forces—economic, environmental, and sociocultural— that affect the community and that must be assessed. Each of these chapters presents appropriate *Healthy People 2000* objectives (U.S. Department of Health and Human Services [DHHS], 1991). At the end of Chapter 3 is a case study by Angela Savage and Anna Pratt showing how economic forces in the community influence decisions about nursing care. Chapter 4 ends with a case study by Jackie Agnew on an environmental health intervention concerning lead poisoning.

Chapter 6 presents community assessment concepts and includes approaches, methods, tools (some of them based on models proposed by other nurse theorists), and an application of community assessment concepts for a fictitious community, "Rudyville," using the Helvie energy theory. The chapter ends with a case study by Christine Elnitsky that uses the Helvie energy theoretical framework to assess a real community—a rural county. Chapter 7 offers concepts of community analysis and community diagnosis and applies them to the assessment data for "Rudyville" presented in Chapter 6.

Part IV covers community planning and interventions. Chapter 8 discusses the planning process; validating the community nursing diagnosis; setting community priorities; and identifying definitions, concepts, principles, and models of community organization. It also presents concepts of community power and politics in planning and useful theories of community change, including multilevel community intervention models. Chapter 9 presents concepts for planning to reach the community aggregate of interest or the community targeted (diffusion theory) and for institutionalizing the community changes implemented following the trial period or completion of funding. It is concluded by a case study by Sondra Riedesel Oppewal on the application of diffusion theory concepts to the dissemination of an arthritis education program. Chapters 10 and 11 discuss concepts concerning use of the mass media, use of the political process, coalition building, empowerment strategies, and the formation of partnerships in community-focused interventions. Two case studies, one on use of the mass media by Bethany Hall-Long and one on use of the political process by Clare Houseman, conclude Chapter 10. Chapter 11 ends with three case studies—two on community empowerment interventions by Laurel Garzon and by Kathleen May and Sandra Ferketich, and one illustrating coalition building by Janie Canty-Mitchell and Sharon Garrett. Chapter 12 discusses interventions with community aggregates, such as nursing centers that provide care for populations of the elderly or the homeless; special mass clinics offering immunizations for preschoolers or flu injections for the elderly or others with chronic illnesses; and interventions in schools and occupational settings. It concludes with a case study by Doris Glick, Barrie Carveth, Sherry Weinstein, and Cynthia Westley on the establishment and operation of a primary care nursing center. Chapter 13, by Jeri Dunkin, presents concepts useful for modifying interventions for use in rural communities.

Part V (Chapter 14) covers evaluation in community nursing. It looks at indicators and methods of measuring community change and methods and approaches in evaluation of community interventions.

REVIEW OF COMMUNITY HEALTH NURSING CONCEPTS

A basic review of community health nursing concepts and philosophy as a foundation for further study of the community is now presented. This should be useful for the nurse who has not studied or worked in community health nursing recently. This review focuses on individuals, groups, and communities. After Chapter 1, the book focuses exclusively on aggregates and communities.

DEFINITIONS OF COMMUNITY HEALTH NURSING

Various definitions of community health nursing have been offered by professional organizations. According to the American Nurses Association (ANA) (1986),

> Community health nursing practice promotes and preserves the health of populations by integrating the skills and knowledge relevant to both nursing and public health. The practice is comprehensive and general and is not limited to a particular age or diagnostic group; it is continual, and is not limited to episodic care. . . . While community health nursing practice includes nursing directed to individuals, families, and groups, the dominant responsibility is to the population as a whole. (p. 2)

In 1981, the Public Health Nursing Section of the American Public Health Association (APHA) defined public health nursing as follows:

> Public health nursing synthesizes the body of knowledge from the public health sciences and professional nursing theories for the purpose of improving the health of the entire community. This goal lies at the heart of primary prevention and health promotion and is the foundation for public health nursing practice. To accomplish this goal, public health nurses work with groups, families, and individuals as well as in multidisciplinary teams and programs. Identifying subgroups (aggregates) within the population which are at high risk of illness, disability, or premature death, and directing resources toward these groups, is the most effective approach for accomplishing the goals of PHN. Success in reducing the risks and improving the health of the community depends on the involvement of consumers, especially groups experiencing health risks, and others in the community, in health planning, and in self-help activities. (APHA, 1981, p. 4)

In 1996, APHA revised the definition as follows: "Public health nursing is the practice of promoting and protecting the health of populations using knowledge from nursing, social and public health sciences" (p. 4).

In 1995, the Association of Community Health Nursing Educators (ACHNE, 1995b) defined community health nursing as

> the synthesis of nursing theory and public health theory applied to promoting and preserving the health of populations. The focus of community health nursing is the community as a whole, with nursing care of individuals, families, and groups being provided within the context of promoting and preserving the health of the community. (p. 2)

Common elements of all definitions include a focus on the entire community or population, the major goals of health promotion and primary prevention, and a community nursing practice based on a body of knowledge from public health sciences and nursing theory. In addition, the APHA (1981) definition identified nursing process as the way to apply the concepts and theories in the community and mentioned working with multidisciplinary teams that include the consumer. It also identified the need to involve people in the community in self-help and in health planning. The importance of these concepts will be reemphasized in Chapter 11.

COMMUNITY HEALTH NURSING VERSUS PUBLIC HEALTH NURSING

Some authors believe that the terms *community health nursing* and *public health nursing* are interchangeable, whereas others assign different meanings to them. For example, participants in the Consensus Conference on the Essentials of Public Health Nursing Practice and Education (Division of Nursing, 1985) made a distinction based on education. They stated that community health nurses have a range of nursing competencies but practice in the community rather than in institutional settings. Thus, the home health nurse who provides care to individuals in the community or the nurse practitioner who provides primary care to individuals in a free clinic and is not concerned about the total community would be a community health nurse. On the other hand, public health nurses have specific educational preparation and supervised clinical experience in a public health setting. Although qualified to function in an official agency, they may choose to work in another setting. Their educational background prepares them to work with individuals or families, but the health of the larger community is their major focus.

For other authors, community health nursing is more than nursing in a noninstitutional setting. For example, in an ACHNE publication edited by Hickman (1990), community health nursing was described as "the synthesis of nursing theory and public health theory applied to promoting and preserving the health of populations" (p. 3). This definition is more like that of the public health nurse in the previous paragraph.

To confuse the issue further, Matuk and Horsburgh (1992) describe public health nursing as a subspecialty of community health nursing in which public health nurses are those employed by official public health agencies, whereas they considered others in the community (in home health, schools, or hospices, for example) to be community health nurses.

In the latest draft of *Scope and Standards of Population-Focused and Community Based Practice,* the ANA (1995) states that, historically, some nurses have used the terms *community health nursing* and *public health nursing* interchangeably, whereas others have considered public health nursing to be a specialty within the broad field of community health nursing. They also state that regardless of the terms, a major focus in defining the specialty has been on the aggregate or population but that in practice a majority of the nurses had been focusing on individuals residing in the community.

GENERALIST VERSUS SPECIALIST

Authors have also differed as to whether community health nursing is a generalized or specialized field of practice. In reality, practice seems to have been cyclic, with a generalized focus at one time and a specialized focus at another. Currently, we seem to be moving from a generalized practice in which a nurse carries a caseload made up of all types of health conditions and all age groups in a variety of settings to a more specialized practice in terms of content area (maternal-child, family planning, sexually transmitted diseases, mental health, family planning), developmental stage (young children, school-age children, elderly), or setting (health department, school, workplace) (Underwood,

Woodcox, Van Berkel, Black, & Ploeg, 1991). This specialization has led to fragmentation of care, increased staffing needs, and higher cost of care provided (Feagin & Alford, 1990).

According to some authors, we should have both generalists and specialists in community health nursing at any given time, and the differentiation of the two should be based on education. This is the position of Dunn and Decker (1990) and the ANA (1995). A draft document by the Public Health Nursing Section of APHA (APHA, 1996) states that generalists are prepared at the undergraduate level of nursing, whereas specialists are prepared at the graduate level. Nurses prepared at the undergraduate level have some knowledge of population-based care, but their primary emphasis is on the individual and family. On the other hand, specialists can perform all functions of the nurse prepared at the undergraduate level, but they also have substantial experience with families and groups, have expertise in the formulation of health and social policy, and are competent to plan, implement, and evaluate health programs. These nurses are population focused.

ACHNE (1995a) defines the specialist role of "community/public health advanced practice nurse" (C/PHAPN) as requiring a master's or doctoral degree and as being the "practice of nursing and public health to achieve specific health outcomes for the community" (p. 13). Thus the focus is on the community or aggregate of the population. Care may ultimately be implemented at the individual and family levels, but the impact is on the total community through community development, community empowerment, and policy formation. This nurse may function in an administrative or clinical role and may be in a public health mandate setting or a setting that serves only a part of the community.

Following Chapter 1, this book focuses on the specialist or advanced practice nurse. Consequently, the term *community health nurse* will be used to refer to this type of nurse.

AGGREGATE- AND COMMUNITY-FOCUSED NURSING

Another area of potential confusion involves the concept of aggregate- or community-focused community health nursing practice. First, *community focused* and *aggregate focused* should be differentiated. Some authors use these terms interchangeably, and others see them as different. From a systems approach (the theoretical approach of this book), either term might be used, depending on how the nurse identified the system of study. For example, a school could be identified either as a community (system) or as a subsystem of a broader community. If the school was identified as the community, the nursing practice would be community focused; if the school was identified as a subsystem of a broader community, the nursing practice would be focused on an aggregate of the community. I prefer to use the term *community focus* for a focus on a total regional community and the term *aggregate focus* for a focus on any high-risk subgroup of a regional population. Thus, practice is community focused if assessment or interventions are directed toward the total community and is aggregate focused if they are directed toward a high-risk subgroup, such as a group of high-risk infants under 1 year of age, unmarried pregnant adolescents, people exposed to a particular event such as a chemical spill, schoolchildren in a particular school, or a subpopulation of industrial workers in a particular work setting. Both approaches are necessary for community health nurses.

Making a distinction between aggregate- and community-focused nursing is more difficult when one is using a multilevel intervention approach (see Chapter 8). In this approach, the goals of the interventions (such as risk reduction interventions to lower the incidence of cardiovascular diseases) may be set for the total community (community focus). But to accomplish these goals, the interventions may focus on individuals, organizations, and the total community as various targets. The targeted subunits of the community could be considered aggregates. The main point is to determine which focus (community or aggregate) is best, depending on where the greatest need for the services can be met in the most cost-effective manner.

COMMUNITY-BASED AND POPULATION-FOCUSED NURSING CARE

Other terms used in the literature that may be confusing are *community based* and *population focused.* The ANA (1995) used both terms in its document titled *Scope and Standards of Population-Focused and Community-Based Nursing Practice.* Population-focused practice, by the ANA definition, is a practice that focuses on populations (community or aggregate) as opposed to individuals. Population-focused practice is based on an assessment of the population, and the nurse who provides care for clients appearing for service without taking actions to gain participation of all who could benefit from the services is not providing population-focused care.

Community-based care is defined by the ANA as care provided outside an institution. This care can be either population focused or individual and family focused. Care provided to a group of people in the community by nurse practitioners, health maintenance organizations (HMOs), private practitioners, home health agencies, and others is individual and family focused unless all people who could benefit are included in the services. More and more care provided in the community is individual and family focused; much of this care is provided by baccalaureate-prepared community nurses. Advanced practice community health nurses, however, should be both community based and population focused.

PHILOSOPHY OF COMMUNITY HEALTH NURSING

Definitions and concepts of a philosophy of community health nursing were developed by Helvie (1991). A summary of this philosophy is presented below:

- Good health and a long productive life are rights of everyone, regardless of race, sex, or sexual preference.
- All people have health learning needs.
- Some clients may not recognize their learning needs or their need for assistance to regain a higher level of wellness.

■ People accept and use information that is useful to them. Thus, knowledge must have meaning.

■ Good health and health care allow a society to live up to its potential and affect the standard of living.

■ Health is one of the competing values of clients and has a different priority at different times.

■ Concepts and values of health will differ depending on the cultural, religious, and social background of clients.

■ Community and individual autonomy may be given different priorities at different times.

■ Clients are flexible and can change with changing internal and external stimuli.

■ Clients are motivated toward growth.

■ Health is a dynamic adjustment of clients to their changing environment.

■ Clients move in different directions along a health continuum at different times.

■ The major function of community health nursing is to assist clients to move toward high-level wellness.

■ This function is accomplished by use of a theoretical framework and a systematic approach.

■ New health knowledge and technology evolve over time to meet changing health needs.

■ By using and participating in developing new knowledge and technology, community health nursing remains an effective force in society.

ROLES IN COMMUNITY HEALTH NURSING

The community health nurse has many roles that are changing and evolving. For example, primary care and some health promotion activities with individuals that have traditionally been part of the role of the community health nurse are being carried out by nurse practitioners in community settings. In addition, health departments have employed increased numbers of health educators who carry out some of the health teaching that was previously part of the nurse's role. On the other hand, some advanced practice community health nurses are becoming more politically active and are taking on a variety of new community-focused roles that will be discussed throughout this book. Some of the current community health nursing roles will be discussed below.

CARE PROVIDER

This role involves assessing, planning, implementing, and evaluating care for clients (individual, family, community) using epidemiological and preventive intervention principles. This role may be carried out in settings such as the home, school, workplace, or clinic. Interventions may involve providing primary care, including physical care and emotional support, or teaching at the individual, family, and community levels.

The assessment and planning phase of the care provider role includes interviewing and counseling. Interviewing differs from counseling in that it involves methods of data gathering, whereas counseling involves methods of problem solving. In interviewing, the nurse may ask broad questions followed by more specific questions to obtain further assessment data. In counseling, the focus is on identifying and clarifying the problem, considering alternative solutions, selecting an appropriate solution, and evaluating the outcome, using a problem-solving approach in which the client is guided throughout the process.

The role of care provider also includes referral when indicated. From an assessment, the nurse may discover health problems that are outside the scope of nursing practice but that require attention. In such instances, the nurse refers the client to other health care providers. For example, a client who is depressed following childbirth might be referred to a mental health service provider; a client who has rats in the backyard might be referred to environmental health; or a client who is out of work and has no source of income might be referred to social services.

NURSE EDUCATOR AND COUNSELOR

In this role, the nurse provides clients with information that allows them to make wise choices and to maintain their autonomy. Education may be carried out with individuals, families, or communities. For example, the nurse may teach a new mother how to bathe her newborn, how to prepare formula, how and when to feed, when to return to the doctor, when to receive immunizations, and so forth. On the other hand, the nurse may use videos to teach a group of prenatal or postpartum clients some of these same skills. Chapter 10 of this book discusses the role of the nurse as a teacher using mass media sources as a community-focused intervention.

In any educational role, the nurse assesses the needs and motivation for learning, develops a lesson plan based on an educational model, and implements the plan. Following the teaching, the nurse evaluates what learning took place by asking for verbal or psychomotor feedback from the client. For example, the nurse may ask the new mother how she prepares the formula or ask her to demonstrate giving the newborn a bath. Feedback may be more difficult to obtain when using mass media or videos and will be discussed in a later chapter.

ROLE MODEL

The community health nurse serves as a role model for clients and other health care professionals. In the home or other settings, clients may identify with the nurse and emulate his or her behavior. For example, when they see the nurse remain calm in a crisis situation, they may adopt this attitude and behavior. Likewise, the mother who is afraid of the newborn may follow the example of the nurse who holds, cuddles, and talks to the child.

The nurse also serves as a role model for other nurses and students. For example, student nurses may identify and role-model some of the behaviors observed by a warm, caring nurse. However, negative role behaviors can also

be adopted, so it is important to identify positive role models in clinical prac-
ticums for students.

CLIENT ADVOCATE

Zerwekh (1991) defines advocacy as "the process of promoting patients'
rights of self-determination" (p. 32). The nurse advocates for clients who are
unable to speak for themselves. Advocacy may take place at the individual,
group, or community level. For example, the nurse may serve as an advocate for
the patient with his or her family, as when a mother tries to toilet train a child
too early and the nurse intervenes. At the family level, the nurse may intervene
with social services when a needy family has been denied financial assistance.

Nurses also serve as advocates for the community. They may organize a
community group to bring their concerns to the attention of local or state legis-
latures. They may also be involved in the political process as advocates for the
community. The role of the nurse as advocate for the community is important
for the advanced community health nursing practitioner and will be discussed
in more detail in the intervention chapters of this book.

The nurse also assists clients to learn the skills and gain the self-
confidence they need to advocate for themselves. This concept will be discussed
further in Chapter 11.

CASE MANAGER

The ANA Council on Community Health Nursing (ANA, 1991) defines
case management as "a health care delivery process whose goals are to provide
quality health care, decrease fragmentation, enhance clients' quality of life, and
contain costs" (p. 7). This role has three dimensions: clinical, managerial, and
financial (Tahan, 1993). The *clinical* dimension involves using the nursing process to assess the client's needs and the factors influencing these needs and
developing a plan to meet the identified needs. The *managerial* dimension involves coordinating the activities of all care providers involved in implementing
the plan of care. The *financial* dimension involves arranging for the most cost-
effective services and care providers to implement the plan of care adequately.

In addition to providing case management to selected individuals and
families, nurses use a case management approach with groups of clients. Anglin
(1993) presents a case management model for use with groups of clients by
agencies and by staff nurses. It is one of the few attempts in the literature to
identify a model for case management with a group of clients. In this approach,
caseload management involves managing a number of clients within a given
time period while also providing optimum services.

COLLABORATOR

Collaboration is the process of making decisions with other people at any
step in the nursing process. It is vital that it take place at the planning stage if
proposed changes are to be implemented. Collaboration always takes place between the nurse and client and may take place with other health care providers

or community workers such as police, fire department personnel, and social services or other city officials.

Collaboration with the client is especially important if the nurse expects changes in the client's behavior, including future independent actions. Dyer (1973) presents an excellent model based on collaboration for ensuring that clients move toward independence. This model starts with building acceptance and trust and moves to sharing of information for the assessment, then to joint goal setting, and eventually to self-control and interdependence on the part of the client. Dyer elaborated on this process and discussed problem areas and resolution of problems. The model is reproduced in Helvie (1991).

DISCHARGE PLANNER

Another role of the community health nurse is that of discharge planner. Discharge planning involves identifying and making plans for the client's needs following discharge from a health care institution. This involves an assessment of the situation into which the client is moving (often a home or other institution) and the needs imposed by this setting as they relate to the patient's condition. In addition, discharge planning involves identifying community resources that are available to assist the specific client. For example, if the client is being discharged to his or her home but is not mobile, the nurse may identify sources of wheelchairs or crutches, find carpenters who will build a ramp for easy access into the home, determine ways to make the home more wheelchair friendly, and find sources for food delivery, part-time homemaker services, financial assistance, or whatever other services may be necessary. These services should be available before discharge.

CASE FINDER

Case finding involves finding clients who need health care and who meet the requirements identified in agency policy or philosophy. This role was mentioned earlier as part of the discussion of caseload management. These clients may need sick care, prenatal care, well-child care, or any other care provided by the nurse's institution.

CHANGE AGENT AND LEADER

Leadership is the ability to mobilize or influence the actions of others. A change agent is anyone who initiates and brings about a planned change. These two roles are closely related. To bring about change—the usual reason for community health nursing care—one must influence and mobilize behavior. Leadership may be exerted with individuals, families, or communities. Most of the rest of this book will focus on the role of the nurse as a leader in the community. Nurses may also initiate change with individuals, families, or communities. For example, the nurse may introduce dietary changes for the diabetic at home, teach low-fat diets to a group of overweight teenagers in a school setting, or assist a community group to obtain necessary services they desire from community leaders by helping them form a coalition.

COMMUNITY CARE PROVIDER AND RESEARCHER

Although the baccalaureate-prepared nurse has beginning skills as a community care provider, this is more often the role of the advanced practice nurse and the subject matter of the remainder of this book. This role involves applying nursing process to the community: that is, assessing, planning, implementing, and evaluating community health problems and solutions. This process can be carried out independently or in combination with other health and community leaders, and the recipient of care (community or subpopulation) is always involved.

Research is another important part of the community health nursing role. This aspect of the role is again more likely to be carried out by the advanced practice nurse. However, the nurse with a baccalaureate degree and experience may identify researchable problems and work jointly with advanced practice nurses on projects or in some instances may carry out a project independently.

NURSES' ROLE IN CARRYING OUT THE *HEALTHY PEOPLE 2000* OBJECTIVES

In 1979, the first surgeon general's report on health promotion and disease prevention was published (*Healthy People;* U.S. DHHS, 1979). The purpose of this report was to identify major national health problems and to set goals for reducing death and disability for different age groups by the year 1990. The major emphasis was on improving the health of the population by individual and collective action such as legislative changes in public and private sectors and promotion of a safe, healthy environment.

In 1980, a second related document was published by the U.S. DHHS (*Promoting Health/Preventing Disease: Objectives for the Nation*). This report set forth specific measurable objectives for meeting the health care priorities established in the earlier report. In these two reports, 15 priorities were identified and categorized according to their emphasis on health promotion (changes in behavioral choices), health protection (changes in environment), and clinical preventive services (access to screening, immunizations, and counseling). The expected gains were identified as broad goals for 1990 to reduce preventable deaths and disability among Americans at major life stages, such as infancy, childhood, adolescence, young adulthood, adulthood, and older adulthood. For example, a goal for child mortality by 1990 was a 20% reduction to 34 deaths per 100,000 children aged 1 to 14.

Examples of individual actions to meet the goals included eliminating cigarette smoking; reducing alcohol abuse; modifying diet to reduce excess calories, fats, sugar, and salt; obtaining moderate exercise; adhering to speed limits and using seat belts; and obtaining periodic examinations to detect signs of major causes of mortality and morbidity, such as hypertension and cancer. In the environmental area, the report directed policymakers to make changes, including legislation to reduce morbidity and mortality caused by air and water pollution, food contamination, accidents, noise, radiation exposure, occupational hazards, and dangerous consumer products.

There were 226 measurable objectives under the 15 priority areas. Priority areas were the following:

- Health promotion
    1. Smoking
    2. Alcohol and drugs
    3. Nutrition
    4. Physical fitness
    5. Stress/violent behavior
- Health protection
    1. Toxic agents/irradiation control
    2. Occupational health
    3. Accident prevention
    4. Fluoridation/dental health
    5. Infectious diseases
- Preventive services
    1. High blood pressure
    2. Family planning
    3. Pregnancy/infant health
    4. Immunizations
    5. Sexually transmitted diseases

Results showed that 32% of the objectives were achieved, 30% showed progress, 15% showed no progress or regression, and 23% were not evaluated because of inadequate data. Notable progress was made in unintentional injury prevention, high blood pressure control, and reduction of cigarette smoking. Improvements were made in the awareness of the benefits of physical activity and exercise, but this did not translate into activity. Poor progress was made in infant mortality and low-birth-weight infants, especially among minority and low-income populations; teenage pregnancies and unintended pregnancies; youth suicide and homicide; drug-related mortality; and the incidence of primary/secondary syphilis, congenital syphilis, measles, and hepatitis B infections. A good overview of outcomes of these goals can be found in McGinnis, Richmond, Brand, Windom, and Mason (1992).

Three areas of needs emerged from these findings. These included the need to focus on minority and low-income populations, the need for broad national participation in developing and implementing national objectives, and the need for adequate data to monitor and manage progress so that there would be no gaps in future data. These and other results guided the philosophy and structure of the *Healthy People 2000* study (U.S. DHHS, 1991).

There were three broad goals for the *Healthy People 2000* project: (a) to increase the span of healthy life for Americans, (b) to reduce the health disparities among Americans, and (c) to obtain access to preventive services for all Americans. The three overall categories of health promotion for groups, health protection for groups, and preventive services for individuals were again used. In addition, surveillance was added to the goals for 2000. Three hundred discrete objectives among 22 priorities to meet these goals were identified. Priorities were similar to those identified in earlier reports, with important additions such as HIV infections. In addition, special populations were identified in 74 of the 300 objectives. An example of objectives for each category follows. For additional objectives, the reader is referred to *Healthy People 2000*. A health promotion area identified was to decrease tobacco use, with objectives for reducing the prevalence of cigarette smoking, deterring the initiation of tobacco use among youth, creating tobacco-free environments, and increasing access to smoking cessation techniques.

An identified health protection area was the safety of food and drugs. Objectives included ensuring the safety of food and drugs by decreasing food-borne infections such as salmonellosis and by decreasing adverse drug reactions, especially among older Americans. A preventive service category included maternal and infant health services. Objectives under this category included increasing prenatal care and reductions in complications of pregnancy, low birth weight, and infant mortality. Objectives for the surveillance category included improved surveillance and data systems, more compatible data sources, expanded systems to collect more information about special populations, and development of surveillance and data systems that would track progress toward identified objectives. Some objectives related to specific content areas will be discussed throughout this book.

PUT PREVENTION INTO PRACTICE

The Public Health Service within the U.S. DHHS designed the Put Prevention Into Practice program to help achieve the goal of improving the delivery of clinical preventive services of *Healthy People 2000*. Services include immunizations, screening tests, chemoprophylaxis, and counseling interventions to prevent or detect diseases during the early stages. The program is a research-based team approach that uses a kit of materials to improve delivery of care. Materials in the kit are used by the care provider, the office or clinic staff, and the recipient of care. Additional information can be found in *Put Prevention Into Practice* (U.S. DHHS, 1995).

NURSES' ROLE IN MEETING THE WORLD HEALTH ORGANIZATION GOAL FOR THE YEAR 2000

The World Health Organization (WHO) has also set a goal for the year 2000. It is "the attainment by all citizens of the world by the year 2000 of a level of health that will permit them to lead a socially and economically productive life," commonly known as "Health for All by the Year 2000" (Basch, 1990, p. 346). This goal is to be implemented by primary health care, which is defined as

> essential health care based on practical, scientifically sound and socially acceptable methods and technology made universally accessible to individuals and families in the community by means acceptable to them, through their full participation

and at a cost that the community and country can afford to maintain at every stage of their development in a spirit of self-reliance and self-determination. It forms an integral part of both the country's health system of which it is the central function and main focus of the overall social and economic development of the community. It is the first level of contact of individuals, the family and the community with the national health system, bringing health care as close as possible to where people live and work, and constitutes the first element of a continuing health care process. (p. 346)

The major components of primary health care as defined by the World Health Organization are (a) health education; (b) environmental sanitation, including food and water; (c) maternal and child health programs, to include immunizations and family planning; (d) community or village health worker employment; (e) prevention and control of endemic diseases locally; (f) appropriate treatment of common diseases and injuries; (g) providing essential drugs; (h) promotion of nutrition; and (i) traditional medicine (WHO, 1978).

Nurses have a primary role in providing many of these components of primary care. Although many of these roles relate to the nurse with an undergraduate degree working with individuals and families, the advanced practice nurse may be involved in implementing health education (see Chapter 10), in implementing activities on behalf of aggregates or the community (see Chapter 10), in assisting aggregates to introduce change on their own behalf (see sections on coalition building and empowerment in Chapter 11), and in assessing and planning community care.

EPIDEMIOLOGICAL AND PREVENTIVE MODELS

DETERMINANTS OF HEALTH AND ILLNESS

Scientists now accept that there is no single cause-and-effect relationship between disease exposure and human illness. Instead, it is believed that multiple interrelated factors culminate in the disease process. The complex disease- or health-producing factors reside in three elements: (a) the disease- or injury-producing agent, (b) the host or humans, and (c) the environment that stands between the host and disease agent. For example, tuberculosis in humans involves exposure to the tubercle bacillus. However, not everyone exposed to this bacillus will contract tuberculosis. Other causal factors that must be present for the disease to occur include environmental factors such as crowding, appropriate temperature, and humidity and host such factors as habits, customs, physical constitution, occupation, fatigue, stress, and nutrition. If tuberculosis is to occur in a human, a combination of these factors must favor the survival of the organism that overpowers the host. A similar process takes place in injuries. For example, in automobile accidents, there are agent factors such as the mechanical condition of the car, window visibility, seat belt availability and use, and tire conditions; host factors such as carelessness, fatigue, worry, and nervousness; and environmental factors such as weather conditions, visibility, and road conditions. If an accident is to occur, there will be a combination of these factors conducive to its occurrence.

Rogers (1960) listed factors in the host, agent, and environment that may influence disease and injury in humans. He stated that the host may be resistant or susceptible to diseases depending on factors such as genetic constitution, nutrition, balance of internal stresses and adaptation, age and sex, physical vigor or fatigue, specific immunity, knowledge and attitudes, and personality. The agent may be virulent or weak depending on factors such as genetic constitution, nutrition, favorable growth conditions, and dosage or intensity of impact. Last, conditions may vary in the environment that brings the agent and host together so that the environment is favorable or unfavorable for a forceful impact. Environmental factors that make a difference include physical conditions such as temperature, humidity, heat, light, shelter, and traumatic hazards; biological conditions such as sanitation, parasites, disease vectors, nutrient value of food available, and crowding; and nonmaterial conditions such as social and cultural patterns and values and emotional forces of many kinds. Rogers's model is reproduced in Helvie (1991).

PREVENTIVE INTERVENTION MODEL

Given that health and illness are processes resulting from the interaction of factors in the host, agent, and environment, it is possible to intervene at various levels in this process. First, because every condition had its origin in other processes, it is possible to interrupt these processes before humans are involved with disease agents so as to influence their health in a positive direction. This is known as *primary prevention* and may involve efforts to increase the resistance of humans, decrease the resistance of the disease agent, or make the environment less favorable for a forceful impact. This is our primary focus in community health and may involve activities such as immunizations, environmental sanitation, or many wellness behaviors that increase the resistance of humans—proper nutrition, exercise, and stress management.

At the community level, the goal of primary prevention is to reduce the incidence and prevalence of illnesses and injuries or to increase wellness behaviors in the population. The interventions throughout this book and the multilevel model of community interventions presented in Chapter 8 are related to community health promotion and disease prevention.

Leavell and Clark (1979) outlined a variety of activities that could be used with individuals, families, and communities at this level of preventive intervention. They separated primary preventive activities into two categories: general health promotion and specific protection. *Health promotion* activities are not directed toward any specific disease but lead to overall good health, whereas *specific protection* activities address specific disease processes. Health promotion includes activities such as health education, nutrition adjusted to the developmental phase of life, adequate housing, recreation and agreeable working conditions, marriage counseling, genetic counseling, and periodic selective examinations. All of the wellness activities would also be placed here. Specific protection includes activities such as specific immunizations, personal hygiene, environmental sanitation, protection from occupational hazards, protection from accidents, use of specific nutrients, protection from carcinogens, and avoidance of allergens.

When primary preventive interventions fail to reach communities or individuals, they experience interaction with the disease- or injury-producing agent, and disease or injury results. Following this interaction, there are two types of interventions. *Secondary prevention* involves early diagnosis and prompt treatment. It is assumed that early intervention will reduce the duration of the illness. Thus, at the community level, the goal of intervention is to reduce the number of days of illness or injury for a significant number of the population affected. Activities at this level of intervention include individual and mass case-finding activities, screening surveys, and selective examinations of the population. This level also involves treatment to arrest the disease process and facilities to limit disability and death. The focus is on both treatment of the person or persons affected and protection of the rest of the community, if appropriate, for such conditions as communicable diseases (Leavell & Clark, 1979).

Tertiary prevention occurs at a later stage in the disease or injury process. The goal for this level of intervention at a community level is to reduce the number of disabilities in the population at risk. Activities at this level include facilities for retraining and education (rehabilitation), use of the rehabilitated in the work setting, full employment of this group if possible, selective placement, and work therapy.

MULTIPLE-APPROACH INTERVENTIONS

In a community, there are usually two major approaches to improving the health of populations. First, given the influence of the health of the individual on the community, certain high-risk groups will become clients either in groups or individually. For example, later in this book, the beliefs, values, and practices of social and cultural groups will be explored because of their influence on the health of these groups, which eventually affects the health of the whole community. The nurse may teach these individuals or groups about a wide range of topics, depending on the assessment and health conditions encountered. Physical nursing care may also be provided.

The second approach involves care for the entire community or large segments of the population. Most environmental health activities, such as food inspection, air and water monitoring, and occupational health surveillance, fall under this approach. All of the interventions discussed later in this book are examples of community-focused interventions. These include teaching through the mass media, introducing change in the legislative process on behalf of the population, building coalitions, forming partnerships to provide more comprehensive community services, and using empowerment concepts. A multilevel community approach discussed in Chapter 8 combines some of these interventions. The two-pronged approach presented here has been effective in providing for community health needs in the past. However, the major community-focused interventions have been carried out by other disciplines. Nurses are beginning to use the community focus to improve the health of the population. This text is an effort to assist community health nurses in that direction.

REFERENCES

American Nurses Association. (1986). *Standards of community health nursing practice.* Kansas City, MO: Author.
American Nurses Association, Council of Community Health Nursing. (1991). *CHN communique.* Washington, DC: Author.

American Nurses Association. (1995). *Scope and standards of population-focused and community-based nursing practice.* Washington, DC: Author.

American Public Health Association, Public Health Nursing Section. (1981). *The definition of public health nursing practice in the delivery of health care.* Washington, DC: Author.

American Public Health Association, Public Health Nursing Section. (1996). *The definition and role of public health nursing.* Unpublished draft.

Anglin, L. (1993). Case management: A model for agency and staff nurses. *Home Health Care Nurse, 10*(3), 26-31.

Association of Community Health Nursing Educators. (1995a). Community/public health advanced practice nurse position statement. *Newsletter, 13*(2), 13.

Association of Community Health Nursing Educators. (1995b). *Perspectives on theory development in community health nursing.* Louisville, KY: Author.

Basch, P. F. (1990). *Textbook of international health.* New York: Oxford University Press.

Division of Nursing, Bureau of Health Professions. (1985). *Consensus conference on the essentials of public health nursing practice and education.* Rockville, MD: U.S. Department of Health and Human Services.

Dunn, A. M., & Decker, S. D. (1990). Community as client: Appropriate baccalaureate- and graduate-level preparation. *Journal of Community Health Nursing, 7,* 131-139.

Dyer, W. G. (1973). The nurse-patient system relationship. In A. M. Reinhardt & M. D. Quinn (Eds.), *Family centered community nursing* (p. 131-144). St. Louis: C. V. Mosby.

Feagin, R., & Alford, R. L. (1990). Public health nursing: Cross-training in core services. *Public Health Nursing, 7,* 52-57.

Helvie, C. (1991). *Community health nursing: Theory and practice.* New York: Springer.

Helvie, C. (1995). A theory for alternative health practitioners. *Alternative Health Practitioner, 1*(1), 15-22.

Hickman, P. (Ed.). (1990). *Essentials of baccalaureate nursing education for entry level community health nursing practice.* Louisville, KY: Association of Community Health Nursing Educators.

Leavell, H., & Clark, G. (1979). *Preventive medicine for the doctor in his community.* Huntington, NY: R. E. Dregos.

Matuk, L., & Horsburgh, M. (1992). Toward redefining public health nursing in Canada: Challenges for education. *Public Health Nursing, 9,* 149-154.

McGinnis, J., Richmond, J., Brand, T. E., Windom, R., & Mason, J. (1992). Health progress in the United States: Results of the 1990 objectives for the nation. *Journal of the American Medical Association, 268,* 2545-2552.

Rogers, E. (1960). *Human ecology and health: An introduction for administrators.* New York: Macmillan.

Tahan, H. (1993). The nurse case manager in acute care settings: Job descriptions and functions. *Journal of Nursing Administration, 23*(10), 53-51.

Underwood, E., Woodcox, V., Van Berkel, C., Black, M., & Ploeg, J. (1991). Organizing public health nursing for the 1990's: Generalist or specialist? *Canadian Journal of Public Health, 82,* 245-248.

U.S. Department of Health and Human Services. (1979). *Healthy people: The surgeon general's report on health promotion and disease prevention* (PHS Publication No. 79-55071). Washington, DC: U.S. Department of Health, Education and Welfare.

U.S. Department of Health and Human Services. (1980). *Promoting health/preventing disease: Objectives for the nation.* Washington, DC: U.S. Public Health Service.

U.S. Department of Health and Human Services. (1991). *Healthy people 2000: The surgeon general's report on health promotion and disease prevention* (DHHS Publication No. 91-50212). Washington, DC: U.S. Public Health Service.

U.S. Department of Health and Human Services. (1995). *Put prevention into practice.* Washington, DC: Government Printing Office.

World Health Organization. (1978). *Report of the International Conference on primary health care, held in Alma-Ata, USSR.* Geneva, Switzerland: Author.

Zerwekh, J. (1991). Tales from public health nursing true detectives. *American Journal of Nursing, 91,* 30-36.

PART II

THEORETICAL FOUNDATIONS OF COMMUNITY HEALTH NURSING

CHAPTER 2

THEORETICAL FRAMEWORK FOR A COMMUNITY FOCUS

OBJECTIVES

1. Discuss energy as a major concept for a theory of community health nursing.

2. Identify concepts used in a theory of community.

3. Explain three concepts of community.

4. Discuss the community as different types of energy.

5. Distinguish between an open and closed system community.

6. Discuss the environments of the community.

7. Distinguish between the positive and negative health effects of community adaptation (balance).

8. Explain different energy needs of communities.

9. Discuss the nurse's role with communities using the theory.

Helvie's energy theory is a systems theory that has evolved over 15 years and was influenced by the early works of Buckley (1967, 1968) and von Bertalanffy (1973). Other nurses who have used a systems approach include Dorothy Johnson (1980), Sister Callistra Roy (1984), Imogene King (1981), and Betty Neuman (1989).

Helvie's energy theory provides the theoretical basis for this text. This theory has been published or presented previously for individuals and families (Helvie, 1979a, 1979b, 1981, 1991, 1994, 1995) and for communities (Helvie, 1981, 1991). Here, the theory will be applied to the community, the focus of this text. This presentation of the theory is adapted from a previous publication (Helvie, 1991). Application examples of the theory will be used throughout the book, and a case study by a nursing leader uses the theory for community assessment. The theory incorporates the four major concepts found in all nursing theories (Torres, 1986). These are humans, environment, health, and nursing. In the context of community, *humans* refers to the community population who receives nursing care. *Environment* refers to both the internal environment of the community (the subsystems such as health, economics, education, and recreation) and the external environment (the supersystem, such as other communities, the state, and nation). *Health* is the health of the community population and is evaluated using statistical data over time. *Nursing* refers to the work of the advanced practice nurse who focuses on the total community or aggregates within a community and who uses nursing process and nursing theory to improve the health of the community.

Theory is knowledge that can be used in practice (Torres, 1986). Riehl and Roy (1980) and Meleis (1985, p. 29) state that theory can be a set of sentences that conceptualize nursing for the purpose of describing and predicting nursing care. The Helvie energy theory of community follows this format.

ENERGY AS AN UNDERLYING CONCEPT

Energy is "the capacity to do work. . . . [It] may occur in the form of heat, light, movement, sound, or radiation. . . . Human energy is usually expressed as muscle contractions and heat production. . . . *Chemical energy* refers to energy released as a result of a chemical reaction, as in the metabolism of food" (*Mosby's Medical, Nursing, and Allied Health Dictionary,* 1994, p. 554).

The reader must consider energy not only in these physical terms but as activity, vigor, or capabilities so that the concept is inclusive enough for a community theory. All living systems within the universe are manifestations of energy that transform other energy (do work) to maintain life. Human energy can be found at any level of life, ranging from atoms, molecules, and cells to individuals, families, and communities. In addition, nonliving objects in the human environment (e.g., automobiles) can manifest energy in that they are able to do work.

Most of the concepts presented thus far relate more to individuals than to communities. The reader may wish to review the energy theory related to the individual (Helvie, 1981, 1991, 1995) as a basis for better understanding this chapter on the energy theory of the community. However, this chapter uses the same format as the theory for individuals and families and can be understood by itself. Some parts of the definition above, such as heat, light, sound, and radiation, are important aspects of a community population's environment. But the theory presented here will go beyond the physical concepts of energy and look at community subsystems such as health, education, and economics as energy subsystems because of the work expended by both the provider and the recipient of services.

Using energy as an underlying concept, one can view the human system (community population) as a changing energy field affecting and being affected through exchanges with all other energies in the environment, whether these are *internal exchanges*—such as those involving air, water, food, or economic, recreational, or health services or labor—or *external exchanges,* such as those involving state and national resources. These exchanges (past and present) and the balance established by them influence the health of the human system (community population) and determine the placement of the community population on a health (energy) continuum. That placement, determined from a nursing assessment (which gathers statistics such as infant mortality rate, exercise rate, and cigarette smoking rate to assess past and present balances and compare them to those of other energy systems such as other communities, states, or the nation), forms the basis for nursing plans, interventions, and evaluations of care.

ENERGY THEORY OF COMMUNITIES

The energy theory as applied to the community consists of the following concepts, which also underlie the theory as it relates to individuals and families (Helvie, 1981, 1991, 1994, 1995). *Human energy system,* in this context, refers to the community.

1. The human energy system is an open system.
2. The human energy system's environment is energy.
3. The human energy system exchanges energy with the environment.
4. The human energy system continually attempts to adapt holistically to energy exchanges.
5. The human energy system's needs vary by time and situation.
6. Adaptation to energy exchanges (community balance) determines the human (community population) level of health.
7. As humans move toward the illness end of a health/illness (energy) continuum, they usually require assistance from others.
8. Community health nurses assist high-risk groups (actually or potentially poor adapters) to maintain or regain efficient adaptation to energies.

AN OPEN SYSTEM

The community is an open system with three types of energy: bound, kinetic, and potential. These energies are located in the community population, community organizations, and community dynamics, all of which must be assessed and which are discussed below.

BOUND ENERGY

The community's bound energy is located in the members of the various organizations in the community subsystems (health, education, transportation, recreation, and others) who are interrelated by interdependence and interactions to accomplish the goals of their particular organization. These organizations in total meet the goals of the community population. The population (bound energy) is also a subsystem of the community and receives the services provided by various organizations as needed.

The community begins with a group of families and individuals (population) located in a specific place at a specific time who decide that it is more beneficial to pool resources and divide tasks. As the number of families and individuals grows and there is need for more assistance from resources outside the home, there will be increased specialization, and a variety of community subsystems will evolve.

Neighborhoods. The urban community is usually composed of several neighborhoods or census tracts. For example, in Virginia Beach, Virginia, are Hilltop, Oceanana, Kempsville, Pembroke, and many other neighborhoods. Each neighborhood has its own history, characteristic family size, social class values and beliefs, economic levels, health problems, and other factors that distinguish it from other neighborhoods. However, its members interact with each other and with members of other neighborhoods and use community resources when needed and thus become an important part of the community through these reciprocal relationships or exchanges (paying taxes, using services, participating in clubs, organizations, socializing).

Neighborhoods may vary from old established areas that have a stable population and a sense of pride, unity, and rapport to those that are relatively new and have a more transient population. A knowledge of the history of a community helps nurses to identify strengths and resources (community leaders, organizational skills) that are useful in mobilizing a community to deal with its health concerns (see community development in Chapter 8).

Community Concepts. Various ways to conceptualize the community (bound energy) are useful in assessing and carrying out plans to improve health conditions. The first way is by using a boundary definition. According to Pearl (1939), population is "a group of living individuals set in a frame that is limited and defined in respect to both time and space" (p. 52). This definition is equally appropriate for a community, where space is defined in political or geographical terms and time is defined in terms of a point in time or an interval of time. A community may be a census tract, a political subdivision, a complete community, a school, an occupational setting, or any other spatial unit. Thus, it is important to identify the unit of service. Within this unit, health problems can be enumerated, health services provided, and health laws enforced. The boundary also defines the unit for taxation for health and other services and identifies the population that must be involved in decision making about health services provided. Using this definition in combination with statistical tools and data, the community health nurse can evaluate changes in population structure, morbidity, mortality, and other health rates between two points in time in a specific geographical area.

A second way to define the community is demographically. The emphasis of this approach is on subgroups of the community (aggregates) who have certain variables (demographics) in common such as age, race, sex, social class, or cultural group factors. Categorization of a population by demographic variables will show an unequal distribution of illnesses or health behaviors in the community and is useful for planning health services and carrying out epidemiological studies. For example, sexually transmitted diseases are more prevalent among young adults, hypertension is more prevalent among African Americans, and alcoholism is more prevalent among middle-aged men. Categorization of a population by demographic variables will identify high-risk aggregates who may become priorities for community health nursing care.

A third way to define community is as a system (basis of theory presented here) with subsystems and supersystems that interact with the community population to establish a dynamic balance. That dynamic balance may move a community population toward or away from health. The internal interrelating parts of a community (subsystems) include health, education, welfare, economics, politics, religion, communication, and transportation. The effects of the dynamics of the subsystem and supersystem on the health of the population will be discussed later in this chapter.

The community health nurse may use any one of these definitions of community at a particular time. For example, the school nurse who assesses the incidence of measles in the school this year (current balance) and compares it with the incidence 5 years ago is using the boundary definition of community: that is, evaluating the health of a population in a specific location at two points in time. In this approach, the nurse is viewing the community as a closed system for comparison purposes, although all living systems are actually open systems. Using the second (demographic) definition, the school nurse may wish to determine whether the children who are absent from school with measles are from the same race, sex, classroom, census tract of the city, or some other variable as a basis for planning nursing care. Using the systems definition of community, the school nurse may teach prevention of the spread of the disease on a local television channel, write an article for the newspaper on measles prevention, or request immunizations from the health department and in these and other ways recognize that the community (school) is an open system from which the nurse may turn to the broader community for assistance.

KINETIC ENERGY

Kinetic energy is the energy of motion—that is, the ongoing role functions and structured patterns of behavior of all members in community organizations. It is also the checks and balances (peer pressures, supervisory evaluations) that maintain the roles that in total meet the organization's and community's goals. Although roles in organizations may be vacated and refilled at different times, those filling roles have been socialized into role expectations so that the role behaviors remain relatively stable over time. When there are attempts to deviate too far from the expected role behaviors, the checks-and-balances phenomenon comes into play. For example, a staff community health nurse has certain roles within the staff nurse subsystem of health and between this subsystem and other subsystems of the community. (Many of these roles were discussed in Chapter 1.) The nurse is responsible to a supervisor for knowing and providing adequate nursing care to clients within the philosophy of the agency and standards of care. This may involve knowing agency philosophy so that the appropriate clients are admitted to service, knowing clients' health needs, having plans to meet these needs, knowing community resources, setting priorities, and having knowledge of health and illness and principles and skills of providing nursing care as appropriate. In addition, this role involves meeting with the supervisor periodically, discussing client problems, and following up on suggestions offered. It also involves additional role behaviors such as participation in immunization clinics, and sexually transmitted disease clinics. Students in educational programs studying community health nursing are socialized into the role and after graduation can assume the appropriate duties with supervision. Thus, the role remains relatively stable. However, if the new nurse decides to admit inappropriate categories of clients as part of case-finding activities or to give bedside care when the agency emphasizes preventive care and teaching, checks and balances may come into play. In this instance, the supervisor may place the nurse on warning and provide certain standards to be met, or colleagues may bring pressure through ignoring, confronting, withholding rewards, or other techniques. If the checks and balances do not work, the nurse may be fired and another nurse hired who better fits the role. As mentioned earlier, relatively stable roles are important for meeting organizational objectives. However, roles may change from time to time. The process whereby this occurs will be discussed later in this chapter.

The nurse (health subsystem) communicates with other community subsystems such as families and population groups (aggregates) to identify and resolve health issues. Assessing and intervening requires relating and communicating, and these skills are developed in educational programs. The nurse also uses these skills when dealing with other community subsystems such as the welfare, education, economic, and recreation subsystems on behalf of the health of the community population.

Patterned role behaviors also include appropriate methods of decision making, lines of authority, and other processes that facilitate the functioning of the nurse. These assist in maintaining stable role behaviors. Agency goals, job descriptions, agency philosophy, policies, and procedures also assist in maintaining stable role behaviors.

Community roles are usually occupied internally (from within the community). However, circumstances may require temporary filling of roles from external sources. For example, during a recent ice storm in Virginia Beach, many electric light wires were broken by ice and fallen trees. Because large numbers of people were without heat and light and the situation was acute, workers came to Virginia Beach from North Carolina and from other parts of Virginia to help restore electricity to those without power. Similar events have happened during recent natural disasters. For example, after a recent hurricane came ashore in Florida, many workers, including community health nurses, went to the area to assist in restoring the community to its previous state. Although kinetic energy is being discussed here, these are also examples of how the community is an open system, as will be discussed later in this chapter.

POTENTIAL ENERGY

Potential energy refers to all of the knowledge, skills, flexible patterns, attitudes, and values of all personnel in community organizations, as well as of the community population who are recipients of services. These are resources (stored energy) created by work (expended energy) that can provide for the future needs of the community. For example, nurses learn (through work) the knowledge and skills required for their roles and these are then available as needed. In addition, other community service people learn their roles before performing them in the community. Potential energy assists the community to meet its changing needs and goals. In addition, the population has some knowledge and skills (potential energy) that will influence health and illness patterns and resources needed by them. For example, some groups know how to care for sick members in their families; know community resources, first aid measures, and other health information; and will need less assistance from community resources than those groups that lack such information.

Communities are open systems because they exchange with their environment. These exchanges take place internally among the subsystems (health, education, recreation) and externally with resources in other communities, the state, or the national government. For example, nurses may request resources from the state to assist with special projects such as mass immunization programs, or they may notify a nearby community of a flu epidemic locally so that the neighboring community can initiate preventive measures to reduce the impact. Thus, even though community health nurses may visualize the community as a closed system for certain aspects of their work (see boundary definition of *community* above), it is an open system.

Communities are able to exchange with the environment and also maintain their structure because there is a greater concentration of energy within the community than between the community and the environment. This concentration of energy is a result of the greater interactions of people and interdependence of roles in the smaller unit.

The community is located between the state (supersystem) and the family (subsystem) in a hierarchy of systems. Because the subsystem and supersystem interact with and influence the system (community), they must be assessed for their effect on health in any community assessment.

THE SYSTEM'S ENVIRONMENT IS ENERGY

The community has both an internal and an external environment. The internal environment is made up of the resources and services of the subsystems of the community, such as health, education, welfare, recreation, political, cultural, social, legal, communications, and economic subsystems, all of which interact with the population and influence health. In addition, the internal environment is made up of a variety of energies, such as air pollutants, water, food, viruses, and bacteria, that also influence the health of the population. Table 2.1 presents some of these energies. It should be noted that the advanced practice nurse is interested in these energies only as they influence the community or aggregates within the community. Polluted air, a food poisoning outbreak in a school, or an increase in viral or bacterial infections in a community would be examples.

The external environment of the community is made up of other communities, the state, and the nation. Exchanges with the external environment also affect the health of the community population by assisting or failing to assist

TABLE 2.1 Selected Energies in the Community

Chemical	Physical	Biological	Psychological
Air pollutants	Airplanes	Animals	Feelings of
Alcohol	Automobiles	Allergens	Anger
Antibiotics	Bullets	Bacteria	Hate
Arsenic	Color	Disease agents	Love
Asbestos	Cosmic forces	Fungi	Rejection
Auto exhaust	Dust, sand	Immunizations	Nonverbal expressions
Candy	Heat	Insect bites	Sociocultural values
Carcinogens	Knives	Plants	Physical closeness or distance of loved ones
Cigarettes	Light	Semen	Prayer
Cleaning agents	Nails	Viruses	Healing
Cosmetics	Physical assault by others		
Drugs—illegal	Radiation		
Drugs—legal	Sound		
Food			
Food additives			
Lead			
Minerals			
Oxygen			
Pesticides			
Vitamins			
Water			
Water pollutants			

SOURCE: Helvie, C. (1991). *Community Health Nursing: Theory and Practice.* New York: Springer Publishing Co. Reproduced with permission.

communities with needed resources, by introducing diseases at various times, or by limiting community autonomy for the benefit of the state or nation. Further discussions of the influence of the external environment on health will be found in the next section of this theory.

A model of the internal and external environments of the community is presented in Figure 2.1. This figure shows the complexity of factors having an influence on the health of the community population.

ENERGY EXCHANGE WITH THE ENVIRONMENT

The community exchanges energy (input/output) with the internal and external environments to which it must adapt throughout its life cycle. Because of the complexity of the exchanges and interactions within and between the com-

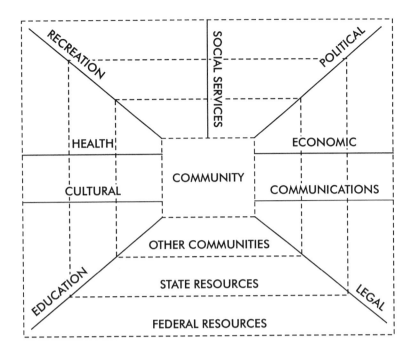

FIGURE 2.1.   The Community and Its Environment (State, Nation)
SOURCE: Helvie, C. (1991) *Community Health Nursing: Theory and Practice.* New York: Springer Publishing Co. Reproduced with permission.

munity and its external environment, it is easier to break these exchanges down into smaller units for study.

INTERNAL EXCHANGES

Some of the environmental exchanges in the community that may affect the population involve factors such as noise; water, air, and soil pollution; food contamination; and radiation effects (see Table 2.1). A variety of exchanges involve services such as garbage collection, providing adequate housing, rat control, air and water purification, noise control, and food inspection, which are provided to the community in exchange for taxes supporting these services. Environmental factors and their potential effects on the health of the community and the services available to prevent the harmful effects are discussed in Chapter 4. Sociocultural and economic forces as they affect community populations and their health are discussed in Chapters 3 and 5. Other interactions between community subsystems that may affect health are discussed below.

Health Exchanges. Exchanges occur between the community population and the community subsystem of health. In any community, there may be a certain proportion of the population with small children, another with school-age children, and another composed of the elderly. Each aggregate will have different needs depending on members' sociocultural and economic backgrounds; their risk behaviors; the diseases prevalent in their age, race, and sociocultural group; and so forth. Many of these groups will have exchanges with the health subsystem. For example, all couples planning to marry must receive a blood test (input), for which they pay a fee (output). When they move into the childbearing years, they will have exchanges with the health subsystem for prenatal care, labor and delivery, and well- and sick-child care, for which they pay a fee or taxes (output). These groups may also receive community health nursing services during these life periods. Throughout the rest of the life cycle, community aggregates may exchange with the health subsystem for preventive services such as immunizations, health teaching, and supervision in various areas (care of the newborn; accident prevention; adequate diet; growth and development, including anticipatory guidance; sex education; the effects of alcohol, tobacco, and stress). Groups may also exchange with community health nurses when there is a need for early case finding and health care such as with unsupervised pregnancies, cases of abuse in families, cases of tuberculosis or other communicable diseases, or needs for sickness or bedside care in the home. Many of these exchanges by the advanced practice nurse involve assessment of and planning for these aggregates in nursing centers or under certain circumstances, such as mass immunization programs (see Chapters 11 and 12) or involve communitywide interventions for or on behalf of the population (see Chapter 10).

Other exchanges between community aggregates and the health subsystem take place in the dentist's office, the doctor's office, the pharmacy, the hospital, or the surgical supply store. These exchanges are for the purposes of obtaining preventive or restorative care, prescribed or over-the-counter medications, and equipment or supplies.

Health care services to community groups may take place in a variety of settings. The environmental services usually take place in various locations throughout the community, such as restaurants, grocery stores, public swimming pools, air-monitoring stations, and neighborhoods. Other services may be provided in schools, industrial settings, clinics, hospitals, health centers, and private practice settings. Some groups may prefer to use alternative sources of health care such as witch doctors or faith healers. The reader is referred to Chapter 5 on sociocultural forces influencing community health for a further discussion of this concept. A simple model of exchanges between the community or aggregates within the community and the health subsystem is presented in Figure 2.2. For example, a group of pregnant women may receive primary, secondary, and tertiary services from health professionals in a variety of settings (input), for which they pay a fee, taxes, or both and also describe symptoms or give a health history (output).

Social Services Subsystem. Community groups may also exchange with the social services subsystem of the community. Some community groups continually exchange with this subsystem because they fail to grow and develop in the area of productivity and thus remain chronically dependent. This chronic dependency has been a concern to the current state and federal governmental officials because of budget shortfalls; recent welfare reforms are discussed in Chapter 4. Other community aggregates exchange with social services on a short-term, temporary basis due to illness, injury, or unemployment. Because social service programs are tax supported, taxes are the recipient's output for

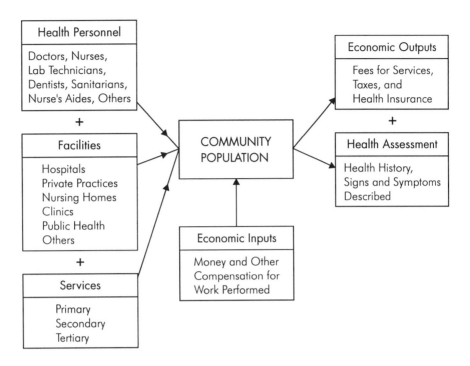

FIGURE 2.2.   Population-Health Subsystem Exchange

services. In exchange, when services are needed, recipients may be eligible for money for food and shelter, medical care, and other basic necessities (input). The advanced practice nurse must be aware of the influence of these services on the health of community aggregates as a basis for planning.

Education Subsystem. Groups also exchange with the education sub-system. Children attend public or parochial schools, and adults may attend college or vocational schools to learn how to cope with the environment. For their education (input), these groups pay a fee for private elementary or secondary school or pay taxes for public schools (output). At the vocational or college level, there is usually a fee charged (output) for education (input), although it may be reduced for in-state residents (taxpayers).

There are also many less formal opportunities for education in the community. Groups may use libraries, neighbors, professionals, and nonprofessionals as sources of information. Groups may receive education from community health nurses in clinic settings, schools, or industrial settings; on the radio or television; or in the newspaper. Because teaching community groups is an important aspect of the advanced practitioner's role, use of mass media as a community intervention is included in Chapter 10. In addition, knowledge of the educational level of the community population or aggregate is important when planning for teaching and will be discussed in Chapter 6 in relation to community assessment.

Economic Subsystem. Another important exchange between groups and a community subsystem is with the economic subsystem. Many of the community's population provide goods or services (output) to the community in exchange for money (input) that is used to pay (output) for items such as housing, food, transportation, education, recreation, and entertainment. In addition, community members pay taxes (output) that pay for other services (input) such as garbage pickup, mail delivery, public education, public health care, and social services. The advanced practice nurse must have a knowledge of the money generated from taxes, how it is allocated, and the influence of these allocations on the health of the population.

Other Exchanges. Groups have exchanges with other community subsystems. They exchange with the legal subsystem for legal advice and for services such as courtroom defense, legal services involving other individuals or organizations, or writing of wills and legal documents. For these services, they pay a fee or obtain services from a tax-supported attorney. They may also exchange with the recreation, transportation, political, or other subsystems.

Interrelation of Exchanges. Exchanges within the community have been separated above for study purposes. However, in reality there are usually many interrelated ongoing exchanges by groups with numerous subsystems. For example, many community people work or attend school and thus exchange with the economic or educational subsystems. However, these contacts may also serve as social exchanges in which friendships develop or as educational exchanges in which they learn from these interactions.

EXTERNAL EXCHANGES

Communities also exchange with other communities, the state, and the nation throughout their life cycles. For clarity, these exchanges will be presented in relation to community subsystems below.

Health Subsystem. One external exchange between the community and its environment is with the health subsystem. For example, if there is a communicable disease such as influenza in a neighboring community or in the state or nation, community health nurses realize that this biological energy may enter their community. Thus, they may establish mass immunization clinics and teach ways to prevent, diagnose, and treat the disease. Education may reach the public by mass media methods such as television, radio, or newspaper. They may also contact state or national organizations such as the Centers for Disease Control for assistance (another external exchange). The advanced practice nurse is always aware of actual or potential changes in the incidence and prevalence of diseases in a community and plans ways to prevent or decrease them.

A second external exchange involving the health subsystem is information. For example, nurses belong to professional organizations and subscribe to professional journals. In addition, they may write articles for professional journals. This writing may influence the practice of others outside their community, or they may apply new knowledge to practice that was gained from reading books or articles or attending meetings originating outside the community. As members of professional organizations, nurses may also attend state or national meetings as delegates or presenters. If they present resolutions or papers at these meetings, they again may influence nursing external to their community. In addition, many pieces of information that are useful in the nurse's assessment of the health of a community may be obtained from these external sources. For example, vital statistics such as morbidity and mortality rates by demographic variables are available from the state and nation and may be useful for comparison purposes. The reader is referred to Chapter 6 for a further discussion of this concept.

Some checks and balances implemented at the state and national levels influence the health of the community. Among those that influence community health nursing are national examinations for licensure, the code of ethics, standards of practice, and procedures for dealing with nurses who do not meet the codes, standards, and established practices.

When the health subsystem of a community lacks resources to deal with actual or potential community problems, it may turn to the state or nation for assistance. For example, if the health subsystem identifies an increased incidence of lead poisoning in children in the community and lacks the financial and human resources for diagnosing, treating, and preventing this problem, it can turn to the state and federal government for assistance (review the concept of the community as an open system, if necessary). During periods of rapid change, it is often imperative for the community to use these exchanges if it is to continue to meet the health needs of its population. For example, during natural or humanly caused disasters, community populations may be endangered, and the health subsystem of the community must seek outside help. Examples include a recent ice storm on the East Coast when many people were without electricity and food because of broken wires and impassable icy roads; several hurricanes that hit populated areas along the East Coast recently; earthquake destruction in San Francisco a few years ago; and riot destruction in several major cities in past years. In each instance, it was necessary to ask for and receive assistance from resources outside the particular community such as the American Red Cross or federal disaster units to restore a favorable balance that would preserve health in the community.

Population Subsystem. The population subsystem (groups of families) also exchanges with the environment (input/output). This takes place through immigration and emigration in relation to a community. These changes—that is, the total population and the demographic variables of the population—can influence the characteristics of the population to be served, including risk factors. They can also influence the morbidity and mortality rates of the population and the need for health services. For example, if many families with young children leave the community and many older people arrive, there may be a change in the services needed (see below, the section "Community Needs Vary by Time and Situation"). Thus, an ongoing assessment of population characteristics, demographic variables, and diseases prevalent by the community health nurse and others is important (see Chapter 6).

The Education Subsystem. The education subsystem (all levels, including both private and public) have exchanges with the environment that are similar to those of the health subsystem. Teachers are influenced by reading journals published beyond the community, they must pass certifying exams and meet certain standards, they can influence national policies and procedures through professional organizations, and they may turn to the state and nation when they lack the resources to deal with problems encountered in education.

Other Exchanges. Other subsystems such as the legal subsystem and the political subsystem also exchange with the environment (other communities, the state, and the nation). The exchanges between the political subsystems of some communities are currently evident where there are efforts to use resources better, such as water or state funding for more equitable education. In some instances, partnerships and coalitions have been established between or within political, health, and other subsystems (see Chapter 11).

In addition, some input into the community consists of basic goods needed by the population. These include food; appliances, such as refrigerators, cars, and air conditioners; clothing; building materials, such as lumber, bricks, and cement; medical supplies and equipment, such as medications, blood pressure cuffs, X-ray machines, and scanners; and materials for heating homes, such as coal, oil, and wood.

The community also provides output in the form of waste products, such as sewage and industrial waste, and goods and services. In relation to goods and services, one community may be an agricultural community and export fruit and vegetables; another may be a coal-mining town that exports coal; another may have a university that prepares and exports teachers, nurses, and scientists. Most communities have multiple exports.

CONTINUAL ATTEMPTS TO ADAPT

Communities must continually adapt to the internal and external exchanges taking place. At any point in time, there is a balance established by community adaptation that can be assessed for its effect on the health of the population. This health effect is particularly noticeable when compared with previous health effects of temporary adaptations or balances (e.g., 5 and 10 years earlier) and with the health effects of state and national balances. These data are obtained from vital statistics.

INTERNAL EXCHANGES AND ADAPTATION

The population engages in internal exchanges to provide for basic needs such as food, shelter, clean air, safe water, and companionship. It also engages in exchanges for education, recreation, entertainment, police and fire protection, and health care, as discussed in the previous section. For these services, there are usually fees or taxes to be paid. These ongoing exchanges between the population and community subsystems require continual adaptation and may influence the health of an aggregate or the community population.

At the same time, there are multiple internal exchanges between subsystems within the community. For example, if a law is passed (legal/political subsystems) requiring immunizations prior to school enrollment, this will involve exchanges between several community subsystems. This program initiated by the legal subsystem may require health personnel (health subsystem) to implement it, school personnel (education subsystem) to evaluate records for compliance, the community's government (economic subsystem) to finance it, and the police to enforce it (legal subsystem). It may also require changes in family practices. Each of these units must adapt to the change introduced. Community health nurses also interact with multiple subsystems such as the political system when intervening on behalf of community aggregates (see Chapter 10); mass media when teaching large segments of the population (see Chapter 10); an aggregate of the population when providing direct services such as mass immunizations programs or coalition building for political clout (see Chapter 11); and educational, recreational, transportation, and other subsystems when carrying out a community assessment or intervening on behalf of the community's health.

EXTERNAL EXCHANGES AND ADAPTATION

Likewise, the community exchanges with the external environment (other communities, state and federal governments) and must continually adapt. For example, the health subsystem of the community may receive money and other resources from the state or federal government on an emergency or ongoing basis to assist in meeting the health needs of the community population. These resources are incorporated into the community's provisions of health care and in combination with local resources (internal) establish a temporary balance (adaptation) of health care depending on the health problems identified and the amount of local, state, and federal funding for health care. The more money available and the fewer health problems identified, the more health care can be provided, and, theoretically, the healthier the community will be. If there is a change in population structure, disease incidence or prevalence, or money available for health services, a new balance must be established (see "The Adaptation and Change Process" below). Other community subsystems also compete for resources, and this will affect the availability of funding for health. Ongoing exchanges (internal and external) establish a community balance that may affect the health of the population in a positive or negative way (see Chapter 3 on economic forces influencing the community).

The community must also adapt to changing illness patterns that may result from exchanges with other communities. For example, a communicable disease in a surrounding community will probably affect the nurses' community and must be dealt with. Prevention and treatment use money from the budget that will then be unavailable for other priorities unless additional money can be obtained from internal or external sources or unless these services can be provided by others in the community such as private doctors.

THE ADAPTATION AND CHANGE PROCESSES

Internal and external exchanges, including internal pressures for and against spontaneous or planned changes, result in periods of equilibrium and disequilibrium that require continual adaptation. The temporary balance (adaptation) established by the community in relation to these exchanges and pressures may move the community toward or away from a healthy level.

Temporary Adaptation. Internally, the community needs periods in which a temporary balance or steady state is maintained and the subsystems are working efficiently to meet the needs and goals of the community. The subsystems, which are interdependent, are composed of organizations and individuals. For example, the health subsystem is made up of hospitals, public health, clinics, private practitioners, group health care organizations, pharmacists, and appliance makers. Individuals function within roles in organizations, and these roles are relatively fixed or patterned at any point in time, as discussed previously. The structure of roles within organizations and the system of rewards and punishment for maintaining appropriate role functions assist the community to maintain a steady state over time.

When change occurs in a community subsystem, other subsystems and the total community will be affected and will thus try to counteract the change to maintain a steady state (one aspect of the feedback process). In the proposed change example presented earlier regarding immunizations prior to school enrollment, the school personnel may refuse to check records, saying they do not have the time; health personnel may say they do not have time to give the immunizations; and families may refuse to obtain immunizations because of religious convictions or may pressure the political subsystem to have the decision reversed. Members of the economic subsystem may say they do not have the money to implement the change. All of these efforts may be to maintain the status quo. In this example, if change is to occur, new plans may be required to overcome the resistance, such as obtaining funding for additional positions in the schools and health subsystems or exempting certain groups from the requirement to obtain immunizations. It should also be remembered that the community is an open system and that a community with limited resources to carry out the program may turn to the state or federal government for assistance.

Change and Growth (Negentropy). Communities need periods of growth (negentropy) in addition to temporary steady states, even though growth periods may produce stress and strain in the community system. These periods are stressful because change leads to new temporary balances (steady states) that may be difficult for some parts of the system. Additional information on this concept is presented in the next section, "The Change Process in the Community."

All subsystems of a community are interrelated, and a change in one will affect some or all of the others as well as the total community. The example above regarding a new requirement for immunizations prior to school enrollment demonstrates this concept. In addition, a change in a subsystem will affect other parts of that subsystem. For example, recently, private doctors in Virginia Beach began seeing pregnant women who were on Medicaid. Care for this group had previously been provided by the health department. Before this change in the health subsystem, community health nurses saw most pregnant clients who were without private resources in the prenatal clinic at the health department and provided a variety of services, including prenatal teaching. After this change was introduced, community health nurses were freed to do other things. Their role changed from clinic care for large numbers of pregnant clients to follow-up home visits for high-risk clients seen by private physicians. They also began to focus on a variety of health promotion activities for which resources had previously been unavailable.

Because a change in one subsystem affects other subsystems and the community as a whole, joint planning and coordination are important to ensure that the needs of the population are being met in the best way possible. These include educational needs, transportation needs, and recreational needs as well as health needs. Joint planning involves frequent communication in meetings, memoranda, or other appropriate ways. It also involves a perception of the need for collaborative planning between members of the health team.

THE CHANGE PROCESS IN THE COMMUNITY

During periods of temporary steady states, the role behaviors of individuals in community organizations become relatively automatic and thus reduce the energy needed to carry out the roles. However, when change is introduced into the community and several subsystems are affected, these role behaviors require conscious efforts, additional energy is needed, and tension rises.

To reduce the tension in the system, certain maneuvers may be tried within and between subsystems. In addition to the maneuvers identified earlier to maintain the status quo, maneuvers to bring about change may include coercing, coaxing, evaluating, mashing, postponing, problem solving, and bargaining. Each of these maneuvers is discussed in Helvie (1991, p. 80). For example, in the immunization example used previously, health personnel might use problem solving and bargaining with school personnel to assist in bringing about change. In this situation, they could work jointly to find personnel to evaluate student records, and health personnel might agree that if school personnel supported this change, those in the health subsystem would support the next change proposed by the school subsystem. Health leaders might also need to work with the economic subsystem to obtain funding for the program. They could present and defend the budget for the program and might gain widespread support for the program with publicity and politicking. Maneuvers might be tried with all subsystems showing resistance until the program (planned change) was passed or abandoned because of too much community pressure. In addition, because the community is an open system, it would be possible to request funding for personnel to evaluate school records, give immunizations, and so forth from the state or national government.

Thus, a subsystem that is committed to a change will work with all other subsystems affected and other resources such as the state and nation to bring about the change (one aspect of self-regulatory processes). If there is too much resistance, people may decide to abandon the change and remain at a steady state (another aspect of self-regulatory processes).

Special-interest groups may also use this approach to bring about change in a community. If they are committed to a certain issue, they may circulate a petition and get the appropriate number of signatures to place the issue on the ballot for voters. They will also politic during this process to gain support. They may also use the mass media (communication subsystem) to gain support by providing information about the change. Or they may go from door to door or visit various leaders for that purpose. They may also build coalitions or partnerships to bring about community changes (see Chapter 11).

Following these maneuvers, change may or may not be introduced into the community. When change does occur, the tension gradually subsides, new patterns of behavior are established, and eventually, behaviors become relatively automatic again. During the movement to the new balance, some energy is lost from the system because of the need to focus consciously on the new role behaviors.

At any point in time, some groups and organizations in the community are content with the status quo, whereas others want change. Although the system (community) remains intact and there is a temporary balance, there is also some stress and strain in the system. In the example presented previously, some families such as the Amish may oppose the immunization requirement because of religious beliefs but may go along with it so that their children can receive an education and because it is strictly enforced. They will, however, experience some stress as a result of the conflict experienced. If many families experience this conflict, they may pressure the political subsystem to reverse the decision. At the same time, others may want to continue the required immunization program. The group who wants change may decide to propose a referendum vote so that the issue is decided by the majority.

Change is often introduced into the community through the political process. At any point in time, there will be established patterns of behavior for populations, but over time, these may change. For example, in my own community, past laws required that only those related by blood or marriage could live permanently in a household. Now this law has changed to allow up to four unrelated individuals in a household. Thus, as society (social subsystem) changes values and beliefs and accepts new behaviors, legal changes may come about at the polls or in courts where lawsuits are decided. Thus, communities do not remain static but change over time as a result of changes initiated by any subsystem. The advanced practice nurse is always aware of community changes and their actual or potential influence on health.

Changes introduced in a community by a subsystem within or beyond the community may affect the health of the population and move it toward or away from a healthy balance. Although community health nurses and others in the health subsystem are health oriented, others in the community may not be. For example, an ongoing concern in Congress and at local levels has been the balance between economic and environmental interests. At times, there are more resources available to deal with environmental problems than there are at other times. Special-interest groups often play a part in these decisions by politicking for purposes other than health. For example, some industries want laws that allow them to continue to discharge waste into waterways or landfills for economic gain, when in reality these practices may have detrimental health effects. There have also been ongoing concerns about such issues as cutting forests for the wood, reducing smog pollution in certain cities, or recycling versus filling of community dumps. Any of these decisions can be detrimental to the health of the population.

ENTROPY IN ADAPTATION

Entropy is the quantity of energy in a system that is not capable of conversion into work. It is always present in the community as the parts continually adapt to change in the process of transformation. However, this loss of energy in a community with efficient subsystems is not detrimental because there is enough energy to go beyond complete disorganization (entropy) to meet community needs and move to new levels (negentropy). For example, new members joining an organization must learn specific role behaviors and must relate to coworkers. During this initial period, the organization is working less efficiently, and some entropy is present. Or new people may have ideas they want to introduce, which means changes for the organization and which may or may not be adopted. During the process of deciding whether to make the changes, parts of the organization may be disrupted and may not function as effectively as usual. In addition, when information about change is initiated from the top of an organization, problems may be created for parts of the system opposed to the change or for those who oppose the methods used to initiate change. At such times, the organization as a whole will not function as effectively.

Various factors in a community may lead to more serious entropy in varying degrees, and this may be temporary or permanent. For example, during a recent holiday weekend in my own community, violence broke out on the resort strip. Looting, vandalism, and other criminal acts followed. This increase in crime could not be handled by the available police, and loss, disorder, and disorganization followed until additional police arrived and other protective devices were put into effect. This entropy was temporary, and although order was restored, many shop owners lost merchandise beyond amounts covered by insurance. Prior to holidays in the following years, a variety of mechanisms were put into effect to prevent a recurrence of this entropy. Such periods of entropy may follow disasters, strikes, or riots when the community is not prepared to counterbalance those disturbances with additional resources (police, health, and so forth).

A more long-term permanent entropy may occur in a community that loses its economic base. In a community with limited job opportunities, the young move away, creating a void for replacing those who retire. This emigration also leads to a lower birth rate and a higher death rate among an aging population. Or a community may experience the closing of its single factory and suffer an economic void. Part of the movement of the military forces and closing of bases around the United States has been of concern to communities who are threatened with loss because of the effect on the economic subsystem of that community. Past examples of complete community entropy were seen in the loss of populations and death of gold rush towns when gold was no longer available or in the area of the Love Canal when the environment became polluted and could not sustain human populations. Whenever the economic subsystem of a community is affected, other subsystems such as health and social services must increase caseloads. When they are unable to do this, the community is subject to population loss and entropy.

EFFICIENT RANGE OF ADAPTABILITY

An efficient range of adaptability for a community is defined as the determined range of adaptability for aggregates or the population in which changes in bound, kinetic, or potential energy may take place but are easily reversible and the system continues to maintain its efficient functioning. For example, in my own community, summer tourism at the oceanfront is big business. During such times, there is a rapid increase in the population (bound energy), but there are hotels available (potential energy) and a variety of restaurants, souvenir stores, recreational opportunities, increased police presence, increased health personnel, and so forth (potential and kinetic energy) to meet the increased demand. Thus, the needs of this increased population are met efficiently, and the community is able to increase its population in the summer and decrease its population during the winter months (an instance of reversible change).

Likewise, because my community is a coastal community, the population is subjected to certain natural disasters that may require changes in bound, kinetic, and potential energies. For example, an increased number of services may be required following disasters such as hurricanes or floods. When the community is able to expand to provide necessary services and contract when these are no longer needed, it is within an efficient range of adaptability.

When federal funding used for various community programs has been withdrawn and the community continues to provide the needed services, it is again within an efficient range of adaptability. Likewise, examples of temporary entropy discussed earlier fall within this category.

When communities are overdependent or underdependent on state and federal assistance for services or are unable to adjust to internal and external exchanges, they move toward entropy. This takes them outside the efficient range of adaptability. At such times, the community may experience increased morbidity and mortality, population loss through emigration, increased crime rates, high teenage pregnancy, and other indications of moving toward entropy. For example, a community that loses its economic base and fails to provide for health care, welfare, and other unmet needs of the population will move outside the efficient range unless it reverses this process.

ENERGY NEEDS VARY BY TIME AND SITUATION

The energy needs of communities change as the population's characteristics, demographics, and structure change. For example, a community with a high proportion of families with small children requires different services than one with predominantly elderly people. Energy needs also vary by the proportion of the population of different sociocultural backgrounds, the racial distribution, economic status, and other demographic variables (see earlier discussion of definitions of community). For example, a working population will have less need for community assistance than one with a high amount of unemployment. A community that has professional schools to prepare nurses, doctors, and other health personnel will have less need for external exchanges for these resources than one without them.

Likewise, communities that are developing or experiencing rapid growth will have different needs than dying communities. In addition, communities experiencing rapid situational changes such as natural disasters will have different energy needs than those without these changes.

NEGENTROPY

Negentropy is energy that can be used by the system for work and is characterized by order and organization. Thus, as a community grows (manifests negentropy), there is increased order and organization: That is, subsystems grow in size and become more organized internally and in their interdependence with other subsystems to deal with the increased population needs. For example, as communities grow, school, health, recreational, and other services increase in size or numbers to meet increased needs. In my own community, rapid growth has led to increased numbers of schools, recreational centers, and increased caseloads at the health department and social services department. These increased demands must be paid for, and thus property and other taxes usually rise.

Whether communities grow, prosper, and become more complex depends on adequate economic, educational, and other opportunities for the population. When these are present, the people living in a community will often remain, and new people will move in. This leads to negentropy. As more and more people immigrate, there is an increased demand for services and material goods, subsystems increase in size, and the community prospers. Or if new needs evolve, there may be a corresponding increase in new services or subsystems. Thus, any time a community is growing, becoming more complex and more formalized or organized, negentropy is present.

ADAPTATION TO ENERGY EXCHANGES DETERMINES LEVEL OF HEALTH

At any point in time, the level of health of the community will be a result of its adaptation to the internal and external energy exchanges. This adaptation or temporary balance can be evaluated by a community assessment when compared with previous community assessments and with the state and nation. Communities may move up and down a continuum ranging from optimum wellness (high energy) to poor health (low or dissipated energy). Although it is not possible to place a community at a specific point on the continuum, it is possible to determine if the current adaptation is better or worse than previous balances established in the community or the balances currently established in other communities.

The community's health is interrelated with family and group health, and as the community moves up or down a health continuum, so do its families and groups. When the community offers adequate services and resources by internal and external subsystem exchanges, the population experiences optimum health. At such times, there are adequate health services (primary through tertiary prevention, as discussed in Chapter 1), sources of financial assistance, recreational opportunities, transportation, economic opportunities, counseling services, and other services to meet the needs of the population. When these services and resources are inadequate, morbidity and mortality rates may rise, and the community may move down the health continuum. For example, a high incidence of unimmunized children; contaminated water; air pollution; high rates of diseases such as cancer, heart disease, and HIV/AIDS; and other factors resulting from inadequate services may move the community down the continuum. At the low end of the continuum would be the community with a complete disruption of services resulting from a natural or humanly caused disaster. In this situation, the community often has contaminated water, limited safe food, and a dislocated population in shelters. These crowded living conditions favor the spread of disease, and the lack of privacy leads to inadequate rest and poor personal hygiene, which may create an increased incidence and prevalence of diseases (concepts defined in Chapter 6).

MOVEMENT TOWARD ILLNESS MEANS COMMUNITIES NEED ASSISTANCE

As communities move toward the illness end of the continuum as determined by a community assessment, they usually require increased internal or external assistance to move them toward a more favorable balance of health. For example, the community identified above in which a disaster has affected the water and food supply and large segments of the population are dislocated to shelters will need assistance to increase the food supply, to make the water supply safe, and to assist the population to make their homes habitable. Other affected subsystems will also need assistance to reverse the process. Thus, a community moving toward the illness end of the continuum will usually need assistance. Sudden loss of employment, rapid population changes due to immigration or emigration, and the introduction of a new disease or environmental pollutant into a community are other examples of factors that may move a community toward the illness end of the continuum (entropy). In each situation, the community's resources may be overtaxed, and the health of the community may be affected. At such times, new resources and services or additional personnel from within or outside the community may be needed to counteract the movement on the health continuum and to move the population toward the efficient range of adaptability.

Even at the wellness end of a continuum characterized by an efficient range of adaptability and balanced energies, the community will need some assistance to remain at that level. For example, the population needs ongoing services such as immunizations; surveillance of diseases, water, air, and food; education about prevention and treatment of illness; and enforcement of laws and regulations to maintain its level of health. Education and surveillance are especially important for those who have not been reached by services previously, including those who have been added to the community through immigration or birth. When a community remains within an efficient range of adaptation, however, it will have a low morbidity and mortality rate when compared with other communities. It will also be better able to deal effectively with minimal changes in health services and personnel when it experiences minor changes in morbidity and mortality and changes in the population structure. Assistance at the wellness end is, however, not as urgent as assistance at the illness end of the continuum.

COMMUNITY HEALTH NURSES ASSIST HIGH-RISK COMMUNITIES

Community health nurses assist high-risk aggregates and communities to remain within an efficient range of adaptability and a state of balanced energies or to regain an improved level of health (move toward the efficient range of adaptability). High-risk groups are aggregates or communities experiencing or with the potential to experience change (developmental or situational) that are deemed least able to adapt to energy exchanges (internal/external), as determined by comparison to established norms. To be the highest priority for community health nursing services, these aggregates or communities should be amenable to interventions with a minimum of time, money, and other resources (see priority-setting models in Chapter 8). These high-risk aggregates change from time to time but are usually the groups identified for nursing services (preventative and curative). The philosophy of the agency will determine which high-risk aggregates are to be seen by nurses. In addition to case finding by nurses for these groups, an assessment and referral system for the specific clients will usually be established. For example, in some health departments, a community health nurse visits prenatal clinics and refers high-risk pregnant clients and newborn children for nursing care.

Many of the interventions used by advanced practice nurses to assist high-risk aggregates or communities will be discussed in Part IV in this book. These include community-focused efforts to strengthen the resources of aggregates or the community, such as the use of mass media for education; use of empowerment and self-help concepts; assistance with coalition building; provision of immunizations for aggregates at special clinics; and provision of services in convenient locations through nursing centers. In addition, community-focused interventions on behalf of aggregates or the community, which will be discussed in Part IV, include interventions such as establishing partnerships, using the political process for change; or dealing with the environment.

USING THE THEORY IN PRACTICE

When used in conjunction with the nursing process, this theory can be applied in practice. A model for this application is presented in Figure 2.3 at the end of this section. Additional applications will be presented throughout the book, including a case study at the end of Chapter 6 using the theory for community assessment.

ASSESSMENT

A community assessment is the first step in assisting community populations with health problems and concerns. Initially, community health nurses assess the effects of past energy exchanges on the health of the community or aggregates (secondary or tertiary prevention) by evaluating the temporary community balance established as it affects health. The effect of this balance on health is determined by (a) evaluating a variety of health indicators in the community, including the incidence and prevalence of diseases by demographic variables and environmental factors such as water, air, and food pollutants, and (b) comparing these data with earlier health data for the community (5 and 10 years previously) and with data from other communities, the state, and the nation to identify whether the community is moving toward or away from health.

In general, data evaluating the community balance will indicate how well the community subsystems (bound, kinetic, and potential energy) are functioning to meet the health needs of the community. For example, an outbreak of hepatitis A in a community may indicate a breakdown in restaurant sanitary conditions and in the enforcement of sanitation measures by health personnel. It may also indicate a decrease in education about hand washing and personal hygiene for restaurant personnel. This breakdown may be a result of inadequate economic resources (internal/external) affecting the teaching and enforcement roles of health personnel, the education of health personnel, the supervision of restaurant staff, or a variety of other factors that favor the survival of the hepatitis virus, which then passes among a susceptible population (see nursing diagnoses below and in Chapter 7).

Community assessment also involves evaluating the community balance in relation to the demographics of the population structure to determine changes resulting from immigration and emigration and changes in developmental levels of aggregates (instances of needs varying by time and situation). For example, an assessment may identify a change from a predominantly middle-class group to a lower-class group or from a predominantly white group to a predominantly African American group. Or the assessment may identify a change from a population made up primarily of families with young children to a population of elderly people living alone. Any of these changes identified by assessment may require a readjustment in providing health services. The advanced practice nurse may be responsible for assessing these data and making decisions about nursing services, but the generalist who is visiting families also has a role in this process. For example, the generalist who works in a census tract might identify population changes in the census tract and resulting gaps in service and would be responsible for presenting this information to the advanced practice nurse (a supervisor or nursing administrator). Following the initiation of new services to meet the deficit, the generalist nurse would take this information to the families in the community who needed the services.

Community health nurses also assess the current energy exchanges between community subsystems and their internal and external environments to determine if future health problems are possible due to shortages of services and resources (and should therefore be targeted by primary prevention). As discussed earlier, a temporary balance will be established within a community between subsystems that may affect aggregates. For example, are television, radio, and the newspapers (communications subsystem) presenting adequate health information? Likewise, are elementary and secondary school personnel presenting adequate health knowledge to students? Can nurses work with key people in the communication subsystem to improve health teaching? Can nurses present information on health and health resources available to the community? Is there accessible (in terms of cost and location) and adequate (all levels of prevention) health care? Are transportation routes located in areas where people lack other sources of transportation? Is there an adequate supply of jobs tailored to the educational background and interests of the population? Are there adequate housing and social services resources? Is there a disease in an adjacent community that may move into the nurse's community and affect the health of the population? These and other questions about the subsystems that may affect the future health of the population or aggregates are assessed.

When community subsystem changes are proposed that will establish a new balance, community health nurses should assess the potential health effect of these changes. For example, when social service caseloads increase as a result of decreased employment and changing eligibility requirements are proposed, the potential effect on health should be assessed. Or if health insurance benefits are reduced for a segment of the population, the effect on obtaining health care should be assessed.

In addition to proposed changes, actual changes in a community may affect health and must be assessed. For example, has a factory closed, putting people out of work? Has a change in leadership in the political subsystem led to decreased funding for health? Has a change in leadership in the communication subsystem led to inadequate health teaching?

In some communities, changes will be counterbalanced with other changes that maintain the balance toward health of the population. For example, a strike in a community may be countered by increased funding in social services, health services, and so forth to meet the changing needs. This increased funding may come from internal or external exchanges (local, state, or national government).

Additional application of this theory will be presented in the next section and in Chapter 6 on community assessment. In addition to a discussion and application of an assessment tool based on this theory in Chapter 6, a community assessment case study by a nurse leader will use this theory.

PLANNING AND INTERVENING

Nursing diagnoses and plans for nursing care for high-risk aggregates and communities are developed following assessment. Nursing diagnoses related to the theory are written in energy terms. For example, an increased incidence of measles among children in a certain school setting could be diagnosed as

> energy deficit related to a high and increasing rate of measles among children in _____ School due to (a) inadequate funding for health personnel and (b) inadequate information of immunizations and prevention, resulting in a measles rate in the school of 9.2 in 1996 compared with 4.2 in 1990 and 5.0 in the state and 5.2 in the nation in 1996. [see Chapter 7]

This would alert the nurse to implement efforts to prevent the spread to others, to teach care of the sick child and how the disease is spread, and to make resources available for preventive or curative care. Teaching might be carried out by sending fliers home to families from school, by placing spot announcements on television, or by getting an article in the newspaper. Other aspects of nursing diagnosis and the framework for writing nursing diagnosis using the energy theory are discussed in Chapter 7.

After nursing diagnoses are written, they are placed in priority categories. This will be discussed further in Chapter 8. Next, goals and objectives are written. Goals are broad and are written in terms of decreasing, increasing, or maintaining energies. For example, a goal related to the diagnosis above would be "Decrease biological energy related to measles." Goals will be discussed further in Chapter 8.

Objectives, also discussed in Chapter 8, are very specific. An example of an objective related to the energy theory will be presented here to provide continuity. For example, in relation to the goal of decreasing chemical energy intake for a group of overweight schoolchildren, some objectives would be the following:

> Client will decrease chemical energy intake, as evidenced by (a) stating the components of a balanced diet for one day by January 1, 1997; (b) selecting a balanced diet from a list of foods by January 1, 1997; (c) demonstrating proper diet by eating a balanced meal in the cafeteria daily beginning January 1, 1997.

Three approaches to intervening for improving community health are used by community health nurses: (a) working with high-risk aggregates or the total population, (b) working with other subsystems of the community on behalf of the population or aggregates, and (c) working with the environment on behalf of the community population. The emphasis of any approach is to improve the health of the population by increasing the resistance of populations to diseases (increasing or decreasing energy exchanges) or to make the environment, including disease agents, less favorable for the forceful impact of disease on the population (altering environmental energies). These approaches will be discussed further in Chapter 10. However, some examples of these approaches follow.

Community health nurses intervene in community populations to improve these populations' resistance before interaction with disease agents occurs (see discussion of primary prevention in Chapter 1). For example, nurses may assist a group of obese adolescents with diet and exercise plans, behavior modification, and other methods to help them reduce their weight and thus prevent diabetes, cardiovascular disease, arthritis, and other chronic illnesses.

Community health nurses also work with subsystems of the community to improve the health of the total population or aggregates. For example, they may teach health information on television programs or write articles for newspapers (communication subsystem), work for changes that improve community health through the political process (political subsystem), or communicate with the recreational subsystem to increase the numbers of recreational facilities or to increase hours when facilities are open. They may also work with the economic subsystem to obtain additional funding for health programs. Several of these community-focused interventions will be discussed in Chapters 10 through 13. In addition, several nursing leaders show how these interventions have been used in practice.

Community nurses also work with the internal or external environment. They may deal with problems in the physical, chemical, or biological environments of the community, or they may approach the external environment (state, nation) for assistance with health programs for the community. Additional information on the physical, chemical, biological, economic, and sociocultural environments of the community is presented in Chapters 3, 4, and 5. In addition, a case study by nursing leaders demonstrates how nurses deal with community forces. Nurses may also work with external environments to prevent the spread of diseases, to influence decisions about nursing and health, and to obtain resources for health care. This concept was discussed earlier in this chapter under external exchanges of a community.

Because the major focus of community health nursing is primary prevention (discussed in Chapter 1), many of our interventions are directed toward wellness. Frequently offered programs for aggregates include those on weight loss, smoking cessation, stress reduction, exercise, and lowering blood pressure.

Following interventions, community health nurses carry out an evaluation process. This process will be discussed in Chapter 14.

ENERGY THEORY MODEL

A model of the energy theory as it is applied through the nursing process is presented in Figure 2.3. This model has been revised from an earlier one that was for individuals, families, and communities (Helvie, 1991, p. 34).

In this model, the energy client is the community or aggregate, the health focus is on aggregates along the health (energy) continuum, including those with a high level of health (within an efficient range of adaptability and with balanced energies) and those with a low level of health (imbalance of energies). The goal of nursing care for the community is to assist aggregates and the community to maintain or regain efficient adaptation.

The method of applying the theory is the nursing process. Initially, the nurse assesses the effects of past energies on the community population and aggregates (morbidity, mortality, and health behavior statistics by demographic variables) and the developmental level of the community (energy needs vary by time and circumstance). Next, the nurse assesses the current energy exchanges (internal and external) and how these affect the health of the population. These population statistics, when compared with standards, identify how well the community is performing in various areas. From this assessment, nursing diagnoses are developed and prioritized on the basis of the observed statistics, behaviors, or other factors when compared with standards or the past observed statistics for the community or those for the state or nation. The format used for writing nursing diagnoses is as follows (see 3 and 4 under "Assess" in Figure 2.3). The community energy balance or deficit (identifying how well the community is doing regarding the particular problem) related to (the problem or behavior and the community or aggregate affected) is due to (community factors that cause the energy balance or deficit) resulting in (the effect of the balanced or deficit energies on the population). An example of this framework was presented earlier.

Plans are written for nursing diagnoses and identify ways of maintaining or regaining balanced energies in the community. Goals are always written in terms of balancing the community's energies in the particular area of concern. An example was presented earlier. The way to accomplish the goal of regaining a community balance is to develop objectives in relation to the effects of the imbalance on the population, as identified in the "resulting in" part of the nursing diagnosis. In the model (Figure 2.3), the four components of objectives are identified and will be discussed in Chapter 8. Interventions follow the establishment of objectives and are directed toward maintaining, increasing, or decreasing energies in the community population or aggregate or the environ-

THE CLIENT	THE HEALTH FOCUS	THE GOAL
Aggregate or Community	Balanced Energies Deficit of Energies	Maintain or Regain Balance of Energies

THE NURSING PROCESS			
Assess	Plan	Implement	Evaluate

1. Community
  a. Balance
  b. Deficit
    (Resulting from past energy exchanges)
 	
2. Energy Exchanges
  a. Balance
  b. Deficit
  c. Basis for exchange
 	
3. Nursing Diagnosis
 	
4. Supported by
  a. Indicators of community performance
  b. Population statistics (effect of community performance)
  c. Population surveys
  d. Standards
	1. Maintain or Regain Balanced Energies
	
	2. Objectives
	  a. Aggregate or community
	  b. Activity
	  c. Time frame
	  d. Standard
	
	3. Planned Activity
		1. Community Plan Energies
		  a. Maintain
		  b. Increase
		  c. Decrease
			1. Goal met
			
			2. Objectives Met
			
			3. Reassess Energies
			
			4. Terminate Process

FIGURE 2.3.   Nursing Process and Community Energy Theory

ment. Following interventions, evaluation determines whether or not objectives were met (see Chapter 14). If these were met, the process is terminated. If they were not met, there is a reassessment, and new plans are developed.

REFERENCES

Buckley, W. (1967). *Sociology and modern systems theory.* Englewood Cliffs, NJ: Prentice Hall.

Buckley, W. (1968). *Modern systems research for the behavioral scientist.* Chicago: Aldine.

Helvie, C. (1979a). A proposed theory for nursing in community health. Part 1. The individual. *Canadian Journal of Public Health, 70*(1), 41-46.

Helvie, C. (1979b). A proposed theory for nursing in community health. Part 2. The family. *Canadian Journal of Public Health, 70*(4), 266-270.

Helvie, C. (1981). *Community health nursing: Theory and process.* New York: Harper & Row.

Helvie, C. (1991). *Community health nursing: Theory and practice.* New York: Springer.

Helvie, C. (1994, May). *Helvie's energy theory of family nursing.* Paper presented at the Third International Family Nursing Conference, Montreal.

Helvie, C. (1995). A theory for alternative health practitioners. *Alternative Health Practitioner, 1*(1), 15-22.

Johnson, D. (1980). The behavioral system model for nursing. In J. P. Riehl & C. Roy (Eds.), *Conceptual models for nursing practice.* New York: Appleton-Century-Crofts.

King, I. (1981). *A theory for nursing: Systems, concepts, process.* New York: John Wiley.

Meleis, A. (1985). *Theoretical nursing: Development and progress.* Philadelphia: J. B. Lippincott.

Mosby's medical, nursing, and allied health dictionary. (1994). St. Louis: C. V. Mosby.

Neuman. B. (1989). *The Neuman systems model: Application in nursing education and practice.* Norwalk, CT: Appleton-Lange.

Pearl, R. (1939). On biological principles affecting populations: Human and others. *American Naturalist, 71,* 50-68.

Riehl, J., & Roy, C. (1980). *Conceptual models for nursing practice.* Norwalk, CT: Appleton-Century-Crofts.

Roy, C. (1984). *Introduction to nursing: An adaptation model.* Englewood Cliffs, NJ: Prentice Hall.

Torres, G. (1986). *Theoretical foundation of nursing.* Norwalk, CT: Appleton-Century-Crofts.

von Bertalanffy, L. (1973). *General systems theory.* New York: Penguin.

PART III

COMMUNITY ASSESSMENT

CHAPTER 3

ECONOMIC FORCES INFLUENCING COMMUNITY HEALTH

OBJECTIVES

1. Define economic concepts.

2. Discuss basic economic theories.

3. Discuss factors influencing the rising cost of health care.

4. Identify the economic concerns of community health nurses.

5. Evaluate current approaches to financing health care.

6. Discuss trends in cost containment.

7. Evaluate proposed plans for increasing the health coverage of the population.

8. Develop a plan for effective health care reform.

9. Justify prevention as an aspect of health care reform.

10. Evaluate the effects of cost containment on health care.

11. Discuss how community health nurses work within the economic subsystem of the community.

THEORETICAL FRAMEWORK

Economics has a tremendous influence on the health of the community population and must be assessed by nurses. In the theory presented in Chapter 2, economics was recognized as one community subsystem that influences and is influenced by other subsystems in a community. Changing relationships between the community subsystems (internal environment) can influence health in a positive or negative way. For example, when adequate funding is provided by local government for health services, it offers a variety of preventive and curative health measures to the population so that the community can move up the health (energy) continuum into the efficient range of adaptability (balanced energies). If this same community experiences a deficit energy balance regarding its economic base through loss of industries resulting in decreased tax revenue for health and other services (such as recreational and social services), these services may decline. At the same time, health insurance that was provided by the industry may no longer be available. This community that is unable to meet the changing needs for increased services (health, social, recreational) will have a population moving toward the illness and entropic end of the health continuum (energy deficits). This change will be reflected in changing health statistics as determined by assessing the community's balance at two different points in time and compared with that of other communities, the state, and the nation. Thus, it is important for nurses to have an understanding of the economic forces that influence the community.

In the 1960s and 1970s, the health care system in the United States was expanding because of unlimited financial resources and an open free market. At the same time, nursing was expanding and assuming increased responsibilities and influence for health. Today, the health care system is moving in the opposite direction, experiencing limited resources, regulatory restrictions, increased competition, and a shift from hospital to community care. Associated with these changes have been diagnostic-related groupings (DRGs), cost containment, managed-care plans, national health insurance proposals, and other developments and concepts that will be discussed later in this chapter.

The current emphasis in health care delivery has thus become one of limiting present and future growth and setting priorities for services within the available resources. In an environment of cost containment, nurses must evaluate community health nursing practices to obtain the most health care with the resources available. To do so, they must understand concepts of economics and the economics of health care delivery. This chapter should provide a foundation for that understanding.

ECONOMIC DEFINITIONS, BASIC CONCEPTS, AND THEORIES

Webster's dictionary (1983) defines economics as the "science that deals with the production, distribution, and consumption of wealth." Health care economics involves the production and distribution of health care resources. In a period of cost containment, distribution of services involves doing the greatest good for the greatest number within the knowledge and resources available.

When money is used for health care, it is not available for other community needs (see theory presented earlier in this chapter and in Chapter 2). Society must decide the extent of health care desired within this framework, given that revenue spent for health care is not available for other services.

ECONOMIC THEORY

Two economic theories are useful in understanding economics: microeconomic and macroeconomic. The microeconomic theory involves the concept of supply and demand. Economists evaluate the supply of goods and services in relation to consumers' income allocation and distribution and how income allocation and distribution influences consumer demands for goods and services.

Supply and demand are closely related, and the increase in one leads to a decrease in the other, with a corresponding influence on price. For example, an increase or oversupply of a product leads to a decreased demand (reduced overall consumption) and lower prices. Conversely, a limited supply of a desirable product will cause an increased demand and a rise in price. This economic theory is useful in understanding price determination, resource allocation, and consumer income and spending patterns at the individual or organization level.

The macroeconomic theory evaluates broad aggregate (group) variables affecting the status of the total economy and is concerned with stability and growth. These broad variables include factors influencing employment, income, prices, and economic growth rates.

HEALTH ECONOMIC THEORY

Health economists use economic theories as a basis for understanding factors influencing the financing and delivery of health services. The large-scale perspective on health care financing that resulted in proposals for health care rationing, national health plans, managed care, poverty of health care, and competition and other concepts is based on macroeconomic theory. These concepts are discussed later in this chapter.

Microeconomic theory may be useful in health economics if health care competition increases in the future to create a change in the balance of supply and demand. Until now, it has not been useful because health care has been a monopoly with a captive consumer market.

HEALTHY PEOPLE 2000 OBJECTIVES

Results of progress toward meeting national health objectives for 1990 (McGinnis, Richmond, Brandt, Windom, & Mason, 1992) showed a disparity in health statistics among social economic groups in the United States, with higher death and illness rates among minorities. This finding was used in *Healthy People 2000* (U.S. Department of Health and Human Services [DHHS], 1991b) to identify the goal of reducing health disparities among Americans. Many of the objectives for the year 2000 focused on specific minorities, and although economics was not specifically addressed, this is a factor in the disparity identified. Higher death and illness rates among minorities may be a result of inadequate diets, inadequate housing, limited or no access to health care, and other conditions based on socioeconomic factors. Specific objectives related to social and cultural populations are identified in Chapter 5, which focuses on social and cultural forces influencing the community.

PAST TRENDS AND COMMUNITY HEALTH NURSING CONCERNS

The reader may ask why the health care system has reached a point of limited growth in its evolution. To answer this question, it is necessary to evaluate the past.

The major factors leading to efforts to control the growth of the health care system has been the rapidly rising costs of health care and the proportion of budgets used for this purpose. One measure of the allocation of money in the federal budget to health care is the percentage of the gross national product (GNP), defined as the total value of goods and services produced in an economy in a year (U.S. DHHS, 1988) devoted to health care. In 1980, health care expenditures accounted for 9.1% of the GNP, whereas in 1990 they accounted for 12.2%, and by the year 2000 they are projected to account for 16% (Sonnenfeld, Waldo, & Lemieux, 1991). The United States spends more than twice as much per person, on average, than any other country in the Organization for Economic Cooperation and Development, which is made up of 15 nations (DeLew, Greenberg, & Kinchen, 1992, p. 151), even though national health expenditures have been rising throughout the world for years (Roemer, 1993, p. 150). The distribution of health care spending in the United States in 1990 was as follows: about 39% for hospital care, 19% for physicians, 8% for nursing homes, 22% for personal health care, and 12% for nonpersonal health care such as construction and research (Levit, Lazenby, & Letsch, 1991).

An interesting side question is, Does this higher cost of health care improve health statistics? The answer is no. For example, in 1989 infant mortality in the United States was 10 infants per 1,000 live births, which was higher than the figure for Australia (8.7), Austria (8.1), Belgium (9.4), Canada (7.2), Denmark (7.5), Finland (6.1), France (7.7), Germany (7.6), Iceland (6.2), Ireland (8.3), Italy (9.3), Japan (4.8), Luxembourg (9.4), the Netherlands (6.8), Norway (8.3), Spain (8.1), Sweden (5.8), Switzerland (6.8), and the United Kingdom (9.0) (Holliday, 1992). At the same time, there were 9.7 perinatal mortality deaths per 1,000 in the United States, a figure higher than that for 15 of the previously mentioned countries. In addition, the life expectancy rate at birth for males in the United States (71.5) was lower than that for 16 of these countries, and for females, the life expectancy rate (78.1) was lower than that for 17 of these countries (Holliday, 1992). When people in the United States were asked about satisfaction with health care in the United States, 10% said minor changes were needed, 60% wanted fundamental changes, and 29% wanted the health care system rebuilt completely. Of 10 countries surveyed (Australia, Canada, France, Germany, Italy, Japan, the Netherlands, Sweden, the United Kingdom, and the United States), only one other country (Italy) surpassed the United States in the desire to rebuild the health care system, and all others were considerably below this percentage (Holliday, 1992).

FACTORS INFLUENCING RISING HEALTH CARE COSTS

Reasons for the increased costs of health care include inflation, technology, unscrupulous practices related to third-party payment, high cost of medical insurance coverage, and changing population characteristics. Inflation in the health care field can be seen in the rising costs of everything from lab and other tests, equipment, and drugs to personnel costs, including the cost of high-priced specialists. Inflation was a major problem between 1950 and 1980, and health costs were even more problematic. By 1990, health care costs were 10% greater than the general inflation rate. Between 1950 and 1987, the population increased by 62%, but the health care cost increased by 4,000%. This amounted to an increase of about 2,000% per person for that period (Office of National Costs Estimates, 1989).

Technology is another factor in rising costs for health care. Physicians and other health care professionals have become dependent on technology for diagnosing and treating clients' health problems. Clients who are knowledgeable about their health concerns also demand the latest technology in their treatment. One of the many examples of increased dependence on technology for diagnosing is the increased use of CT scans and ultrasound. In an 11-year period, use of inpatient CT scans increased 400%, and ultrasound and angiocardiography increased threefold (U.S. DHHS, 1988). Although it is difficult to determine the exact amount of increase in health care costs that can be attributed to technology, Raffel and Raffel (1989) reported on one study that attributed one fourth of the increase to technology. The U.S. Department of Commerce (1993) reported that the per capita expenditure per year for health care rose from $143 in 1960 to $2,868 in 1991. This rise in per capita expenditures was probably involved in several factors listed in this section.

A third factor related to increased costs of health care is the unscrupulous practices of health personnel related to third-party payment. Consumers have made increased demands for care because they have been buffered from actual costs. In addition, because someone other than the client has been paying, there has been an attitude that funding for care is unlimited. Physicians, hospitals, nursing homes, and others have known that they would be paid regardless of costs and have therefore been more likely to request additional costly lab or other services or to order costly equipment, medications, or other treatments. According to DeLew et al. (1992, p. 159), the third-party system has allowed providers to add more services or to bill for higher levels of service to increase their revenue. Recently, several television programs have shown that millions of dollars are lost each year because of the failure of Congress to specify cost containment measures with equipment, medications, and other treatments for Medicaid and Medicare patients. Health care fraud is estimated at more than $80 million yearly (White House Domestic Policy Council, 1993).

Advertising by attorneys, fees contingent on settlements, and other methods have led to increased lawsuits against health personnel, especially physicians. Thus, malpractice health insurance has risen drastically and has increased health care costs. Many physicians practice defensive medicine: That is, they order unnecessary diagnostic and other procedures out of fear of malpractice suits. The American Medical Association (1990) estimated that 3% of all health spending is used for defensive medicine. A last factor influencing rising health care costs is changing population characteristics. The population in the United States increased by almost 25% between 1970 and 1991 (U.S. Department of Commerce, 1993). This growth has led to increased demands for service. There is also a growing population of individuals aged 65 and older in the United States, and they require more health care than younger persons. In 1988, 12.4% of the population was 65 or older, and it is projected that by the year 2030 this age group will make up 22% of the total population (U.S. DHHS, 1991a). People over 85 are projected to be the fastest-growing population, and their number is expected to increase sevenfold by the middle of the 21st century (*Senior Power*, 1987; U.S. DHHS, 1990). However, this population has more health problems and uses more health care services. This population has 80% of all chronic diseases, some of which limit activities. Conditions may include arthritis, diabetes, heart disease, hypertension, and hearing and visual impairments (Burke & Walsh, 1992). Although people over 85 make up just over 12% of the population, they are responsible for 19.6% of physician visits. In addition, hospital stays for this group are longer with age and occur more often than with younger populations.

DIMINISHED HEALTH CARE FOR POPULATION SEGMENTS

Cost containment has resulted in limited access to or reduction in health care services for segments of the population. Those most affected include the elderly, poor children, and the medically indigent. This latter group includes those who lack health insurance, are ineligible for federal health care assistance, and lack resources to pay for their own care. Between 1980 and 1985, the percentage of Americans without health insurance rose 45%, with about 37 million people in the United States without health insurance (Johnson, 1990; White House Domestic Policy Council, 1993). According to Relman (1987), the under- and uninsured make up 15% to 20% of the population. In 1990, 35.7 million Americans (almost 17%) under the age of 65 were reported to have no insurance benefits (Institute of Medicine, 1996). In most instances, those who are uninsured are in the workforce. For example, Short, Monheit, and Beauregard (1989) stated that 75% of the uninsured were employed or dependents of an employed individual, and the White House Domestic Policy Council (1993) placed this figure at 85%. Those employed are often in companies that do not offer health insurance for low-paid employees. Lack of insurance and low-paying jobs should make them eligible for federally funded health care. However, according to the U.S. Department of Commerce (1993), less than half of the population below the poverty level is served by Medicaid, the federal and state health program for the indigent. In addition, because of the high cost of coverage, many self-employed people are without insurance. There is also a population with some coverage but not enough to meet major emergencies. According to Rowland and Salganicoff (1994), the underinsured make up 17% of the population.

Access to care is particularly problematic for the poor and elderly. Many are uninsured. If insured, these groups are often covered by Medicaid or Medicare, and fees for service may be predetermined. Because these fees may be limited in amount, more and more physicians do not accept these clients. In addition, when these clients are hospitalized, their stays are shortened. According to Warden (1993), Medicare reductions of fees for physician's office visits has led to reductions in the proportion of Medicare patients seen by physicians: 8% reduction in 1990 and 12% in 1993. Furthermore, patients with predetermined fees are 43% more likely to be discharged from the hospital in an unstable condition with a higher risk of dying.

These two issues—rising health care costs and the lack of access to care for segments of the population—are of concern to community health nurses. To understand what can be done to resolve these concerns, the reader needs a background in methods of financing health care and proposals suggested for changes. Concepts on financing and proposals for health care reform follow.

HEALTH CARE FINANCING METHODS

APPROACHES TO FINANCING HEALTH CARE

There are two basic approaches to financing health care: retrospective and prospective reimbursement.

The traditional approach to reimbursement for health services was *retrospective reimbursement,* in which a fee was paid after services were rendered. The name for this approach was *fee for service* (FFS), and its disadvantage was that unnecessary office visits could be scheduled or procedures performed because they were reimbursable. When services were reimbursed by a government or insurance source, neither the client nor the health care provider was accountable for cost containment.

Prospective reimbursement evolved in 1983 as a cost containment method. It is a method in which rates are predetermined for a specific health care program or set of services. Prospective payment, initiated by the federal government for Medicare patients, was based on a set of predetermined fees for services for clients who fell into specific DRGs. Thus, providers received fees for services based on fixed rates that were determined in advance.

PAYMENT SYSTEMS

There are basically two payment systems for health care: direct client payment and third-party payment. These may use either retrospective or prospective reimbursement.

DIRECT CLIENT PAYMENT

In direct client payment, the consumer pays the provider for the service. This is the FFS approach discussed earlier. Direct client payment may involve payment for services when there is no insurance coverage or when there are exclusions in insurance plans. For example, plans that cover only major medical insurance may leave individuals without coverage for physician office visits, prescriptions, dental care, and eyeglasses. According to Feldstein (1993), consumers pay about 5.5% of hospital care costs, 19% of physician care costs, and 72% of the cost of medications. Consumers may also be required to pay fees until a certain deductible has been reached. Some insurance policies also require a certain copayment from consumers. Direct client payment has decreased and currently accounts for less than the other sources of health care payment. The U.S. Department of Commerce (1993) stated that in 1960 about 50% of the health care expenditure was paid by clients, whereas in 1991 this figure was reduced to 19%.

THIRD-PARTY PAYMENT

This method of payment is payment to the health care provider by some-one other than the recipient of care. It is called *third party* because the payer organization is outside the provider-recipient relationship. There are two basic types of third-party payment sources: private insurance companies (private sector) and government health plans (public sector).

Private Insurance. Private insurance is of three types. First, there are non-profit insurance plans operating under special state laws that allow the company exclusive rights to the whole or part of the state and to a specific type of insurance. Examples of companies operating under this plan include Blue Cross, Blue Shield, and Delta Dental. Specificity is demonstrated by the following: Blue Cross sells insurance that usually covers hospitalizations, Blue Shield usually covers medical and outpatient expenses, and Delta usually covers dental expenses. In my own state, Virginia, Blue Cross, Blue Shield is one option offered to state employees. Second, there are private commercial stock companies with stockholders that sell health insurance nationally, such as Aetna, Connecticut General, and Travelers. These are for-profit companies. A last type of private insurance company is mutual companies that have a national market. Examples in this category include Metropolitan Life, Mutual of Omaha, and Prudential.

Private health insurance may also be provided to employees through independent health plans. These include health maintenance organizations (HMOs) and self-insurance plans offered by businesses, medical groups, and others. Most of these plans are localized and may consist of insurance only or insurance and health care. According to Rooney (1990), more and more companies are turning to self-insurance plans as a cost-saving measure.

In 1990, 74% of the U.S. population had coverage from private health insurers. Of this group, 61% received coverage through an employer, whereas 13% received it by direct purchase of nongroup coverage (U.S. Bureau of the Census, 1991).

Because of the cost of health insurance, employers are taking actions to decrease costs. These efforts include sponsoring more preventive and health promotion activities for employees to reduce illnesses, using health care services that cost less, requiring more financing of health care by employees, using preferred provider agreements to negotiate reduced prices for care, and using self-funding insurance plans (Rooney, 1990).

Government Health Care Plans. The second type of third-party reimbursement is government- or publicly funded health programs. The major health insurance programs of the government are Medicare and Medicaid, which consume the largest amount of revenue of the government's health programs.

Medicare provides mandatory federal insurance for all Americans over the age of 65 and for some disabled Americans. It is a result of a Social Security Act Amendment in 1965 and is the "single largest health insurer in the country, covering about 13 percent of the population, including virtually all the elderly 65 years of age or over (31 million people) and certain persons with disabilities or kidney failure (3 million people)" (DeLew et al., 1992, p. 152). These same figures for recipients of Part A of the Medicare program were reported by the U.S. Department of Commerce (1993).

Medicare has two parts: Part A and Part B. Part A provides inpatient hospital services, including a semiprivate room, laboratory work and X rays, meals, medications, nursing care, supplies and equipment, and operating and recovery room services. Medicare is provided to all participants in the social security program and does not require a fee for the insurance. Limited nursing home and home care may also be provided. There is no coverage in nursing homes beyond 100 days. The services of physicians, nurses, and occupational and speech therapists in the home as well as a major proportion of the cost of home equipment are covered.

Part B is a supplemental health insurance that covers the services of physicians, nurses, or others working under the direction of a physician. It also covers outpatient and emergency room services, physical and occupational therapy, lab and ambulance services, and outpatient psychiatric services. This insurance is optional and requires an additional premium from the recipient. According to the U.S. Department of Commerce (1993), about 96% of people under Part A also receive Part B benefits. The recipient is responsible for paying a deductible and a percentage of the cost of services.

Medicare pays about half of the elderly person's health care costs. Long-term nursing care, outpatient prescribed medications, and routine eye care are excluded. In addition, a deductible and copayment are usually required with care. As a result, "About 68 percent of Medicare beneficiaries have private supplemental health plans . . . and an additional 9 percent have Medicaid" (DeLew et al., 1992, p. 153).

Medicaid was also a result of the Social Security Act Amendments of 1965 and provides health services for certain elderly who cannot pay Part B of Medicare, for selected families with dependent children, for the blind, and for the permanently and totally handicapped. It is jointly funded by the federal and state governments. Services provided may vary from state to state, but certain federally mandated programs are required. These include inpatient and outpatient hospital care; physician care; skilled nursing; family planning; home health care; and early and periodic screening, diagnosis, and treatment (EPSDT) for eligible children who are less than 21 years of age.

Eligibility for Medicaid is based on low income as well as on being elderly, blind, disabled, pregnant, or the parent of a dependent child. According to DeLew et al. (1992), "Mothers and children comprise about 68 percent of Medicaid recipients, the elderly 13 percent, the blind and disabled 15 percent, and others 4 percent" (p. 153). Medicaid is the only government health care program that finances long-term nursing home care. According to the U.S. Department of Commerce (1993), less than half of the people in the United States with incomes below the poverty level were covered by Medicaid. Those excluded would include low-income segments of the population such as homeless men and homeless women without children.

Another insurance program offered by the government is CHAMPUS, a program of health services for dependents of active-duty or retired military personnel. This program pays for inpatient services when these are not available through army or navy hospitals and for outpatient services. Services provided require a deductible and copayment.

In addition, the federal government offers direct health services to certain populations. These include services to military personnel and their dependents, veterans, and Native Americans.

COST CONTAINMENT REIMBURSEMENT TRENDS

Cost concerns have led to changes in reimbursing and delivering care. These changes are significant for community health nurses because they affect the types of nursing services that will be provided, including the scope of independent nursing practice. Roemer (1993) outlined four major concepts of cost containment worldwide:

1. Influencing the behavior of clients about seeking care (e.g., charging clients copayments or other fees or to require a referral by a general practitioner in order to access a specialist)
2. Deliberately limiting health care resources (e.g., limiting hospital construction by governmental bodies, the number of students in medical schools, or the amount of drugs allowed into a country)
3. Influencing health care providers' reimbursement (e.g., substituting DRG reimbursement for FFS)
4. Influencing the performance of professions (e.g., peer reviews of physicians that may lead to disciplinary action if care is inappropriate) (p. 150)

MANAGED CARE

Managed care became popular in the late 1980s and 1990s. It is a system for providing care while minimizing costs. It may involve procedures such as second opinions before surgery, preauthorization for hospital admissions, concurrent review of care, outpatient surgery, and testing requirements to reduce unnecessary or inappropriate care (Thorpe, 1990). Types of organizations using managed care include HMOs and preferred provider organizations (PPOs).

HEALTH MAINTENANCE ORGANIZATIONS

Health maintenance organizations provide comprehensive care through a defined network of providers in exchange for a prepaid fixed monthly premium. They usually provide more coverage without a copayment or deductible than other insurance plans. There is also an emphasis on prevention, health promotion, and ambulatory care as cost-saving measures (DeLew et al., 1992). All inpatient and outpatient care is provided for a predetermined fixed rate. Care outside of the network will not be reimbursed except in an emergency.

HMOs have been growing. Kenkel (1989) reported more than 604 HMOs in the United States in 1989, with 32 million people enrolled. In 1992, 15% of the American population was enrolled, numbering near 37 million (Porter, Ball, & Kraus, 1992). This growth has resulted from government subsidies, cost containment efforts, and official encouragement.

Major characteristics of an HMO are (a) a contract between the HMO and consumers or "enrolled population"; (b) a premium, usually monthly, covering all services, which is paid by the enrollee; and (c) professional providers, contracted by the HMOs, who deliver services to the enrollees (Rapoport, Robertson, & Stewart, 1982).

HMOs have used a variety of patterns. In one pattern, the HMO builds its own facilities, hires physicians, nurses, and other personnel and provides all services to the enrollees. Another pattern is to provide some services to enrollees and contract for the remaining services.

PREFERRED PROVIDER ORGANIZATIONS

PPOs also provide managed care. A PPO is a system of physicians, hospitals, and health-related services that agree to provide health care at fixed discounted prices through a contract with a third-party payer organization. PPOs use formal standards to select providers and carry out utilization reviews (DeLew et al., 1992) to contain costs. Care is obtained by enrollees for no additional cost or for minimal costs. If care is sought outside the network, it is reimbursed at a fixed rate and the recipient must pay the remainder of the cost.

PPO enrollment has been increasing. Participants of medium and large employer health plans grew from 1% enrollment in 1986 to 10% in 1989 (U.S. Department of Labor, 1990).

In both plans, more expensive services such as hospitalization are avoided when possible. Cost containment efforts have been criticized by some as decreasing the quality of care. Results of studies have been contradictory (Gravely & Littlefield, 1992; Krieger, Connel, & LoGerfo, 1992; Reis, 1990). In a recent issue of the *Virginian Pilot* (Bristow, 1996), a physician discussed the health hazard of the "gag" clause in managed care. The gag clause forbids physicians from telling clients anything that might undermine confidence in the insurance plan even if the doctor believes the information could save the patient's life. For example, if a patient is diagnosed with a condition for which federal agencies recommend treatment by physicians who have had previous experience with the condition and none are available in the provider network, the physician is unable to discuss this with the patient. Insurance companies are ordering physicians to keep information about essential procedures, facilities, and medical specialists not included in the health plan from patients, and the American Medical Association's Council on Ethical and Judicial Affairs has found the "gag clauses unethical and a violation of the patient-physician relationship" (Bristow, 1996, p. A12).

RATIONING OF HEALTH CARE

Because cost containment has not been completely effective in controlling health care costs, there have been efforts to control the use of services and technologies. Control of such services is not a new concept because the uninsured who did not qualify for federal programs have always been denied services. In the past, private insurers have also engaged in rationing to exclude those enrollees who were at the greatest risk of health problems (Warden, 1993).

However, new and costly technologies have led to deliberate attempts to limit care to certain individuals or groups. For example, new technologies such as organ transplants have led to committees' or individuals' making decisions about who is eligible for these procedures. Thus, it is predominantly the insurer or health care provider who is unilaterally making decisions about rationing to save money. Rationing can affect the quality of services and raises ethical questions such as the following:

1. Knowing that certain lifestyle behaviors such as smoking are health hazards, should individuals who participate pay higher insurance premiums or be excluded from health services for diseases related to those behaviors?

2. Should a younger person needing a specific procedure that is expensive take precedence over an elderly person?

3. Should someone who is basically healthy but needs specialized care be a priority over another who needs the same care but has a potentially terminal disease such as HIV/AIDS?

PROPOSED PLANS FOR INCREASED COVERAGE OF THE POPULATION

Despite private and public insurance and cost containment plans, more than 37 million Americans still have no health insurance or assistance with health care costs and cannot pay for health care services (Ginsburg & Prout, 1990). In addition to this lack of access to care, questions have been raised about quality of care resulting from cost containment measures. Some changes have been proposed to resolve these concerns. These include universal coverage with a single payer and a national health care plan.

SINGLE-PAYEE UNIVERSAL HEALTH COVERAGE

With single-payer universal coverage health insurance, all citizens would be eligible for health care, and coverage would be provided by a single payer. The single payer, the government, would replace all health insurance companies in the United States. National health insurance has been debated for many, many years, with peaks of interest in the 1960s, the mid-1970s, and the early 1990s. Piecemeal legislation for social security recipients in the 1960s resulted from attempts to pass a national health insurance plan. Although Medicare reached only a small percentage of the population, it was the first national health insurance program in the United States. Other efforts to extend this insurance have been debated in Congress. From these discussions, four major areas of controversy emerged. These included the public-private mix of health insurance involvement, the financial responsibility that consumers should share for coverage, the amount of costs and quality control of the program, and the impetus of a national plan for health care reform (Somers & Somers, 1977). According to Somers and Somers (1977), the ideal national health insurance program would include the following components: (a) universal coverage for all people, (b) financing from multiple sources to be channeled through one source, (c) a comprehensive and balanced structure of benefits, (d) incentives for cost containment, (e) controlled competition in underwriting and administering the program, (f) feasible and appropriate options for consumers, (g) simple administration of the program, (h) flexibility, and (i) acceptability to consumers and providers. The Older Women's League (1993, p. 1) added the following guidelines for a universal single-payer system: (a) universal access regardless of employment status; (b) comprehensive care covering prevention, diagnostic, and treatment services, including mental health; (c) long-term home or institutional care; (d) choice of providers; (e) cost containment; and (f) public funding by a progressive financed plan and public administration.

According to Young (1993), polls indicate that the majority of Americans would prefer a government-financed health insurance program, and Blendon, Leitman, Morrison, and Donelan (1990) reported considerable support for a single-payer plan: In a 1989 study, 61% of the American people stated that they would prefer a Canadian-style health care system in the United States. Accountability for cost savings, quality of care, and access to care are the major advantages of such a single-payer plan. This approach would also simplify administrative paperwork and would eliminate inequities in the health care system. Despite the advantages and support, the program has not become a reality.

HEALTH CARE REFORM EFFORTS

Most people in the United States agree that health care reform is needed. As mentioned earlier, cost containment measures have not been completely effective in stabilizing rising health care costs, and 37 million people are without health care. Thus, any program should reduce the rising health care costs and provide access to health care for all people.

At the turn of the century, the American Association for Labor Legislation advocated state insurance programs to cover health care for all non-work-related illnesses and injuries. Since this initial attempt at health care reform, there have been many efforts to introduce legislation for change in the system. Although these attempts at overall reform have been unsuccessful, Medicare and Medicaid are examples of selected reform.

From a worldwide perspective, the United States does not do well in terms of access to health care for its citizens. According to Roemer (1993), in 1990, social security or equivalent health care protection was provided by 70 world countries to some or all citizens. In 34 countries, mainly industrialized, the coverage is universal or nearly so. In the remaining 36 countries, which are all developing countries except the United States, coverage is only partial. Thus, the United States lags behind other industrialized countries in providing universal health care to its citizens.

HEALTH CARE REFORM PROPOSALS

Health care reform proposals fall mainly into two groups: proposals to reform financing of health care and proposals to reform the health care delivery system. Plans to reform the financial basis of care do not recognize the need for change in the organization of health care delivery, whereas health system reform proposals would change the structure of health care delivery. In 1993, Congress introduced seven health care reform proposals, of which three proposed changes in the structure of health care delivery and four basically proposed changes in the financing of care.

PROPOSALS FOR REFORMING HEALTH CARE FINANCING

Various suggestions for financing health care have been advanced that would make care more accessible for all. Some of these are presented here. One proposal suggested that employers provide insurance for all employees and that the government provide for those who are unemployed and unable to pay. Another proposal was to expand Medicaid eligibility criteria for those in need of health insurance and to allow those above eligibility levels to pay for insurance on an income-based sliding scale. Another suggestion was to tax employees for employment insurance benefits and to use this money to pay for insurance for those who were without employer-provided insurance (Feldstein, 1993).

PROPOSALS FOR REFORMING HEALTH CARE DELIVERY

There are two basic suggestions for reform in health care delivery systems, and a conflict in values exists between two groups of advocates for these changes. One group values the managed-competition model; the other values universal coverage or the single-payer plan. Universal coverage would involve restructuring of the health care system, whereas managed care involves some changes but lacks the broad restructuring of the universal coverage plan.

Managed-Competition Model. The managed-competition model encourages competition in a free marketplace and advocates the right of recipients to choose the type of health care desired. According to Merline (1993), managed competition would achieve cost containment due to free market competition and would increase access to care as it moved away from governmental regulation. In this approach, accountability for the success of the plan resides with the insurance industry.

Under this system, clients would choose between competing privately owned and for-profit health insurance plans. According to Young (1993), these companies would "compete for managed care contracts from large employers and group purchasers known as 'health insurance purchasing cooperatives' (HIPC's)" (p. 945). In other words, insurers would compete for large-scale contracts from networks or employers, individuals, and governmental agencies (Duerksen, 1993; National League for Nursing [NLN], 1993). The HIPCs would be regional or statewide organizations composed of employers and individuals that could demand favorable rates because of their size and purchasing power. HIPCs would require the meeting of federal guidelines and the inclusion of mandated benefits of plans that they selected (Merline, 1993). Other features of this plan include (a) reports to consumers on quality of care provided, (b) penalties for companies screening out high-risk enrollees to achieve a better risk pool, and (c) guaranteed coverage of all who apply. Most plans include government subsidies for low-income people who cannot afford premiums (Citizen Action, 1994), but part or all of the existing Medicaid program would be eliminated.

Universal Health Care Model. The universal health care model was discussed earlier in this chapter. This is the model of care proposed by the American Public Health Association (APHA). In *The Nation's Health* (APHA, 1995), a proposed policy statement suggested reaffirming support for legislation for universal, comprehensive health care; single-payer financing; political action; and strengthening of public health programs.

NURSING'S PROPOSAL FOR HEALTH CARE REFORM

A coalition of nursing organizations developed a proposal for a national health care program in 1991. Members of the coalition included the American Nurses Association, the American Association of Colleges of Nursing, the Association of Community Health Nursing Educators, the National League for Nursing, and the National Association of School Nurses.

This plan focused on cost containment and the provision of quality care through strategies such as (a) case management, (b) consumer and provider incentives for cost savings, (c) control of the growth of health systems through planning and allocation of resources, (d) reimbursement tied to the outcomes of care as demonstrated by research, (e) choice of providers for health care consumers, and (f) control of administrative costs (American Association of Colleges of Nursing [AACN], 1991). More specific features of the proposal included (a) a defined package of services that included primary and preventive care; (b) universal access to care; (c) implementation of the program in steps, with priority given to the care of pregnant women and children; (d) financing through governmental and private sources by taxes and employee and individual contributions; (e) continuation of private insurance but with mandated minimum benefits; (f) optional purchase of additional services, if desired; and (g) mandated private or public insurance for employees by employers.

The program financing would be by a combination of private and public sources. The poor would receive standardized services through a program provided by the government that could also be purchased by employers and individuals. Although private insurance companies would continue to provide plans, they would be required to provide minimum standardized benefits. Employers and individuals could also purchase additional services.

A follow-up document by the NLN (1992) looked at changes needed in nursing education to prepare for health care reform. Changes suggested included (a) significantly increased numbers of advanced practice nurses who can provide primary care in a variety of settings; (b) a shift in emphasis for all nursing education programs (graduate and undergraduate) to prepare nurses who are community based and community focused; (c) increased numbers of community nursing centers used by students as model clinical sites; (d) increased numbers of faculty prepared to teach community-based, community-focused nursing; and (e) a shift in the emphasis of nursing research to the study of community and aggregate health promotion and disease prevention.

CLINTON'S PROPOSAL FOR HEALTH CARE REFORM

President Bill Clinton's proposal for health care reform, presented in 1993, did not pass. However, it would have provided coverage for all Americans and legal immigrants for expenses such as hospital care, emergency services, physicians' and other health professionals' services, pregnancy-related services, hospice and home health care, ambulances, outpatient lab tests, and prescription drugs. It included a long-term care program for disabled people, free preventive care, and initial limited coverage of dental care, eye care, and mental health care, to be expanded by 2000. It also proposed a new Medicare benefit for prescription drugs that would be partially funded. Employers could provide more than the standardized package, but by the year 2000 these benefits would be taxed. Recipients would be offered a choice between fee for service, an HMO, or a combination of the two.

By this proposal, most Americans would enroll in a regional group called an *alliance* (see discussion of health insurance purchasing cooperatives with information about the managed care model) that would negotiate the price of coverage with health plans, offer a range of services, and collect premiums from employers and individuals. People under Medicare would continue under Medicare but could later join an alliance. Medicaid patients would be enrolled in alliances. All Americans would be issued a national health identification card to gain access to care. Costs for the plans would be based on a combination of employer and employee fees and government subsidies.

EFFECTIVE HEALTH CARE REFORM REQUIREMENTS

Several requirements for effective health care reform have been advocated. The Clinton administration, which proposed health care system reform recently, identified the following: choice, quality, responsibility, savings, security, and simplicity (White House Domestic Policy Council, 1993). *Choice* involves choice of health care providers by care recipients and in some instances a choice of a health care plan, although this is not considered in the proposal for single-payer plans. *Quality* refers to high-quality care, including preventive and curative care, that is research and theory based. *Responsibility* refers to the responsibility for quality, cost-effective health care assumed by all involved people so that the system is not abused by physicians, hospitals, clients, or others. *Savings* involves cost containment measures to reduce or eliminate the rising costs of health care. *Incentives* should be included for plans with the least expensive care providers and settings consistent with quality and other cost saving measures. *Security* refers to the accessibility of care for all Americans regardless of employment or other demographic variables. *Simplicity* involves making a system of reimbursement that is simple and requires minimal administrative time.

TABLE 3.1 Health Expenditures by Purpose, United States, 1988: Amount in Billions of Dollars and Percentage Distribution

Purpose	Billions ($)	%
Hospital care	211.8	39.2
Nursing home care	43.1	8.0
Physician services	105.1	19.5
Dental services	29.4	5.4
Other professional services	22.5	4.2
Home health care	4.4	0.8
Drugs and medical supplies	41.9	7.8
Eyeglasses and medical equipment	10.8	2.0
Other personal health care	9.3	1.7
Program administration	26.3	4.9
Public health activities	15.9	2.9
Health science research	9.9	1.8
Facility construction	9.5	1.8
All purposes	539.9	100.0

SOURCE: U.S. Department of Health and Human Services (1990).

PREVENTION: A PART OF HEALTH CARE REFORM

Prevention should be a part of health care reform because without prevention, there is no guarantee of improved health of the American population. Baker et al. (1994) stated that making administrative tasks simpler and providing access to care for all Americans will not do much "to influence the true determinants of ill health: unsafe environments, unhealthy personal behaviors, and biologic, genetic, and socioeconomic factors," which account for "more than 1 million deaths per year and untold levels of preventable morbidity and expensive (avoidable) health care in the United States" (p. 1277). The authors argued that the health of the public could best be improved by broadening the focus of lawmakers, private insurance companies, physicians, hospitals, and other organizations to include public health systems.

According to Salmon (1995), the current U.S. health care system focuses mainly on the interaction of biology and medical technology. Thus, the emphasis is on the interaction of disease agents and humans at the secondary level of intervention (sick care) and technology available to deal with illness, with little or no emphasis on primary prevention or public health. Table 3.1, on the percentages of the budget spent on health care, bears this out. It shows that in 1988, public health activities accounted for 2.9% of the total national budget, whereas illness care (hospital care, nursing home care, physician services, dental services, other professional services, home health care, drugs and medical supplies, eyeglasses and medical equipment, and other personal health care) accounted for about 88.6%. In 1993, "Less than 1% of the aggregate amount for all health care was spent on population-based public health activities" (Salmon, 1995, p. 5).

There have been some efforts to broaden concepts of health care to shift its focus more toward prevention for policy formulation purposes. *Healthy People 2000* (U.S. DHHS, 1991) and earlier related reports broadened the framework of health to include inherited biological, environmental, and behavioral risks as determinants of health. These reports also focused on keeping people healthy rather than on caring for the sick. Other studies and reports that have focused on health and that may have had an influence on policy include the Medical Outcomes Study (Stewart & Ware, 1992), which included well-being among the indicators of health; a "health field concept" policy proposal by the Canadian Department of National Health and Welfare that included biology, environment, lifestyle, and health care as major elements (Lalonde, 1974); and an epidemiological model of health policy proposed by Dever (1976) that included lifestyle and environment among other health indicators.

Using a broad framework of health determinants, Salmon (1995) identified eight essential elements of a satisfactory health system: (a) universal coverage, with clinical preventive services excluded from cost sharing; (b) financially rewarding health plans that keep populations healthy; (c) a system of evaluating and reporting activities of health plans that focuses on achieving healthy outcomes for clients; (d) an integrated system of health information for reporting to insurance companies and clients; (e) a prepared and geographically distributed force of health care providers; (f) health-related research support, including preventive and epidemiological research as well as health services and behavioral, and social sciences research; (g) ability to deliver coordinated, comprehensive care to populations who are underserved; and (h) strengthening of the health and governmental systems with a web of population-based, basic public health activities.

We often look at prevention in terms of whether the gains in health are reasonable for the cost incurred. Simmons (1993) presented a table of the cost of treatment for diseases that are preventable based on data from *Healthy People 2000*. For example, 500,000 deaths from heart disease and 2,884,000 bypass surgeries annually (at a cost of $30,000 per person for the first year) could have been avoided with adequate preventive care, according to Simmons. Cancer causes 510,000 preventable deaths annually and 1 million new cases of cancer annually; the high costs of lung cancer treatment ($30,000/person for the first year) and cervical cancer treatment ($29,000/person for the first year), for example, could be avoided by preventive care. Every year, 23,000 low-birth-weight babies die and 260,000 low-birth-weight babies are born; their neonatal intensive care may cost $10,000, and other care for them may cost $31,000 for the first year. Simmons also presented data on cost of treatment by year for preventable diseases and conditions related to alcoholism, injuries, and inadequate immunizations.

In addition, Simmons (1993) presented three models for use of financial resources in preventive health care: investment, insurance, and consumption. In the investment model, the cost-effectiveness of the outcome is weighed against today's cost of preventive interventions. Thus, the outcomes as well as the expenditures for providing the services are considered and compared. Expenditures may include both direct costs (screening tests and provider time) and indirect costs (time spent with activity such as exercise or class attendance). Outcomes may be reported as single outcomes, such as years of life saved, or as combined outcomes, such as results from a quality-of-life scale. The model is used to help decision makers focus on services that provide the most or best outcomes for the money invested. This model of cost-effectiveness analysis of preventive services has been used for lead poisoning detection, cholesterol monitoring, cervical cancer screening, and mammography screening (Simmons, 1993).

The other models, insurance and consumption, are alternative models of economic decision making. The insurance model states that future potential negative outcomes can be avoided by spending in the present. The focus is on the avoidance of negative future outcomes and involves pooling funds in anticipation of a low probability event.

In contrast to the other two, the consumption model says that prevention is an expenditure that provides benefits today, such as the feeling of well-being following physical exercise. The emphasis is on active prevention in which individuals receive an immediate positive response to the output of time, energy, and money in an effort to change behavior. Other cost-effectiveness models will be presented in Chapter 14.

Salmon (1995) also advocated including public health in health care reform, stating that "a system that addresses personal care alone simply will not be capable of assuring the health of the people of this country" (p. 2). To ensure successful health care reform, the personal care system and public health system must work together to include preventive and health promotion activities, early interventions, and cost-effective care.

POTENTIAL EFFECTS ON HEALTH OF COST CONTAINMENT

There is a delicate balance between cost containment and quality of care as they affect health and health patterns. Some cost containment measures may influence quality because illnesses will increase or illness care will become more expensive. For example, Roemer (1993) reported an experiment in California in which patients on Medicaid were charged a $1 copayment because officials considered the number of physician visits to be excessive. Thereafter, office visits decreased and a savings was realized. However, after a few months, hospitalizations increased when compared with those of a control group who did not pay a copayment. The cost for this care exceeded that paid for office visits.

A second effect of cost containment was reported in the *Washington Post* in 1995 (Bloodman, 1995). It was reported that the average length of stay for childbirth dropped from 4 days in 1970 to 24 hours in 1995. At the same time, there was an increase in jaundice, dehydration, and other serious problems of infants that required readmission.

Another effect of cost containment was reported in the *New York Times* (Fein, 1995). After budget cuts led to layoffs in New York city hospitals, there was an increase in decubitus ulcers and late medication delivery to patients.

Duffy and Farley (1995) looked at the effect of financial incentives and changing hospital structures on services provided by hospitals. Using data from a variety of sources, they studied 150 of the most frequently performed procedures on inpatients from 1980 to determine what had happened by 1987. They found that (a) 36 of the 150 procedures were used 40% less in 1987 than in 1980; (b) patients receiving one of these 36 procedures as inpatients in 1987 were more severely ill than patients receiving one of the procedures in 1980; and (c) rates of decline in use of procedures were considerably greater for Medicaid patients. Three factors contributed to the decreased use of procedures on inpatients: (a) a shift in care from inpatient to outpatient settings, (b) new technologies, and (c) pressure from reimbursement sources and utilization review policies.

FEDERAL LEGISLATION AND HEALTH

Current federal legislation may also affect health for segments of the population. The Welfare Reform Bill, signed into law in 1996, basically mandates the following (although there are exceptions to each aspect of the bill): (a) limits lifetime welfare to 5 years and requires the head of households to find work within 2 years or lose benefits; (b) denies most welfare benefits, including food stamps, to legal immigrants; (c) requires at least half of all single parents on welfare in each state to be working by 2002 or denies the state some of its federal funding; (d) limits the food stamp program to 3 months in a 3-year period for childless adults between ages 18 and 50; (e) denies cash aid or food stamps to convicted drug felons; and (f) requires school attendance and living with parents as a requirement for teenage mothers to receive benefits (Church, 1996).

The National Coalition for the Homeless (1996) has argued that the impact of H.R. 3734 is to move Americans off welfare and into homelessness. The Urban Institute (Zedlewski, Clark, Meier, & Watson, 1996) has estimated that the welfare changes may place 2.6 million more people below the poverty line, including 1.1 million children. In addition, they have predicted that one fifth of all families with children will see their incomes fall by about $1,300 per year. They have stated that about half of the families affected currently work and that four of five of the affected families have incomes below 150% of the poverty level. The 1996 poverty level for a family of three is $12,980, and 150% of poverty-level income for this same family would be around $19,470. In addition, the 14.5% of the population (about 38.1 million people) who currently live below the poverty line would be affected (U.S. Bureau of Census, 1996).

ECONOMIC FORCES AND COMMUNITY HEALTH NURSING

Community health nurses work with the economic subsystem of the community regularly. At the non-advanced-practice nurse level, the economics of individuals and families are assessed as a basis for planning a variety of interventions. If income is inadequate to support the family, a variety of changes may be suggested, such as food budgeting, obtaining food stamps, thrift shopping for clothing, obtaining free medical care, moving to cheaper housing, and disposing of one's car and using public transportation.

The community health (advanced practice) nurse is also involved with the economic subsystem but at the level of the total community or community aggregates. An assessment of the community population and statistics will often identify aggregates with inadequate incomes to provide for basic needs or without access to health care. For example, groups of the poor and elderly may lack resources to obtain adequate housing and a variety of other basic necessities. In addition, the homeless and certain other low-income groups are ineligible for health care.

Educational programs in high-risk neighborhoods with these segments of the population may focus on traditional issues such as budgeting for food and housing, sources of medical care, food stamps, and other service programs. However, the advanced practice nurse may also present topics such as how to contact legislators, how to form coalitions to resolve problems, and how to obtain corrective measures in rented apartments.

Nurses also interact with the economic and other community subsystems as part of an assessment to determine the influence of these subsystems on health. For example, nurses always evaluate local and state funding for health services and other sources of funding for additional services. They assess transportation to determine if it is accessible to segments who rely on it for work and other activities. They also assess recreational, social service, and other subsystems impinging on populations. When services are deficit, the economics of bringing services up to an acceptable level should be assessed.

Interventions regarding economics include education, as identified earlier, and political action. Community health nurses may need to meet with legislators to present a case for additional funding for more immunizations for an increased infant population or to advocate for a national health program that will allow all people access to care.

At times, community health nurses must plan care for increased numbers of aggregates with no increase in funding or must continue to provide care when funding has been reduced. Again, an assessment and prioritizing of needs is necessary as a basis for deciding on appropriate interventions. In some situations, partnerships with hospitals and other organizations have been established so that money is available and care can continue to be provided. Several of these partnerships will be discussed in Part IV. At other times, a shift in the site and financing of care may be necessary. For example, in my own community, local physicians recently began seeing pregnant clients on Medicaid in their offices. This population had previously received care at the local health department. This shift in funding and personnel freed nurses to provide nursing care to the most high-risk pregnant clients and to add community-focused preventive care services within the existing funding and staffing constraints.

At the very end of this chapter is a case study by two community health nursing leaders, a community health nurse manager, and a community health nurse supervisor and adjunct professor in the Virginia Beach Health Department in which they discuss how they have dealt with economic forces in their community. This case study should assist the reader in applying the concepts presented in this chapter to aggregates and the community.

Case Study 1

Economic Changes and the Worksmart Health Department

ANGELA B. SAVAGE
ANNA L. PRATT

The cross-currents of societal changes in the mid-1990s have brought profound challenges for local health departments. More than ever, the ability of local health officials to maintain what has been customary service to their communities faces uncertainty. Curtailment of funding levels has caused a retrenchment as officials make hard choices about how to make the most of dwindling resources. Administrators confronted with these challenges find themselves in uncharted waters for the most part. Their task of getting the most out of each remaining dollar of funding has demanded new formulas that include partnerships with private medical providers and other community health groups. New choices about how to commit remaining resources to serve a growing population—and where to cut services—has forced administrators to examine new stratagems, often requiring considerable ingenuity and diplomacy. Even the basic missions of local health agencies are being called into question.

As the body politic hunts for cost-cutting targets, the health department that may only recently have been a last refuge of sickness care for the poor is shedding its role as healer as it searches for its place in a sea of change. With uncertain resources in its future, it is looking back to its core values. Once again, traditional prevention services are held up as the model that public health will follow into the 21st century.

The broad societal trend of cost containment and its spin-off effects, including the absorbing of Medicaid clients by managed-care providers, reassignments of resources at the local level, and occasionally, staffing reductions, all combine to affect service delivery to the community. Because these tides of change are already being felt in quick succession at the local level of public health, it will be useful to examine one such local agency that we will call the Worksmart Health Department in the imaginary community of Waterville. This agency will provide the model to help examine some real issues faced in a day-to-day community-based public health department.

We will start with a look at the Worksmart Health Department's nursing program and its traditional role in its community. This model health department will serve to demonstrate how changes in federal and state funding for health care affected the Worksmart Health Department and how the department met the particular challenges. Included are decisions on (a) shifting allocations of services, such as development of public-private partnerships; (b) changes in direction away from health care on demand and toward community-based education and prevention services; and (c) a final section on what the new realities will demand for the future, including new criteria for staffing that emphasize community involvement in creative new ways.

The driving engine of many changes—economic changes—will be dealt with in a more general way to emphasize the local agency's role in its quest to continue to meet the needs of Waterville residents. It is important for the reader to keep in mind that although "Worksmart" and "Waterville" are fictitious names, the situations presented are based on real-life occurrences. Some other details have also been changed for the sake of clarity in presenting situations, so the model presented should be not presumed to reflect point-by-point the experiences of a particular agency.

A SENTINEL TO ACTION

The Institute of Medicine (1988) document, *The Future of Public Health,* warned of the state of disarray in public health. It concluded that the nation had lost sight of its public health goals and had slackened its public health vigilance nationally. In Congress, national health care reform was being discussed and debated. Momentum was building for those who had long claimed that paying for "sick care" was breaking the bank of the health care system. "Prevention is by far cheaper" went the argument, and there was more talk of health care coverage paying for prevention. Public health practitioners were concerned about the shift in practice into providing primary care to underserved, vulnerable populations, serving as part of their "safety net." It seemed that this shift might result in public health's forfeiting its traditional role of protecting and promoting the public's health and preventing disease.

Beginning in the late 1980s, changes began to occur in state Medicaid. In addition, many poor pregnant women and their infants and children were not insured by the government's safety net. National data on the health of women and children (i.e., statistics on infant mortality rate and low birth weight) were worse than for many Third World countries. Increasing Medicaid eligibility standards was viewed as a strategy to improve access to care for the most vulnerable groups: pregnant women and their babies. Supporters of this plan argued that the health status of this underserved group would be improved.

When it was decided to implement the proposed strategy, beginning in 1988, Medicaid eligibility criteria changed, resulting in more pregnant women qualifying for Medicaid coverage for prenatal care. It was hoped that more pregnant women would enter prenatal care in the first trimester because they would have a payment source. Increased numbers of Medicaid clientele did not mean a concurrent increase in reimbursement dollars. The result was that in the 1980s, public health clinics struggled financially to provide primary health care to pregnant women receiving Medicaid. Some health departments were actually providing this costly prenatal care at a loss, putting even further demands on stressed budgets. When the reimbursement rates finally did increase in the early 1990s, private obstetricians came forward, even recruiting pregnant women with Medicaid into their practices.

As a result of uncontrolled rising Medicaid costs incurred by the state budget, more changes in Medicaid occurred in the mid-1990s. By controlling access to care, Medicaid managed-care systems were seen as a way to control ever-increasing Medicaid expenditures. State by state, people insured by Medicaid were required to enroll with a managed-care provider by January 1, 1996. One requirement made of Medicaid providers was ensuring their Medicaid managed-care patients access to 24-hour care. Health departments were not able to meet that requirement on their own. Worksmart, a Medicaid provider in those years, met that stipulation through entering into a fee-based contractual arrangement with a local hospital in a nearby city to provide pediatric services to Medicaid-enrolled children.

Another strategy to contain costs was the creation of leaner, more efficient workforces at all levels of government. The impetus for "downsizing," "right-sizing," and "re-engineering," well-known and daunting phrases, was being felt in the health departments. "Public-private partnerships" became the key phrase and the call to action as the only effective way to maximize ever-shrinking resources. Clearly, leaders were saying that no one group could do it all; there was synergy and increased potential in joining resources. Public health departments began to invite hospitals, private physicians, nonprofit agencies, voluntary organizations, and citizen-based groups to the meeting table. Their shared purpose was working together to improve the health of communities. The health departments and private health care providers were challenged to develop a new relationship, one characterized by collaboration and cooperation, each sharing their strengths and expertise, each expanding into new knowledge, skills, and abilities. The predominant questions were these: Would such a partnership evolve? More important, would it work?

PUBLIC HEALTH NURSING PROGRAM: THE WAY IT WAS

In the 1960s and 1970s, the public health nurses of the Worksmart Health Department functioned in the traditional role of "visiting nurses." The department was minimally involved with clinical services; the main focus of service delivery was on school- and home-based services and health education. None of the hospitals in Waterville provided outpatient clinical services. Thus, poor residents needing primary care and specialized services attended clinics conducted by general hospitals in a nearby city.

The nursing programs did include small maternity clinics, well child care, family planning, childhood immunizations, and the control of tuberculosis and general communicable diseases, including venereal disease. Nurses made home visits to provide maternal and child health education/anticipatory guidance, teach accident prevention, stress the importance of regular well child care, and evaluate the progress of children with handicapping conditions who were enrolled in the Crippled Children's Program. Public health nurses also visited tuberculosis patients to monitor their treatment. In those years, elderly residents, served through the Home Health Program, received home-based skilled and health maintenance nursing care. The goal of those services was to enable senior citizens to remain in their own homes as long as possible. Public Health Nurses also visited people recently discharged from mental health institutions to evaluate their progress in the home and community setting.

When possible, revenue was collected for Home Health Services from Medicaid and Medicare payments. Local revenue generation was not yet a necessary part of the budget process.

During those years, the Worksmart Health Department gradually increased clinical services. Concurrently, federal block grants encouraged health departments to expand clinical services because health care needs of indigent populations were unmet elsewhere. Private providers were not accepting "Medicaid patients" in their practices. Therefore, serving community residents, either in the clinics or in the home, became the role for the health department. The increased health department services, beginning in the mid-1970s, resulted in the need to increase staff to deliver those services. Specialized staff were needed to ensure delivery of appropriate and competent care to this population, many of whom presented higher health risks. Laboratory staff, pharmacists, and board-certified physicians were hired, funds to support them coming from federal grants and from Medicaid and other collected fees. Added fiscal staff were necessary to keep up with increased demands associated with grant management and the Medicaid billing process.

This trend of increasing services and staff to meet the demands of an ever-growing Medicaid population in Waterville continued until the late 1980s. At that time, collecting fees from clients for services delivered became critical to supporting and continuing clinical services and staff. Medicaid reimbursements continued to lag behind actual cost of care.

But the climate of public support for publicly funded health care policies was changing. With the advent of the 1990s, sentinel changes in allocation of resources for local health departments, notably funding, were well underway.

STAFF AND FUNDING

During the early 1970s, the core of the Worksmart Health Nursing Department, directed by one nurse manager, was composed of 3 nursing supervisors, 30 public health nurses, 1 nurse practitioner, and 1 nursing assistant. A physician served as the local health director, and that leadership continues to the present. Federal funding and revenues allowed the department to grow so that by 1990, the nurse manager was responsible for a staff of 5 nursing supervisors, 45 public health nurses, and 4 nursing assistants. Three nurse practitioners, 1 public health outreach worker, 1 health educator, WIC nutritionists, and office support personnel also fell under the nurse manager's organizational/functional control. That staffing level was maintained until the mid-1990s, when a governmental downsizing action, described more fully in a later section, significantly reduced numbers.

The funding for the Worksmart Health Department budget comes from 55% state funding allocated annually by the state legislature and 45% city matching funds. This is known as "the cooperative budget." These monies often include specialized grants and allocations. Family planning grants (Title X) have been a part of Worksmart's budget for many years; maternal and child health (Title V) grants followed. In later years, grants funded chronic disease prevention programs, childhood injury prevention, and childhood immunizations.

A population explosion in Waterville with no corresponding update in state-funding formulas left the Worksmart Health Department with a relatively small budget and staffing per capita. When measured with other health departments throughout the state, Worksmart Health Department administrators found they were losing ground in the effort to maintain service levels. The local budget grew through grants and revenue collections, not through sufficient state-funding allocations. Critical to remember is that although Worksmart's nursing staff did grow, even that increase did not keep pace with population growth.

Between 1980 and 1990, the population of Waterville grew by 130,870 people. In 1990, census exceeded 393,000 people, and 1995 population estimates were placed at higher than 410,000. In the early 1990s, Medicaid cases increased by greater than 150% and Aid to Families With Dependent Children (AFDC) cases increased by greater than 75%. The "working poor," chronically ill adult residents who lack health insurance, are still Waterville's vulnerable population: Private health care providers are not yet willing to significantly serve them, resources of the existing "free clinic" are overburdened, and the health department cannot afford to provide primary care to these individuals. Their care remains an unmet need and challenge for the community.

THE NEW REALITIES

The countless unknowns and endless changes beginning in the late 1980s and continuing into the 1990s had significant financial implications for the Worksmart Health Department. Following is a chronology of how the department responded to a public health system in chaos.

In the late 1980s, the Worksmart Health Department experienced its first funding reduction. More than half of the state dollars supporting the nonmandated dental program were removed from the state legislature's allocation. The removal of those funds meant a loss of the 45% city match. An equivalent reduction in dental staff occurred, which meant that the department needed to reprioritize service delivery. Strategic planners chose to focus on the dental health of economically needy children who qualified for service. As with indigent adults with chronic general health problems, adults needing dental care lacked a resource.

This funding crisis jolted the sense of job security among part-time staff members. Although no additional funding losses were anticipated, two part-time nurses chose to seek more secure employment in other agencies. Administrators decided to maintain clinical services status quo, with all remaining staff "tightening their belts." Although the threat of such state-funding reductions had loomed in previous years, nothing had ever materialized. This was the first message that the historically "dependable" state and local dollars were clearly in jeopardy. Earning revenue now became critical to the local budget process, essential to continuing programs and to staff.

In the late 1980s, the previously dependable revenue from the Home Health Program began to decrease. More and more private home health agencies moved into Waterville and competed with the local health department's Home Health Care Program for the market. Again, it was time for the health department to critically evaluate its role: If the private sector was now going to meet the home care needs of city residents, was it appropriate and affordable for the health department to compete with or duplicate that service? A difficult decision was made: Worksmart would stop its Home Health Program, a historical service to public health nursing.

Meantime, the infant mortality rate in Waterville exceeded the rate for the state in the late 1980s. Improving this statistic became a focus of the health department, a direction supported at the state level. One state strategy to improve birth outcomes was to develop Medicaid funding for "baby care providers."

Worksmart decided to participate in this case management program. Through this initiative, high-risk pregnant women received individualized care and services, aimed at promoting healthy pregnancies and preventing poor outcomes. Worksmart's home health nurses, already skilled in home-based care and assessments to the elderly, were now available to provide those services in the Baby Care Program. They attended workshops to gain related knowledge, skills, and abilities.

It became evident that many factors that defined a pregnancy as high risk were social in nature (e.g., substance abuse, child care issues, and domestic violence). It was critical that interventions be family oriented. Thus, in addition to the nurses' needing education about the physiological aspects of high-risk pregnancies, they also needed to be educated about socioeconomic factors. Networking with a wide variety of community human service agencies was necessary to provide broad individualized care and services to pregnant women and their babies and small children.

Initially, nursing staff turnover in these positions was high, leading to repeated vacancies, hiring, and orientation of new staff members. Remaining staff members worked hard to maintain continuity of care. Because the practice of public health had been primarily clinic-based for 10 to 15 years, nurses had become unaccustomed to and uncomfortable with community-based service delivery. They also voiced feelings of discouragement and burnout. The social situations that they encountered were more overwhelming than they had anticipated; they experienced a sense of "culture shock." They had a repeated sense of professional failure when their efforts to assist patients were met with nonacceptance, hostility, and continuance of the very behaviors (substance abuse) that placed the pregnancies and the unborn babies at high risk. Through mutual support and training in concepts such as behavior change and the individual's self-responsibility for health, the nurses recognized and accepted the realistic limitations of their interventions. In addition, they realized that setting short-term goals, with a high degree of patient involvement, led to a greater sense of success, served to develop trust, and acted as building blocks for acceptance of health teaching.

Now, in 1996, case management has been a regular service of the Worksmart Health Department for 4 years; turnover of nursing staff has stopped, and instead of viewing their jobs as frustrating, nurses once more feel a sense of satisfaction, accomplishment, and success in helping women and their families.

Because Medicaid reimbursement levels were finally increased, negotiations began between the department and the local obstetricians to explore the development of a partnership in prenatal care. Private obstetricians in Waterville began to market to the pregnant women receiving Medicaid. They also contacted the health department, offering to provide care for all these women in the city. Worksmart viewed this star-tling shift as positive: The local private medical community was starting to take a more active role in the health care of needy pregnant women. After the health director set the stage by meeting with the obstetricians to draft the general plan, the nursing department developed and finalized the details. Nurses met with the physicians and their staffs to learn what the doctors wanted from the health department in this partnership and to describe the services, skills, and expertise that the department brought to the table. Both partners identified areas where services, knowledge, skills, and abilities needed enhancement. The result was the creation of a system in which these partners collaborate to provide care to high-risk pregnant women, infants, and children up to 2 years of age. By choice, pregnant women can attend the department's maternity triaging clinic. During their first clinic visit, they receive a pregnancy risk assessment by a nurse practitioner or physician; a nutrition assessment and, if eligible, enrollment into the WIC Program (a federally funded supplemental food and educational program for pregnant and lactating women, infants, and children); and basic laboratory studies. After that appointment, those women receive office-based prenatal care with the private doctor, and depending on their high-risk status, they may also be referred to public health nurse case managers. The small number of pregnant women who do not qualify for Medicaid continue prenatal care with the health department, also being referred to case managers if they present with or develop complications of pregnancy. The only reimbursement for this service is direct payment from those clients, on a sliding scale.

When she receives a referral, the public health nurse makes a home visit to assess the pregnant woman, her risk factors, and her family. The nurse and the doctor maintain communication about the patient and work with the woman and her family to promote a healthy pregnancy and baby. Medicaid reimburses the health department for these case management services.

Gradually, this referral system allowed the Worksmart Health Department to significantly downsize its prenatal clinic program. However, this presented a new, dual-headed problem for Worksmart: Although the budget was relieved of the costly prenatal program, Medicaid revenue followed the Medicaid pregnant women out of the health department to private care providers.

The demand on Worksmart's budget from that program had eased, but less revenue was being earned. A health department is a service agency, depending on staff to provide its services. If a budget cannot support the staff, reducing staff is a strategy to explore; it became necessary for Worksmart to make that difficult decision. Because the prenatal services had reduced in magnitude and scope, related specialty staff were no longer needed. Administration succeeded in placing those staff members in other employment. The department had successfully survived a major shift in its services.

The opportunity now presented itself for the department to explore strengthening preventive services: Staff members who were previously absorbed with maternity clinic services were now available. More strategic planning led to the formation of a team of professionals whose focus would be delivering health promotion and risk-based prevention education at various sites in Waterville. This new team was created in the early 1990s, about the same time that national health care reform was proposing that health departments needed to return to their original mission: protecting and promoting the health of the public and preventing disease through their core functions of assessment, assurance, and policy development.

Nurses in the department were offered the opportunity to work on this new team. Those demonstrating skill and motivation to provide community-based programming were chosen. Worksmart was viewed as a pioneer in the state because it had dedicated staff resources specifically for health promotion. Traditionally, community-based health education programs have been developed and implemented primarily, often solely, by degreed health education specialists. Now, public health nurses were being assigned to provide community-based health promotion, using their clinical expertise and enhancing their health education skills. Staff and programs were beginning to be funded once again through a combination of grant monies and the cooperative budget. This self-directed work team is supported by one nursing supervisor with experience in team building and health education. The department's management team approved the team's developing its mission statement, which reflected the state's mission of public health: healthy people in healthy communities.

Team priorities, service goals, and program activities were also carefully focused. Program areas that make up the core of the team include (a) dealing with cardiovascular disease, (b) dealing with breast and cervical cancer, (c) childhood injury prevention, (d) childhood immunizations, (e) prevention of tobacco use by youth, (f) prevention of sexually transmitted diseases to include HIV and AIDS, and (g) supporting agencies whose mission is violence prevention. Some of the priorities were related to already established and operating grant-funded programming, and others reflected national and local health concerns and initiatives.

Each team member maintains a broad base of key contacts within Waterville, both in the private and public sectors. Networking and collaborating with other human service agencies has become a cornerstone of the team. Members serve on coalitions and advisory boards. Their knowledge of risk-based disease prevention education, skills in coalition building and collaboration, and expertise with developing partnerships with community resources are well-known and sought by staff in other Waterville agencies.

The team answers requests for service and also markets its programs to target populations and the general community, depending on required program directions. Community-needs assessments were conducted and results provided direction for programming. Team members focus on delivering services to high-risk target populations identified in the city. Having a firm understanding of their mission and goals, team members are empowered to make decisions to pursue contacts, develop programs, and deliver services. They also collaborate and coordinate with other health department services (e.g., WIC) to maximize the range of appropriate services brought to residents. Neighborhood-based community centers, private homes, homeless shelters, schools, churches, businesses, and a mobile van are among the many different sites where services are delivered. Team members are clearly aware of each other's assignment area and the team focus and purpose; they are alert for opportunities to involve each other in programming and service delivery when appropriate. Programs are consistently evaluated to assess impact and effectiveness.

The Worksmart Health Department met yet another challenge in the mid-1990s associated with state government's goal of becoming smaller and more efficient. In 1995, the nursing department was significantly affected: More that 20% of its staff left employment through a government downsizing initiative. Public health nurses, nurse practitioners, one full-time physician, and several clerical support staff took advantage of the state's early retirement workforce reduction incentive plan. At the state level, these positions were abolished; the locality could not refill them unless it could convince the state employment office that they were "critical to the continued operation of the overall department." Remaining staff members faced two major stressors: the loss of many friends and the knowledge that they would have to answer service demands with fewer teammates.

When it seemed that no one could cope with more change, another occurred. Around 1994, Worksmart's child health clinics began to experience the effects that the Medicaid managed-care system was having on its AFDC clients. In 1995, the Medicaid managed-care system required Medicaid-covered patients to come under the care of a managed-care provider. Pregnant women had already made that shift; the remaining population consisted of infants and children on Medicaid. Worksmart needed to decide its future as a Medicaid care provider. Clinical services had suffered a dual assault: the significant decrease in nursing and physician staff directly working in clinical services due to downsizing and the now upcoming loss of clients and, with them, Medicaid revenue should the department discontinue being a Medicaid provider. Multiple questions needed answers:

- If the department continued to be a Medicaid provider, who would staff child health clinics?
- Was continuing to offer pediatric services affordable, appropriate, or even necessary now that Medicaid infants and children would have access to service through Medicaid managed-care systems?
- Was it time for the department to provide child health care to only the uninsured?
- Because only minimal revenue collection from that client group was likely, could the department even afford that service?
- What would happen to those uninsured children if the department discontinued child health services?

Once again, strategic planning meetings were held to determine the future direction of the health department. Philosophical issues related to Worksmart's role in the community surfaced, and more hard questions needed answers:

- Which services must be maintained because no other health care provider in the city would provide them?
- What group(s) would be affected by a decision to stop selected services and what might those effects be?
- Of the services the department could afford to maintain, at what level could they be provided?
- Which services must absolutely be deferred to the private health care providers in the community?

The health director met with the private pediatricians in the community to explore their willingness to provide care to uninsured children if Worksmart stopped that service. Responding that their caseloads were at capacity, community pediatricians declined to add these uninsured patients to their practices. Traditionally, uninsured infants and children are viewed as a challenging, multiproblem population, not cost-effective for physicians in private practice to manage. Therefore, the strategic planners decided to continue abbreviated child health clinics, focusing care to uninsured infants and children. Physician services were collaboratively arranged with another community care provider.

Because the number of child health clinics had declined, the remaining nurses were available to address other community needs of public health significance. The incidence of teenage pregnancy was high in Waterville so that a decision to expand family planning services to that age group was appropriate and one that the department could afford due to continued grant support. Only 66% of the city's children from birth to 2 years of age were found to be adequately immunized according to their age. Therefore, making childhood immunizations a priority for the department and reassigning additional nurses to that service was certainly appropriate and again affordable due to federal funding for vaccines and staff.

Another significant change that the Worksmart Health Department endured, due to downsizing its pediatric clinics, was a decision to close a service site. This site was an original office of Worksmart when the department first began to serve Waterville. It had been the home office to staff for many years. Its closure represented the end of an era in public health in Waterville. Staff members were consolidated at the remaining sites, and once again, they regrouped, formed new work teams, and went on about their business: providing public health services to residents of Waterville.

Public health will no doubt continue to change as the nation tries to create a health care system for all citizens. With all of the data indicating that the number of people lacking health care insurance will only continue to increase, one unsettling, unanswered, and critical question remains: Who will serve as their safety net?

The public health workforce is resilient, and its flexibility will enable it to meet the challenges of change. Public health nurses must possess unique skills and expertise in epidemiology and community-needs assessments, in collaborating and networking with community resources, in coalition building, in prevention, and in risk-factor-related health promotion. By maintaining our focus on the mission of public health, healthy people in healthy communities, public health will not only survive change but will also flourish as we return to our origins and explore new challenges.

REFERENCE

Institute of Medicine, Committee for the Study of the Future of Public Health. (1988). *The future of public health.* Washington, DC: National Academy Press.

REFERENCES

American Association of Colleges of Nursing. (1991). *Nursing's agenda for health care reform: Executive summary.* Washington, DC: Author.

American Medical Association. (1990). *The cost of medical professional liability in the 1980's.* Chicago: Author.

American Public Health Association. (1995). *The nation's health: APHA members suggest policy statements to the association.* Washington, DC: Author.

Baker, E., Melton, R., Strange, P., Fields, M., Koplan, J., Guerra, F., & Satcher, D. (1994). Health reform and the health of the public: Forging community partnerships. *Journal of the American Medical Association, 272,* 1276-1282.

Baltimore County Association of Senior Citizen Organizations. (1987). *Senior power: America's newest untapped natural resource.* Towson, MD: Author.

Blendon, R., Leitman, R., Morrison, I., & Donelan, K. (1990). Satisfaction with health systems in ten nations. *Health Affairs, 9*(2), 185-192.

Bloodman, S. (1995, June 27). Discharge too soon? Doctors across the country are alarmed by an increase in complications in newborns who have left the hospital after one day. *Washington Post,* Health Section.

Bristow, L. (1996, February 14). "Gag" clauses are health hazardous: Another view. *Virginian Pilot,* p. A-12.

Burke, M., & Walsh, M. (1992). *Gerontologic nursing: Care of the frail elderly.* St. Louis: Mosby Year Book.

Church, G. (1996, August 12). Ripping up welfare. *Time Magazine,* pp. 18-22.

Citizen Action. (1994, January). Comparison of key congressional health care reform bills—1993. *The Nation's Health,* pp. 14-16.

DeLew, N., Greenberg, G., & Kinchen, K. (1992). A layman's guide to the health care system. *Health Care Financing Review, 14,* 151-169.

Dever, G. (1976). Epidemiological model for health policy analysis. *Social Indicators Research, 2,* 2-4.

Duerksen, S. (1993, January 10). Getting a grip on jargon of a national health plan. *San Diego Union Tribune,* p. B-3.

Duffy, S., & Farley, D. (1995). Patterns of decline among inpatient procedures. *Public Health Reports, 110,* 674-683.

Fein, E. (1995, June 18). At hospitals, budget cuts are forcing big layoffs. *New York Times,* p. 25.

Feldstein, P. (1993). *Health care economics.* Albany, NY: Delmar.

Ginsburg, E., & Prout, D. (1990). Access to health care. *Annals of Internal Medicine, 112,* 641-661.

Gravely, E., & Littlefield, J. (1992). A cost-effective analysis of three staffing models for the delivery of low-risk prenatal care. *American Journal of Public Health, 82,* 180-184.

Holliday, J. (1992). *The National Health Service transformed: A guide to the health reforms.* Manchester, UK: Baseline.

Institute of Medicine. (1996). *Employment and health benefits.* Washington, DC: National Academy Press.

Johnson, P. (1990). A national health insurance program: A nursing perspective. *Nursing and Health Care, 11,* 416-418, 427-429.

Kenkel, P. (1989). HMO profit outlook begins to brighten. *Modern Healthcare, 28,* 21.

Krieger, J., Connel, F., & LoGerfo, J. (1992). Medicaid prenatal care: A comparison of use and outcome in fee-for-service and managed care. *American Journal of Public Health, 82,* 185-190.

Lalonde, M. (1974). *A new perspective on the health of Canadians.* Ottawa, Ontario: Ministry of Health.

Levit, K., Lazenby, C., & Letsch, S. (1991). National health expenditures, 1990. *Health Care Financing Review, 13*(1), 29-54.

McGinnis, J., Richmond, J., Brandt, E., Windom, R., & Mason, J. (1992). Health progress in the United States: Results of the 1990 objectives for the nation. *Journal of the American Medical Association, 268,* 2545-2552.

Merline, J. (1993, April 5). What is "managed competition"? *Investor's Business Daily,* pp. 1-3.

National Coalition for the Homeless. (1996). *Welfare repeal: Moving Americans off welfare, into homelessness.* Washington, DC: Author.

National League for Nursing. (1992). *An agenda for nursing education reform: In support of nursing's agenda for health care reform. A draft.* New York: Author.

National League for Nursing. (1993, April). The financing of health care reform. *NLN's Health Care Update,* pp. 1-2.

Office of National Costs Estimates, Office of the Actuary. (1989). National health expenditures, 1987. *Health Care Financing Review, 10,*(2), 109-122.

Older Women's League (1993). Speak up on universal health care. *The OWL Observer, 13*(1), 1.

Porter, M., Ball, P., & Kraus, N. (1992). *The Interstudy competitive edge.* Excelsior, MN: Interstudy.

Raffel, M., & Raffel, N. (1989). *The United States health care system: Origins and functions.* New York: John Wiley.

Rapoport, J., Robertson, R., & Stewart, B. (1982). *Understanding health economics.* Rockville, MD: Aspen.

Reis, J. (1990). Medicaid maternal and child health care: Prepaid plans vs. private fee-for-service. *Research in Nursing and Health, 13,* 163-171.

Relman, A. (1987). The National Leadership Commission on Health Care. *New England Journal of Medicine, 317,* 706-707.

Roemer, M. (1993). *National health systems of the world* (Vol. 2). New York: Oxford University Press.

Rooney, E. (1990). Corporate attitudes and responses to rising health care costs. *AAOHN Journal, 38,* 304-311.

Rowland, S., & Salganicoff, A. (1994). Lessons from Medicaid: Improving access to office-based physician care for the low income population. *American Journal of Public Health, 84,* 548-549.

Salmon, M. (1995, April). Public health policy: Creating a healthy future for the American public. *Family and Community Health,* pp. 1-11.

Short, P., Monheit, A., & Beauregard, K. (1989). *National Medical Expenditure Survey: A profile of uninsured Americans.* Rockville, MD: National Center for Health Services Research.

Simmons, S. (1993). The economics of prevention. In R. Knollmueller (Ed.), *Prevention across the life span: Healthy people for the twenty first century.* New York: American Nurses Association.

Somers, A., & Somers, H. (1977). *Health and health care: Policies in perspective.* Germantown, MD: Aspen.

Sonnenfeld, S., Waldo, D., & Lemieux, J. (1991). Projections of national health expenditures through the year 2000. *Health Care Financing Review, 13*(1), 1-27.

Stewart, A., & Ware, J. (Eds.). (1992). *Measuring functioning and well-being: The Medical Outcomes Study approach.* Durham, NC: Duke University Press.

Thorpe, K. (1990). Health care cost containment. In A. Kovner (Ed.), *Health care delivery in the United States.* New York: Springer.

U.S. Bureau of the Census. (1991). Poverty in the United States: 1990. *Current Population Reports* (Series P-60, No 175). Washington, DC: Government Printing Office.

U.S. Bureau of the Census. (1996). Income, poverty, and valuation of noncash benefits: 1994. *Current Population Reports* (Series P60-189). Washington, DC: Government Printing Office.

U.S. Department of Commerce. (1993). *Statistical abstracts of the United States, 1993.* Washington, DC: Government Printing Office.

U.S. Department of Health and Human Services. (1988). *Health: United States* (DHHS Publication No. PHS 89-1232). Washington, DC: Author.

U.S. Department of Health and Human Services. (1990). International comparisons of health care financing and delivery. *Health Care Financing Review, 11*(4), 30.

U.S. Department of Health and Human Services. (1991a). *Aging in America: Trends and projections* (Publication No. 7C OA-28001). Washington, DC: Government Printing Office.

U.S. Department of Health and Human Services (1991b). *Healthy people 2000: National health promotion and disease prevention objectives. Summary report.* Washington, DC: Government Printing Office.

U.S. Department of Health, Education and Welfare. (1985). *Health: United States* (DHEW Publication No. PHS 86-1232). Washington, DC: Author.

U.S. Department of Labor, Bureau of Labor Statistics. (1990). *Employee benefits in medium and large firms, 1989* (Publication No. 2363). Washington, DC: Government Printing Office.

Warden, C. (1993, July 2). Is health care rationing next? It might control costs but patients will suffer. *Investigator's Business Daily,* pp. 1-3.

Webster's new universal unabridged dictionary. (1983). New York: Simon & Schuster.

White House Domestic Policy Council. (1993). *Health security: The president's report to the American people.* Washington, DC: Government Printing Office.

Young, Q. (1993). Health care reform: A new public health movement. *American Journal of Public Health, 83,* 945-947.

Zedlewski, S., Clark, S., Meier, E., & Watson, K. (1996). *Potential effects of congressional welfare legislation on family incomes.* Washington, DC: Urban Institute.

C H A P T E R 4

ENVIRONMENTAL FORCES INFLUENCING COMMUNITY HEALTH

OBJECTIVES

1. Discuss *Healthy People 2000* objectives that relate to environmental health.

2. Discuss five areas of environmental concerns that influence the health of human populations.

3. Identify the effects of physical factors, such as radiation, noise, solid waste, and accidents on population health.

4. Identify the effects of biological environmental problems, such as infectious diseases, insects, rodents and other animals, and plants, on population health.

5. Discuss the effects of chemical environmental problems, such as metals and metallic compounds, chemicals in air, and chemicals in the water, on population health.

6. Discuss the effects of the psychosocial environment, such as violence in the home and community, on population health.

7. Discuss the effect of the mechanical environment on health.

8. Describe the community health nurse's role in promoting environmental health.

THEORETICAL FRAMEWORK

In Chapter 2, a theoretical framework for this book was presented. This framework identified internal exchanges between the community population and its environment. Aspects of the environment identified included the physical, biological, chemical, and psychosocial. These and others will be discussed in this chapter.

INTRODUCTION

> The very first canon of nursing, the first and last thing upon which a nurse's attention must be fixed, the first essential to the patient, without which all the rest you can do for him is as nothing, with which I have always said you may leave all the rest alone, is this: TO KEEP THE AIR HE BREATHES AS PURE AS THE EXTERNAL AIR WITHOUT CHILLING HIM. (Nightingale, 1859, p. 8)

Florence Nightingale believed the environment was so important to health that she made air in the patient's room the first canon of nursing. In her *Notes on Nursing,* she also discussed ventilation and warmth of air, light, noise, and cleanliness of the room. Thus, she placed a major emphasis on the influence of the environment on health.

A contemporary document stressing the environment's importance on health is *Healthy People 2000* (U.S. Department of Health and Human Services [DHHS], 1991). This document, which was discussed in Chapter 1, includes 16 objectives related to the environment. These will be discussed later in this chapter.

A beginning idea of the extent of harmful effects of the environment on health can be found in the number of people who have been forced to leave environmentally unfit areas. It is estimated that more than 15 million people worldwide have left areas because of environmental problems related to chemical contamination, nuclear disasters, desertification of previously arable land, and inundation of coastal areas due to the melting of the polar ice caps (Zuk & White, 1990).

The important influence of the chemical environment specifically and the need for further research on its effects on humans is asserted in a report by the U.S. DHHS (1991), which states that

> the most difficult challenges for environmental health today come not from what is known about the harmful effects of microbial agents; rather they come from what is not known about the toxic and ecologic effects of the use of fossil fuels and synthetic chemicals in modern society. (p. 66)

Currently, it is estimated that 72,000 chemicals are used in commerce, excluding food additives, drugs, cosmetics, and pesticides. The majority of these chemicals have had limited testing for their effects on the health of humans and on the environment.

A variety of environmental factors influence human health. Some of these were identified in the model in Table 2.1 in Chapter 2. Microorganisms such as bacteria, fungi, and viruses may cause communicable diseases. Plants may cause accidental poisoning or allergic reactions. Water pollution, air pollution, or both, causing a variety of health problems, may be a result of industrial or auto emissions or "sick air" in poorly ventilated buildings. These and other environmental factors contribute to health problems in populations and are a national focus for interventions as a result of objectives identified in *Healthy People 2000.*

ENVIRONMENT AND *HEALTHY PEOPLE 2000* OBJECTIVES

Sixteen objectives from *Healthy People 2000* (1991) are related to environmental health. These cover the following risks, diseases, conditions, and needs: asthma; serious mental retardation among schoolchildren; infectious waterborne diseases; chemical poisoning outbreaks; high blood lead levels of young children from exposure to lead-based paint, the threat of radon in homes, and the need to inform home buyers of these two hazards; toxic chemicals in air, water, and soil; solid waste contamination; the need for safe drinking water, habitable lakes, and improved air quality; hazardous waste sites; learning to use recyclable materials; and monitoring of sentinel diseases.

Most objectives for *Healthy People 2000* are written in terms of reducing, increasing, or establishing. For example, the objective for asthma is to reduce asthma hospitalizations to less than 160 cases per 100,000 population. The objective for radon testing in homes was written to increase to 40% the proportion of homes tested for radon and found to pose minimal risk or modified to reduce risk. The objective for tracking diseases was written as follows: Establish and monitor plans to define and track sentinel environmental diseases in at least 35 states. These objectives allow for evaluation in the year 2000.

ENVIRONMENTAL PROBLEMS

Environmental concerns having an effect on health fall under five major categories: physical, biological, chemical and gaseous, mechanical, and psychosocial factors. These will be discussed below, along with the community nurse's role related to each hazard. A model specific to these factors is presented in Table 4.1. The reader is also referred to Table 2.1.

PHYSICAL FACTORS

Physical factors in the environment may lead to diseases, disability, and death. Those discussed below include radiation, noise, solid waste, toxic waste, and accidents.

RADIATION

Radiation is energy in motion that occurs as waves or particles (H. Blumenthal, 1985). The major forms of radiation-producing health hazards are ionizing and nonionizing radiation.

Ionizing Radiation. Ionizing radiation is energy transferred through electromagnetic waves or subatomic particles causing ionization. During this process, atoms gain or lose electrons to become electrically charged. Ionizing radiation creates a variety of health effects in humans.

TABLE 4.1 Categories of Environmental Energies in Community

Physical	Biological	Chemical and Gaseous	Mechanical	Psychosocial
Radiation	Infectious agents	Metals and metallic compounds	Vibration stress	Societal violence
Noise	Insects	Chemicals in air and water	Repetitive motion	Spouse abuse
Solid waste	Rodents and other animals		Lifting	Child abuse
Toxic waste	Plants			
Accidents				

There are many sources of ionizing radiation. It occurs naturally in soil and rocks, especially volcanic rocks. It also results from radon, a radioactive gas caused by the breakdown of radium in soil or building materials or well water. Radon gas may be inhaled or attached to dust particles, damaging lung tissue and causing lung cancer. It cannot be seen, smelled, or tasted. Radon is responsible for 55% of all exposures to ionizing radiation and accounts for an estimated 5,000 to 20,000 deaths each year (Koren, 1991). Murdock (1991, p. 12) says radon is the second leading cause of lung cancer in the United States, and the Environmental Protection Agency (EPA, 1990, p. 11) estimates that 7% of all American homes (4 million) have elevated radon levels. Cosmic radiation, another natural source of ionizing radiation, comes from the sun and accounts for 8% of all exposure (Moeller, 1992). According to Moeller (1992), more than 80% of all human exposure to ionizing radiation is from natural sources.

Artificial ionizing radiation results from X rays and a variety of nuclear power industrial processes. Medical and dental X-ray procedures account for about 11% of all exposures to artificial radiation, and nuclear medicine treatments account for 4% more (Moeller, 1992). Although research data are contradictory on the health effects of medical irradiation, some researchers have found a relationship between diagnostic X rays and multiple myeloma and breast cancer. Others have found no relationship of X rays with diseases such as leukemia and non-Hodgkin's lymphoma. Other sources of artificial ionized radiation include smoke detectors using americium, glazes on fiesta ware, and tobacco (Moeller, 1992).

Nuclear radiation can also be detrimental to health in high doses but accounts for a small proportion of radiation exposures. According to Moeller (1992), ionizing radiation from nuclear industrial processes accounts for 3% of all exposures. However, when accidents occur involving nuclear power, they can be damaging. For example, acute exposures of 300 to 600 rem (measure of biological damage to humans from radiation) may cause 50% fatality within weeks of the exposure, and a 5,000-rem exposure may lead to death within hours.

Although most people are not exposed to large doses of ionizing radiation, long-term exposure to low levels may produce cumulative health effects. According to Gibbons (1991), for employees of nuclear plants, the risk of death from cancer increases almost 5% for every rem of long-term radiation exposure.

Some things can be done to detect and prevent exposure to naturally occurring radiation. Alpha-tract or charcoal canister types of radon detectors are effective for detection, and information on detection and removal of radon from buildings is available in guides from state health departments or the Centers for Disease Control in Atlanta.

Nurses should teach populations at risk about testing for radon and about resources available for removing the source from homes or other buildings. This can be accomplished by using mass media sources (see Chapter 10). They should also participate in the political process to advocate building standards that safeguard populations from radon and other harmful radiation.

Some things can be done to control exposure to artificial radiation. Standards for exposure set by the International Commission on Radiological Protection (ICRP) recommended cumulative exposure limits of less than 100 mrem ($\frac{1}{1,000}$ of a rem) per year over a 5-year period for the public and 2 rem per year for occupational exposure. Nurses should teach the public about the sources of exposure in hospitals and doctor's and dentist's offices, the standards established to prevent overexposure, and the hazards of excessive exposure. They should also participate in the political process to encourage setting and enforcing safe standards for nuclear reactors. Lack of response to public pressures for change may lead to nurses' assisting in coalition building with community aggregates.

Nonionizing Radiation. Nonionizing radiation does not transfer energy as it passes through matter and does not, therefore, result in ionization (H. Blumenthal, 1985). Nonionizing radiation may occur in the following forms: electric and magnetic fields, ultraviolet radiation, visible light, and infrared radiation.

Electric and magnetic fields result mainly from high-voltage lines but may also be produced by electric blankets, toasters, microwave ovens, hair dryers, televisions, and video display terminals (VDTs). Although the health effects from these sources of radiation are not well-known, it is believed that fatigue, headache, blood dyscrasia, cataracts, memory loss, decreased fertility, genetic defects, and arrhythmias may result from chronic exposure to microwave radiation and that headache, eyestrain, visual disturbances, cataracts, and genetic defects can be health effects of long-term use of VDTs.

Another type of nonionizing radiation is ultraviolet radiation. These waves of light energy are beyond the visual field of humans and occur in sunlight, fluorescent lights, and sunlamps. Activities of humans are currently increasing the amount of ultraviolet radiation in the environment. Many gases generated on earth, particularly chlorofluorocarbons (CFCs), are destroying the protective layer of ozone in the stratosphere that protects the earth's population from harmful ultraviolet radiation. These gases are routinely used in refrigerators and air conditioners (freon), aerosol sprays, and cleaning agents. Annually, 750,000 metric tons of CFCs are used worldwide (Elmer-Dewitt, 1992, p. 64). Ozone depletion is a health hazard expected to result in an increased incidence of skin cancer, accelerated skin aging, increased eye cataracts, mutations in DNA, weakening of the immune system, and unfavorable climatic conditions and crop production.

Some efforts have been made to prevent further depletion of the ozone layer. International agreements target a phaseout of CFC use by the year 2000, and the United States had hoped to cease its production by 1996 (Lemonick, 1992, p. 60); however, as of this writing, the goal had not yet been accomplished. Because of ozone depletion, nurses should advise populations at risk of measures to reduce their exposure to ultraviolet radiation. These include wearing sunglasses, protective clothing, and sunscreen when outside for long periods of time. In addition, time in the sun should be minimized between peak hours (10 a.m. to 3 p.m.), and sunbathing should also be minimized. In addition, the use of ultraviolet beds for tanning should be discouraged. Mass media may be used to reach target populations.

Other nonionizing radiation includes visible light and infrared light. Visible light includes sunlight, artificial light, and laser beams. Retinal burns from looking at the sun, eyestrain from inadequate lighting, and laser burns of the retina or skin are reported health effects. The sun and heating appliances such as stoves produce infrared radiation that may cause skin burns, cataracts, heat exhaustion, and heat stroke.

Nurses should teach ways to prevent harmful health effects of nonionizing radiation. Looking directly at the sun should be avoided, and sunglasses should be worn when outside. Adequate inside lighting should be used when reading, writing, or carrying out other activities. Heat exhaustion and heatstroke should be avoided by maintaining adequate water and salt intake and by limiting time in the sun or near heat-producing appliances. Teaching may be carried out by mass media methods (see Chapter 10).

NOISE

"Noise is discordant sound which results from nonperiodic vibration of air" (Baetjer, 1965, p. 758). Noise pollution is "a noise level in an environment that is uncomfortable for the inhabitants" (Anderson, 1994, p. 1077). There are many sources of noise pollution in urban areas, including construction activities, diesel trucks, airplanes, power mowers, people, radios, and televisions. Health hazards are determined by the level, frequency, and length of exposure to noise and may include hearing loss, stress-related conditions, mental illness, social maladjustment, and pathological conditions such as atherosclerosis and heart disease.

The level of noise is measured in decibels (dB), and the dB scale is based on a power of 10. Each increase of 10 dB is equal to an increase in intensity times 10. Thus, 40 dB is 10 times as intense as 30 dB, and 50 dB is 10 times as intense as 40 dB. Humans can hear within a range of 120 dB; that is, the difference between the loudest or faintest noise is 120 dB. Usually, the danger level for hearing loss is 80 dB. The standard set by the Occupational Safety and Health Association (OSHA) for sound levels in the workplace is an average level of 90 dB in a 24-hour period. However, sound levels of much lower intensity may cause gastrointestinal, cardiovascular, or neuroendocrine disturbances (Salazar, 1987). No standard has been set for sound levels in the community, but it is known that a jackhammer measures 100 dB and a live performance of a rock band 110 dB. Other common community sounds and their levels include loud thunder 120 dB, loud motorcycle 110 dB, subway train 105 dB, truck or bus 90 dB, heavy street traffic 80 dB, ordinary conversation from 3 feet away 60 dB, and a vacuum cleaner 50 dB.

As identified earlier, noise level damage is a result of the frequency and duration as well as the intensity of the noise. Thus, one might tolerate the noise level of 90 dB for 8 hours a day without hearing loss, but just over an hour a day at 105 dB would cause loss (Auerbach, 1985). In the workplace, approximately 10 million Americans are exposed to potentially harmful noise levels (McCunney, 1992, p. 1121). Federal efforts to regulate industrial noise began in 1955. Hearing loss is one of the most common and most preventable problems in industry. It may be gradual, and often the worker is unaware of this loss until it is severe.

In an industrial setting, the nurse performs a variety of functions related to noise. Initially, the nurse assesses workers for hearing losses and their environment for noise sources. She or he carries out audiometric exams, refers workers with questionable audiometric results or hearing complaints to a physician, teaches workers about industrial noise and protective measures, and supplies workers with and enforces use of protective devices. In the community, the nurse may also teach those exposed to noise about protective devices or ways to drown out intermittent noises that may disrupt sleep or other activities. Two appropriate ways to deal with intermittent noise include soft music or a "sleep mate," available at many department stores. This appliance makes a continuous noise like an electric fan and has various sound levels. Nurses may also work with the politicians using the political process to pass ordinances related to noise levels.

WASTE DISPOSAL

There are two major categories of waste: solid waste and toxic waste.

Solid Waste. Referring to solid waste, DiChristina (1990) says, "Each American tosses 4 pounds of stuff daily, or more than half a ton a year. As a nation, it adds up to 179.5 million tons annually—enough to fill a convoy of ten-ton garbage trucks more than 145,000 miles long" (p. 57).

Basically, two methods have been used to dispose of solid waste: burning or dumping. Until recently, burning was commonly done in fireplaces, leaf piles, and rubbish heaps. Most communities now ban open burning, although many metropolitan areas and industries use highly efficient incineration techniques rather than or in addition to landfill disposal. When incineration is used as an addition to landfill, it can reduce the amount of refuse to be dumped by 90%, thereby extending the length of use of the landfill. Although a modern incinerator requires a high initial investment and is expensive to operate, it is an efficient and carefully designed unit that maximizes the combustion of solid waste and minimizes the emission of pollutants.

Dumping is the disposal of wastes in open dumps, landfills, or oceans. Open dumps are land areas where garbage and waste materials are dumped with little consideration for the site. They have become breeding grounds for rats, flies, mosquitoes, and other scavengers. Flies and rodents attracted to dumps may transmit diseases, and mosquitoes, which also transmit diseases, may breed in water accumulating in cans and other vessels. Diseases transmitted by flies and rodents include typhoid, dysentery, tularemia, plague, leptospirosis, salmonellosis, murine typhus, and trichinosis. Mosquitoes transmit malaria, yellow fever, dengue, and hemorrhagic fever. In addition, air pollution and water pollution problems have been common. In 1976, the Resource Conservation and Recovery Act was passed and required that open dumps be closed or upgraded to landfills. It also prohibited the establishment of any new open dump sites.

Landfills are an improvement over open dumps because waste is covered periodically with layers of earth, thereby minimizing air pollution and accessibility to rats, flies, and mosquitoes. Care should be taken in the placement of landfills to avoid surface and groundwater contamination. Landfill is the major method of permanent disposal of nonhazardous waste in the United States. In my own community, which is at sea level, waste is placed on top of the ground and covered with layers of earth, thus producing a modified landfill. When one such site became high enough, it was opened as a recreational facility and aptly called Mount Trashmore.

Open dumping is a third method of waste disposal. The ocean has been used by nations of the world as a dump for everything from garbage to toxic chemicals and radioactive materials. In 1933, a U.S. Supreme Court decision prohibited the dumping of municipal waste in the ocean, but other forms of waste continued to be dumped there. In 1972, the U.S. Ocean Dumping Act was passed. This has resulted in drastic decreases of industrial waste dumping, but some dumping continues. About 54 nations, including all major maritime nations, agreed to stop dumping certain types of chemical, biological, and nuclear waste into the ocean by 1975. Despite these measures, the ocean is still polluted with unacceptably high quantities of harmful waste products, such as degradable and nondegradable plastic products and toxic chemicals.

Although some European countries have recognized the value of and have implemented recycling for years, this is a relatively new method of dealing with solid waste in America. However, as landfills become saturated, recycling is becoming an attractive alternative. Many materials that are filling up landfills, such as paper, textiles, aluminum, glass, rubber, steel, scrap iron, and lubricating oil, can be recycled. Communities in America are beginning to recycle on a voluntary or mandatory basis. Community health nurses should be advocates for this preferred method of disposal, either through teaching groups or through working with the political process.

Toxic Waste. Toxic waste includes radiological and chemical waste. With the use of nuclear power, nuclear weapons, and nuclear medicine (discussed briefly above) came radioactive wastes that needed to be processed, safely disposed of, and stored. Underground tanks or deep pools at nuclear plants store temporarily most of the radioactive waste. Long-term disposal proposals have included outer space, underground salt mines, land beneath the Antarctic ice caps, and the sediments of the deep ocean floor. Safe disposal is still being debated.

Chemical toxic waste is a by-product of the improved standard of living in America resulting from plastics, detergents, new pesticides, synthetic fabrics, and other products. Although chemicals in the environment are discussed later in this chapter, the waste from these products is briefly mentioned here to provide continuity. In 1962, Rachel Carson, in a book titled *Silent Spring*, brought attention to the effects of chemicals on the environment. This led to the formation of the environmental movement. It has been estimated that 6 billion tons of hazardous waste have been generated in the United States since World War II. More than 90% of it came from chemical, petroleum, and metal-related industries (Miller, 1992). Potential health hazards have been created by improperly protected disposal sites, and in 1988 the EPA (1990) identified about 1,200 sites that were especially hazardous. These were placed on a list of national priorities.

Hazardous waste threatens human health in various ways. These include direct exposure resulting from accidents during transport to a disposal site or exposure at or near the site, polluted air exposure resulting from improper incineration, contaminated groundwater from leaching or runoff of waste, and contaminated food from biological magnification of toxic chemicals. The EPA reports that more than 40 million people live within 4 miles of hazardous waste sites that threaten the health of humans, and about 4 million people live within 1 mile of such sites (Chiras, 1994, p. 462).

Health reactions to toxic waste may occur shortly after exposure or may be a long-term consequence. For example, immediate harmful effects may be experienced from exposure to certain common chemicals such as arsenic and cyanide, which are poisonous; from sulfuric or hydrochloric acids, which burn the skin; or from sodium hydroxide or ammonia gas, which irritates the lungs. Although the long-term effects of exposure to toxic waste are not well-defined, it is believed to lead to problems such as mental depression, birth defects, depressed immunity, and lowering of intelligence. One study of long-term effects involved a group eating mercury-contaminated fish who developed health concerns years later. These included symptoms of brain and nerve damage, congenital defects, and death of some of those exposed.

Nurses may teach the danger of toxic and other wastes and may work with the political process to pass and enforce safe disposal of waste products. In addition, they may help groups who live near such dangerous sites to form coalitions to bring pressure on appropriate politicians and others who can help reduce the dangers.

ACCIDENTS

Although many accidents are preventable, they represent a major cause of death for all ages and are the leading cause of death in the population between 1 and 37. For people of all ages, they represent the fifth leading cause of death. Accidents kill more people than homicide in the 15- to 24-year-old population (National Safety Council, 1994, p. 7). Motor vehicle accidents, falls, drowning, and fires are the most common sources of accidents. Males have higher death rates from accidents than do females at all ages. Others at highest risk are "the young and elderly, the poor, minorities, and rural residents" (Spradley & Allender, 1996, p. 136).

A downward trend in accidental death rates has been seen in the 1990s (National Safety Council, 1994). This reduction has been attributed to factors such as lower rates of alcohol use, changes in speed limits, and increased seat belt use (U.S. DHHS, 1991, p. 19).

Because many accidents are preventable and community health nurses advocate prevention and health promotion, this is an important area of education. Nurses may participate in school programs, civic leagues, women's clubs, or business groups or on mass media channels to advocate the use of seat belts, child safety seats, and helmets when riding on motorcycles. These are all advocated in *Healthy People 2000,* which sets a goal of increasing the use of seat belts, inflatable safety restraints, and child safety seats to 85% from 42% in 1988. Another goal is to increase the use of helmets by motorcyclists from 60% in 1988 to 80% and by bicyclists from 8% in 1988 to 50%.

Nurses can also present programs for school or other groups or on mass media sources on home accidents and safety. Topics might include home surveys (a) to reduce fire hazards (improper storage of combustible materials, improper use of heaters, malfunctioning smoke detectors, or child-accessible matches; (b) to prevent falls by assessing for lighting and railings or loose toys on stairs, loose rugs, gates across stairways if small children are present, and nonskid mats in bathtubs; and (c) to prevent accidental poisoning or injury by assessing for chemicals such as prescribed or over-the-counter medications or cleaning products accessible to small children and sharp instruments, such as razors, knives, and scissors, or farm equipment, in accessible locations. Nurses can also teach first aid and CPR classes and present information on community resources available in emergencies.

BIOLOGICAL ENVIRONMENTAL PROBLEMS

Biological problems are caused by living organisms in the environment. Those of concern to community health nurses are infectious agents; insects, rodents, and other animals; and plants.

INFECTIOUS AGENTS

Some infectious agents are transmitted by contact with an infected person; others are transmitted through the environment. Because the emphasis of this chapter is on environmental influences on health, infectious agents transmitted from person to person will be omitted.

Water is a primary vehicle for infectious agents. It has been estimated that water serves as the vehicle for 80% of the communicable diseases throughout the world due to unsafe drinking water for approximately 2 million people. Although sanitation and water treatment in the United States have limited waterborne diseases, they still exist, and an increase in waterborne diseases has been noted since 1955. Moore et al. (1993) found 34 waterborne diseases in 17 states that resulted in 17,000 cases of illness in 1991 and 1992.

Unsafe water usually is a result of improper sewage treatment and improper solid waste disposal (see above). About 30% of the population uses septic tanks for waste disposal, and some of this waste enters groundwater. Sewage systems prevent contamination of groundwater, but excess demands in some communities have led to inadequate sewage treatment. Untreated sewage may also contaminate the water supply. For example, in San Diego, untreated sewage from Tijuana, Mexico, contaminated both the groundwater and surface water.

Improper handling of solid waste may also contaminate the water supplies. This results from biological pathogens carried from solid waste sites to a water supply by rain.

Improper disposal of medical waste such as needles and syringes contaminated with blood or other body waste has also posed a biological hazard. Although medical waste disposal is supposed to be strictly regulated, waste has been found on beaches as a result of apparent illegal ocean dumping. Medical waste has also been found with solid waste.

Although water is the primary vehicle for biological hazards, some are transmitted by air. Improper cleaning of heating and cooling units allows these units to serve as breeding grounds for microorganisms (Briasco, 1990). The organisms that are then spread when the unit is in use are believed to cause diseases such as Legionnaires' disease (Benenson, 1990).

INSECTS, RODENTS, AND ANIMAL SOURCES

Insects. Insects such as flies, cockroaches, mosquitoes, and ticks carry diseases. Fly bites may cause filariasis, river blindness, sleeping sickness, kala-azar, tropical ulcer, cutaneous leishmaniasis, and other diseases. Cockroaches are not a significant source of disease in the United States. Mosquitoes transmit malaria, filariasis, encephalitis, yellow fever, and dengue. In 1985, D. S. Blumenthal (p. 37) estimated that more than 200 million people were infected with malaria worldwide. Yellow fever is not a major problem in the United States. Preventive efforts include eliminating still water in which mosquito eggs hatch and develop, eliminating flies and mosquitoes from homes, and wearing protective clothing and insect repellent when outside.

Ticks transmit several diseases to humans, including Lyme disease, Q fever, relapse fever, Rocky Mountain spotted fever, and tularemia. Following a bite, symptoms may include nervousness, loss of appetite, tingling, and headache. These may be followed by muscle pain and, occasionally, by respiratory failure. Some ticks carry a neurotoxin in their saliva that may cause ascending paralysis beginning in the legs when the person is bitten. Symptoms may disappear after the attached tick is removed. Removal by forceps is facilitated by placing a drop of ether or alcohol on the tick or coating it with nail polish.

Lyme disease has received much attention and is an acute inflammatory infection caused by the tick. It occurs throughout the United States. Symptoms manifest in recurrent episodes and usually last about a week. There may be a week to several weeks between symptom episodes, and these decline in severity after 2 or 3 years. Symptoms specific to this disease include chills, fever, headache, malaise, skin eruptions, and joint inflammation and swelling similar to arthritis (Goldstein et al., 1990).

There are a couple ways to reduce the chances of contact with ticks. The most important one is to avoid areas such as woods or parks that are considered high risk for ticks. If avoidance is not possible, wearing long-sleeved shirts and long pants of a light color and using insect repellent may help. People leaving high-risk areas should also examine themselves carefully and remove any ticks found on the body. These areas of concern can be taught to high-risk groups by community nurses.

Rodents and Animals. Rats and other rodents are the source of several diseases in populations, of which plague is the most serious and widespread.

Other diseases spread by rodents include leptospirosis, salmonellosis, murine typhus, trichinosis, and other parasites and infections. Plague is spread by the bite of a flea from a rodent infected with the bacillus *Yersina pestis* and may occur in shepherds, farmers, ranchers, and hunters. Bubonic plague is the most common type of plague, with symptoms caused by an endotoxin released by the bacillus. These include painful enlarged lymph nodes in the axilla, groin, or neck; temperature often rising to 106° F; prostration with a rapid thready pulse; hypotension; delirium; and bleeding into the skin from the superficial blood vessels.

Preventive measures include inoculation with plague vaccine, which confers partial immunity; improved sanitary conditions; and the eradication of rats and other rodent reservoirs of the bacillus to prevent outbreaks.

Other animals also transmit diseases. Some of the most well-known diseases are anthrax, brucellosis, and rabies. Anthrax affects primarily farm animals (cattle, goats, pigs, sheep, and horses) and is caused by the bacterium *Bacillus anthraces*. Humans may contract the disease when a break in the skin is in touch with an affected animal or its hide. This may result in skin lesions followed by internal hemorrhage, muscle pain, headache, fever, nausea, and vomiting. Anthrax most often affects shepherds, farmers, butchers, hide handlers, and veterinarians. A vaccine is available for high-risk groups.

Brucellosis is another disease primarily of animals that may affect humans. It is caused by the bacillus *Brucella abortus suis* and may be transmitted to humans through a break in the skin or from contaminated milk or milk products. It is seen most often in farmers, shepherds, veterinarians, and lab and slaughterhouse workers. Symptoms include fever, chills, sweating, malaise, weakness, anorexia, weight loss, headache, muscle and joint pain, and an enlarged spleen. Although the disease may be acute, it is more often chronic, and symptoms recur over a period of months or years.

Rabies is transmitted from animals (skunks, bats, foxes, dogs, raccoons, and cats) to humans by infected blood, tissue, or most often, saliva. Within 10 days to 1 year after being infected, humans develop symptoms of fever, malaise, headache, paresthesia, and myalgia. Severe encephalitis, delirium, muscle spasms, seizures, paralysis, coma, and death may occur within a few days after the initial symptoms. Rabies is usually a fatal disease, and human survival requires treatment to be started before the virus reaches the nervous system. Rabies has become an increased health threat in Virginia and other nearby states.

Preventive measures against rabies include prophylactic immunization and control of domestic animals, elimination and avoidance of wild animals that act as a reservoir of infection, and immediate first aid for any animal bite. Nurses should teach the importance of immunizations for animals and work with the political process to encourage the development and enforcement of immunizations and leash laws. They can also teach signs and symptoms of rabies and encourage immediate treatment of animal bites.

PLANTS

Plants are another source of biological hazards to humans resulting from accidental poisoning (ingesting poisonous plants) or from allergies to plants.

Many plants found in homes, yards, or neighborhoods are poisonous. Prevention involves eliminating poisonous plants from the home or yard, teaching children to avoid eating plants, and supervising small children closely. Because treatment may vary depending on the type of plant involved, nurses should also teach groups about resources for use when poisoning occurs, such as poison control centers and emergency units in the community.

Plant allergies include conditions such as asthma, hay fever, and other reactions to weed, tree, or other pollens as well as to poison oak and poison ivy. Allergies often result in a variety of nasal and eye reactions similar to those of a cold. Poison ivy and poison oak lead to localized vesicular eruptions with itching and burning. The main preventive measures are elimination of the poisonous plants from the environment.

CHEMICAL AND GASEOUS ENVIRONMENTAL FACTORS

"Since 1950, more than 65,000 new chemical compounds have been introduced into common use in the western world, the majority of which (84 percent) have not been tested for human toxicity" (Pope, Snyder, & Mood, 1995, p. 3). Chemicals may be inhaled, ingested, or absorbed. Chemicals discussed below include metals and metallic compounds, chemicals in air, and chemicals in water.

METALS AND METALLIC COMPOUNDS

Metals and metallic compounds, including lead, mercury, arsenic, and cadmium (see Table 4.2), pose a threat to community populations. Lead can be found in soil, water, air, or dust and paint chips in older homes. Air sources of lead include vehicle emissions, industrial processes, decomposition of solid wastes, and stationary source fuel combustion, such as burning coal to generate electrical power. Lead in the air from vehicle emissions has been drastically reduced as a result of the use of unleaded gas. Between 1979 and 1988 the amount of lead expelled into the air yearly declined 89% (Moeller, 1992). Lead in paint chips has been reduced because of the elimination of lead-based paint use in residences beginning more than 40 years ago (Farfel & Chisolm, 1990). However, older homes still contain lead-based paint, and an estimated 17% of children in the United States under the age of 5 have blood lead levels high enough to cause decreased intelligence and retarded growth. This figure increases to 40% for children in poverty (Committee on Advances in Assessing Human Exposure to Airborne Pollutants, 1991). Painting over walls previously painted with lead-based paint has not been effective. The current procedures of removing this paint by burning or sanding may result in lead in the dust. The most recent federal effort to reduce lead poisoning is the EPA's lead disclosure regulation. This gives buyers or renters the right to ask for copies of test results on paint and gives them 10 days to determine the potential risks and to inspect the property before being bound to a contract ("Lead Paint Warnings," 1996).

text continues on page 110

TABLE 4.2 Environmental Agents, Their Sources and Potential Exposures, and Their Adverse Health Effects: Metals and Metallic Compounds, Hydrocarbons, Irritant Gases, Chemical Asphyxiants, and Pesticides

Agent	Exposure	Route of Entry	System(s) Affected	Primary Manifestations	Aids in Diagnosis[a]	Remarks
Metals and metallic compounds						
Arsenic	Alloyed with lead and copper for hardness; used in manufacturing of pigments, glass, pharmaceuticals; by-product in copper smelting; used in insecticides, fungicides, rodenticides, tanning	Inhalation and ingestion of dust and fumes	Neuromuscular	Peripheral neuropathy, sensorimotor	Arsenic in urine	
			Gastrointestinal	Nausea and vomiting, diarrhea, constipation		
			Skin	Dermatitis, finger and toenail striations, skin cancer, nasal septum perforation		
			Pulmonary	Lung cancer		
Arsine	Accidental by-product of reaction of arsenic with acid; used in semiconductor industry	Inhalation of gas	Hematopoietic	Intravascular hemolysis: hemoglobinuria, jaundice, oliguria, or anuria	Arsenic in urine	
Beryllium	Hardening agent in metal alloys; special use in nuclear energy production; used in metal refining or recovery	Inhalation of fumes or dust	Pulmonary (and other systems)	Granulomatosis and fibrosis	Beryllium in urine (acute); beryllium in tissue (chronic); chest X ray; immunologic tests such as lymphocyte transformation may also be useful	Pulmonary changes virtually indistinguishable from sarcoid on chest X ray

TABLE 4.2 Continued

Agent	Exposure	Route of Entry	System(s) Affected	Primary Manifestations	Aids in Diagnosis[a]	Remarks
Cadmium	Electroplating, solder for aluminum; metal alloys, process engraving; nickel-cadmium batteries	Inhalation or ingestion of fumes or dust	Pulmonary Renal	Pulmonary edema (acute); emphysema (chronic) Nephrosis	Urinary protein	Also a respiratory tract carcinogen
Chromium	In stainless and heat-resistant steel and alloy steel; metal plating; chemical and pigment manufacturing; photography	Percutaneous absorption, inhalation, ingestion	Pulmonary Skin	Lung cancer Dermatitis, skin ulcers, nasal septum perforation	Urinary chromate (questionable value)	
Lead	Storage batteries; manufacturing of paint, enamel, ink, glass, rubber, ceramics; used in chemical industry	Ingestion of dust, inhalation of dust or fumes	Hematologic Renal Gastrointestinal Neuromuscular CNS Reproductive	Anemia Nephropathy Abdominal pain ("colic") Palsy ("wrist drop") Encephalopathy, behavioral abnormalities Spontaneous abortions (?)	Blood lead, urinary ALA, zinc proto-porphyrin (ZPP), free erythrocyte protoporphyrin (FEP)	Lead toxicity, unlike that of mercury, is believed to be reversible, with the exception of late renal and some CNS effects
Mercury (elemental)	Electronic equipment; paint; metal and textile production; catalyst in chemical manufacturing; pharmaceutical production	Inhalation of vapor; slight percutaneous absorption	Pulmonary CNS	Acute pneumonitis Neuropsychiatric changes (erethism); tremor	Urinary mercury	Chemical form has a profound effect on its toxicology, as is the case for many metals. Effects of mercury are highly variable. Though inorganic poisoning is primarily renal,
Mercury (inorganic)		Some inhalation and GI and percutaneous absorption	Pulmonary Renal CNS	Acute pneumonitis Proteinuria Variable	Urinary mercury	elemental and

Agent	Uses/Sources	Route of absorption	Target organ	Clinical effects	Biological monitoring	Comments
Mercury (organic)	Agricultural and industrial poisons	Efficient GI absorption, percutaneous absorption, and inhalation	Skin CNS	Dermatitis Sensorimotor changes, visual field construction, tremor	Blood and urine mercury, but questionable sensitivity	organic poisoning are primarily neurological. The responses are difficult to quantify, so dose-response data are generally unavailable. Classic tetrad of gingivitis, sialorrhea, irritability, and tremor is associated with both elemental and inorganic mercury poisoning; the four signs are not generally seen together. Many effects of mercury toxicity, especially those in CNS, are irreversible.
Nickel	Corrosion-resistant alloys; electroplating; catalyst production; nickel-cadmium batteries	Inhalation of dust or fumes	Skin Pulmonary	Sensitization dermatitis ("nickel itch") Lung and paranasal sinus cancer		
Zinc oxide[b]	Welding by-product; rubber manufacturing	Inhalation of dust or fumes that are freshly generated		"Metal fume fever" (fever, chills, and other symptoms)	Urinary zinc (useful as an indicator of exposure, not for acute diagnosis)	A self-limiting syndrome of 24-48 hours with no apparent sequelae
Hydrocarbons						
Benzene	Manufacturing of organic chemicals, detergents, pesticides, solvents, paint removers; used as a solvent	Inhalation of vapor; slight percutaneous absorption	CNS Hematopoietic Skin	Acute CNS depression Leukemia, aplastic anemia Dermatitis	Urinary phenol	Note that benzene, like toluene and other solvents, can be monitored via its principal metabolite

TABLE 4.2 Continued

Agent	Exposure	Route of Entry	System(s) Affected	Primary Manifestations	Aids in Diagnosis[a]	Remarks
Toluene	Organic chemical manufacturing; solvent; fuel component	Inhalation of vapor; percutaneous absorption of liquid	CNS Skin	Acute CNS depression; chronic CNS problems such as memory loss Irritation dermatitis	Urinary hippuric acid	
Xylene	A wide variety of uses as a solvent; an ingredient of paints, lacquers, varnishes, inks, dyes, adhesives, cements; an intermediate in chemical manufacturing	Inhalation of vapor; slight percutaneous absorption of liquid	Pulmonary Eyes, nose, throat CNS	Irritation, pneumonitis, acute pulmonary edema (at high doses) Irritation Acute CNS depression	Methylhippuric acid in urine, xylene in expired air, xylene in blood	
Ketones (acetone; methylethyl ketone—MEK; methyl n-propyl ketone—MPK; methyl n-butal ketone—MBK; methyl iso-butyl ketone—MIBK)	A wide variety of uses as solvents and intermediates in chemical manufacturing	Inhalation of vapor; percutaneous absorption of liquid	CNS PNS Skin	Acute CNS depression MBK has been linked with peripheral neuropathy Dermatitis	Acetone in blood, urine, expired air (used as an index for exposure, not diagnosis)	The ketone family demonstrates how a pattern of toxic responses (that is, CNS narcosis) may feature exceptions (i.e., MBK peripheral neuropathy)
Formaldehyde	Widely used as a germicide and a disinfectant in embalming and histopathology, for example, and in the manufacture of textiles, resins, and other products	Inhalation	Skin Eye Pulmonary	Irritant and contact dermatitis Eye irritation Respiratory tract irritation, asthma	Patch testing may be helpful for dermatitis	Recent animal tests have shown it to be a respiratory carcinogen. Confirmatory epidemiological studies are in progress

Trichloroethylene (TCE)	Solvent in metal degreasing, dry cleaning, food extraction; ingredient of paints, adhesives, varnishes, inks	Inhalation, percutaneous absorption	Nervous Skin Cardiovascular	Acute CNS depression; peripheral and cranial neuropathy Irritation, dermatitis Arrhythmias	Breath analysis for TCE	TCE is involved in an important pharmacologial interaction. Within hours of ingesting alcoholic beverages, TCE workers experience flushing of the face, neck, shoulders, and back. Alcohol may also potentiate the CNS effects of TCE. The probable mechanism is competition for metabolic enzymes
Carbon tetrachloride	Solvent for oils, fats, lacquers, resins, varnishes, other materials; used as a degreasing and cleaning agent	Inhalation of vapor	Hepatic Renal CNS Skin	Toxic hepatitis Oliguria or anuria Acute CNS depression Dermatitis	Expired air and blood levels	Carbon tetrachloride is the prototype for a wide variety of solvents that cause hepatic and renal damage. This solvent, like trichloroethylene, acts synergistically with ethanol

TABLE 4.2 Continued

Agent	Exposure	Route of Entry	System(s) Affected	Primary Manifestations	Aids in Diagnosis[a]	Remarks
Carbon disulfide	Solvent for lipids, sulfur, halogens, rubber, phosphorus, oils, waxes, and resins; manufacturing of organic chemicals, paints, fuels, explosives, viscose rayon	Inhalation of vapor, percutaneous absorption of liquid or vapor	Nervous	Parkinsonism, psychosis, suicide; peripheral neuropathies	Iodine-azide reaction with urine (nonspecific because other bivalent sulfur compounds give a positive test); CS_2 in expired air, blood, and urine	A solvent with unusual multisystem effects, especially noted for its cardiovascular, renal, and nervous system actions
			Renal	Chronic nephritic and nephrotic syndromes		
			Cardiovascular	Acceleration or worsening of atherosclerosis; hypertension		
			Skin	Irritation; dermatitis		
			Reproductive	Menorrhagia and metrorrhagia		
Stoddard solvent	Degreasing, paint thinning	Inhalation of vapor, percutaneous absorption of liquid	Skin	Dryness and scaling from defatting; dermatitis		A mixture of primarily aliphatic hydrocarbons, with some benzene derivative and naphthenes
			CNS	Dizziness, coma, collapse (at high levels)		
Ethylene glycol ethers (ethylene glycol monoethylether—Cellosolve; ethylene glycol monoethyl ether-acetate—Cellosolve-acetate; methyl- and butyl-substituted compounds such as ethylene glycol monomethyl ether—Methyl Cellosolve)	Ethers used as solvents for resins, paints, lacquers, varnishes, gum, perfume, dyes, and inks; acetate derivatives are widely used as solvents and ingredients of lacquers, enamels, and adhesives. Exposure occurs in dry cleaning; in plastic, ink, and lacquer manufacturing; and in textile dying, among other processes	Inhalation of vapor, percutaneous absorption of liquid	Reproductive, CNS, renal, liver		Adverse effects of ethylene glycol ethers primarily associated with ethylene glycol monomethyl ether (Methyl Cellosolve)	
			Hematopoietic	Pancytopenia fatigue, lethargy, nausea, headaches, anorexia, tremor, stupor (from encephalopathy)		
			CNS			

104

Substance	Uses	Route	Organ/System	Effect	Diagnostic tests	Remarks
Ethylene oxide	Used in the sterilization of medical equipment, in the fumigation of spices and other foodstuffs, and as a chemical intermediate	Inhalation	Skin Eye Respiratory tract Nervous system	Dermatitis and frostbite Severe irritation; possibly cataracts with prolonged exposure Irritation Peripheral neuropathy		Recent animal tests have shown it to be carcinogenic and to cause reproductive abnormalities. Epidemiological studies indicate that it may cause leukemia in exposed workers
Dioxane	Used as a solvent for a variety of materials, including cellulose acetate, dyes, fats, greases, resins, polyvinyl polymers, varnishes, and waxes	Inhalation of vapor, percutaneous absorption of liquid	CNS Renal Liver	Drowsiness, dizziness, anorexia, headaches, nausea, vomiting, coma Nephritis Chemical hepatitis		Dioxane has caused a variety of neoplasms in animals
Polychlorinated biphenyls (PCBs)	Formerly used as a di-electric fluid in electrical equipment and as a fire retardant coating on tiles and other products. New uses were banned in 1976, but much of the electrical equipment currently used still contains PCBs	Inhalation, ingestion, skin absorption	Skin Eye Liver	Chloracne Irritation Toxic hepatitis	Serum PCB levels for chronic exposure	Animal studies have demonstrated that PCBs are carcinogenic. Epidemiological studies of exposed workers are inconclusive

Irritant gases [c]

Substance	Uses	Route	Organ/System	Effect	Diagnostic tests	Remarks
Ammonia	Refrigeration; petroleum refining; manufacturing of nitrogen-containing chemicals, synthetic fibers, dyes, and optics	Inhalation of gas	Upper respiratory tract	Upper respiratory irritation		Also irritant of eyes and moist skin

TABLE 4.2 Continued

Agent	Exposure	Route of Entry	System(s) Affected	Primary Manifestations	Aids in Diagnosis[a]	Remarks
Hydrochloric acid	Chemical and manufacturing; electroplating; tanning; metal pickling; petroleum extraction; rubber, photographic, and textile industries	Inhalation of gas or mist	Upper respiratory tract	Upper respiratory irritation		Strong irritant of eyes, mucous membranes, and skin
Hydrofluoric acid	Chemical and plastic manufacturing; catalyst in petroleum refining; aqueous solution for frosting, etching, and polishing glass	Inhalation of gas or mist	Upper respiratory tract	Upper respiratory irritation		In solution, causes severe and painful burns of skin and can be fatal
Sulfur dioxide	Manufacturing of sulfur-containing chemicals; food and textile bleach; tanning; metal casting	Inhalation of gas, direct contact of gas or liquid on skin or mucosa	Middle respiratory tract	Bronchospasm (pulmonary edema or chemical pheumonitis in high dose)	Chest X ray, pulmonary function tests[d]	Strong irritant of eyes, mucous membranes, and skin
Chlorine	Paper and textile bleaching; water disinfection; chemical manufacturing; metal fluxing; detinning and dezincing iron	Inhalation of gas	Middle respiratory tract	Tracheobronchitis, pulmonary edema, pnuemonitis	Chest X ray, pulmonary function tests	Chlorine combines with body moisture to form acids, which irritate tissues from nose to alveoli
Ozone	Inert gas-shielded arc welding; food, water, and air purification; food and textile bleaching; emitted around high-voltage electric equipment	Inhalation of gas	Lower respiratory tract	Delayed pulmonary edema (generally 6-8 hours following exposure)	Chest X ray, pulmonary function tests	Ozone has a free radical structure and can produce experimental chromosome aberrations; it may thus have carcinogenic potential

Agent	Source/Use	Route	Target organ	Effects	Diagnostic tests	Comments
Nitrogen oxides	Manufacturing of acids, nitrogen-containing chemicals, explosives, and more; by-product of many industrial processes	Inhalation of gas	Lower respiratory tract	Pulmonary irritation, bronchiolitis fibrosa obliterans ("silo filler's disease"), mixed obstructive-restrictive changes	Chest X ray, pulmonary function tests	
Phosgene	Manufacturing and burning of isocyanates and manufacturing of dyes and other organic chemicals; in metallurgy for ore separation, burning, or heat source near trichloroethylene	Inhalation of gas	Lower respiratory tract	Delayed pulmonary edema (delay seldom longer than 12 hours)	Chest X ray, pulmonary function tests	
Isocyanates (toluene diisocyanate—TDI; methyleme diphenyl-diisocyanate—MDI; hexamethylene diisocyanate; and others)	Polyurethane manufacture; resin-binding systems in foundries; coating materials for wires; used in certain types of paint	Inhalation of vapor	Predominately lower respiratory tract	Asthmatic reaction and accelerated loss of pulmonary function	Chest X ray, pulmonary function tests	Isocyanates are both respiratory tract sensitizers and irritants in the conventional sense
Asphyxiant gases Simple asphyxiants (nitrogen, hydrogen, methane, and others)	Enclosed spaces in a variety of industrial settings	Inhalation of gas	CNS	Anoxia	O_2 in environment	No specific toxic effect; acts by displacing O_2
Chemical asphyxiants						
Carbon monoxide	Incomplete combustion in foundries, coke ovens, refineries, furnaces, and more	Inhalation of gas	Blood (hemoglobin)	Headache; dizziness, double vision	Carboxyhemoglobin	

TABLE 4.2 Continued

Agent	Exposure	Route of Entry	System(s) Affected	Primary Manifestations	Aids in Diagnosis[a]	Remarks
Hydrogen sulfide	Used in manufacturing of sulfur-containing chemicals; produced in petroleum production; by-product of petroleum product use; decay of organic matter	Inhalation of gas	CNS Pulmonary	Respiratory center paralysis, hypoventilation Respiratory tract irritation	PaO_2	
Cyanides	Metallurgy, electroplating	Inhalation of vapor, percutaneous absorption, ingestion	Cellular metabolic absorpt enzymes (especially cytochrome oxidase)	Enzyme inhibition with metabolic asphyxia and death	SCN in urine	
Pesticides						
Organophosphates (malathion, parathion, and others)		Inhalation, ingestion, percutaneous absorption	Neuromuscular	Cholinesterase inhibition, cholinergic symptoms: nausea and vomiting, salivation, diarrhea, headache, sweating, meiosis, muscle fasciculations, seizures, unconsciousness, death	Refractoriness to atropine; plasma or red cell cholinesterase	As with many acute toxins, rapid treatment of organophosphate toxicity is imperative. Thus, diagnosis is often made based on history and a high index of suspicion rather than on biochemical tests. Treatment is atropine to block cholinergic effects and 2-PAM (2-pyridine-alsoxine methiodide) to reactivate cholinesterase

Agent	Route of exposure	System affected	Signs and symptoms	Laboratory tests	Comments
Carbamates (carbaryl [Sevin] and others)	Inhalation, ingestion, percutaneous absorption	Neuromuscular	Same as organophosphates	Plasma cholinesterase; urinary 1-naphthol (index of exposure)	Treatment of carbamate poisoning is the same as that of organophosphate poisoning except that 2-PAM is contraindicated
Chlorinated hydrocarbons (chlordane, DDT, heptachlor, chlordecone [Kepone], aldrin, dieldrin, uridine)	Inhalation, ingestion, percutaneous absorption	CNS	Stimulation or depression	Urinary organic chlorine, or p-chlorophenol acetic acid	The chlorinated hydrocarbons may accumulate in body lipid stored in large amounts
Bipyridyls (paraquat, diquat)	Inhalation, ingestion, percutaneous absorption	Pulmonary	Rapid massive fibrosis, only following paraquat ingestion		An interesting toxin in that the major toxicity, pulmonary fibrosis, apparently occurs only after ingestion

SOURCE: Reprinted with permission from *Principles and Practice of Environmental Health*, A. B. Tarcher, Ed. Copyright 1992 by Plenum Publishing Co.

a. In most cases, occupational and medical histories are the most important aids in diagnosis.

b. Zinc oxide is a prototype of agents that cause metal fume fever.

c. The less water soluble the gas, the deeper and more delayed its irritant effect.

d. Pulmonary function tests are useful aids in diagnosis of irritant effects if the patient is subacutely or chronically ill.

Lead, nickel, mercury, arsenic, cadmium, and other metals may also be found in contaminated drinking water. These metals, when present in soil or in improperly processed solid waste, may enter the water supply. Lead and copper can also enter the water supply from lead or copper pipes in older homes.

Lead-poisoning symptoms include headache, irritability, weakness, abdominal pain, vomiting, and constipation. Convulsion, coma, and paralysis may occur in later stages. Mercury poisoning includes symptoms of listlessness and irritability, followed by recurrent rashes; photophobia; a pinkish coloration of fingertips, nose, hands, and feet; pruritus; severe perspiration; and a burning sensation in and desquamation of hands and feet. Neuritis, mental apathy, and loss of deep-tendon reflexes may also be present. Chelation therapy is used for both lead and mercury poisoning.

Symptoms of acute arsenic poisoning include nausea, vomiting, diarrhea, severe burning of the mouth and throat, and acute abdominal pain. Weakness, prostration, muscle aches, desquamation and hyperpigmentation of the trunk and extremities, and linear pigmentation of fingernails are symptoms of chronic poisoning. Within 10 minutes, cadmium poisoning produces symptoms of nausea, vomiting, diarrhea, and prostration. Other sources of exposure, route of entry, systems affected, primary manifestations, and aids in diagnosis for these and other metals are listed in Table 4.2.

Nurses should teach high-risk groups about (a) the danger of poisoning from heavy metals, especially lead; (b) ways to remove the sources of contamination; and (c) signs and symptoms of exposure. They should also teach resources for care. In addition, they may work with the political process to pass laws regarding removal of lead-based paint from buildings, or they may work with groups subjected to lead-based paint in public housing to form coalitions to force landlords to remove lead-based paint.

CHEMICALS IN AIR

Chemicals and gaseous materials contaminate air and contribute to health problems of populations. Air pollution is a result of one or more chemicals in the air that are in high enough concentrations to harm plants, animals, or humans (Miller, 1992). Air pollution occurs indoors and outdoors and is measured in terms of the pollutant standards index (PSI) for outdoor or ambient air. Ratings are categorized as follows: 100 to 200 is unhealthy; 200 to 300 is very unhealthy; and more than 300 is hazardous to health. A very unhealthy rating may lead to significant symptom aggravation with decreased exercise tolerance in people with heart or lung disease and may lead to widespread symptoms in healthy populations. At such times, elderly persons with these diseases should remain indoors and reduce activities. A hazardous health rating may lead to premature onset of certain diseases and decreased exercise tolerance in healthy people. If the condition worsens, there may be premature death of the ill and elderly and adverse symptoms from normal activities among healthy people. Under these conditions, elderly people with heart or lung conditions should remain indoors and avoid physical activity and healthy people should avoid outdoor activity. When conditions are at their worst, all people should remain indoors with windows and doors closed and with minimal physical activity (Turk & Turk, 1988). Routinely monitored pollutants include carbon monoxide, ozone, sulfur oxides, volatile organic compounds, nitrogen oxides, lead, and particulates (Moeller, 1992).

Some progress in controlling pollutants has been made. Most measured air pollutants declined between 1979 and 1988. In addition, there was a large decrease (more than 50% to 22%) in the proportion of the population who lived in counties exceeding the EPA standards for major air pollutants. However, the levels of volatile organic compounds such as benzene, formaldehyde, and vinyl chloride increased by 2% (Moeller, 1992). In addition, in 1992, EPA standards were violated at least once in areas inhabited by 54 million people (U.S. DHHS, 1993).

Sources of pollution include automobile emissions, industrial processes, and consumer goods. Technological advances in auto design have decreased that source of pollution, and the Clean Air Act has had an effect on industrial pollution; the act was passed in 1963, expanded in 1970, and amended in 1990. Amendments included specific mandates related to the control of air contaminants and to the enforcement of regulations. The penalty for noncompliance increased, and the process for imposing penalties was simplified, making it easier to ensure compliance with state and EPA regulations. Consumer products such as paint, nail polish remover, and aerosols are not regulated, however, and continue to pollute the environment.

Outside air pollution may affect health. Respiratory symptoms, eye irritation, fatigue, headache, and occasionally, death may be the result. Death most often occurs in the elderly and persons with respiratory diseases.

Indoor air pollution can also be a health concern. As many as 150 hazardous chemicals will be found in an average American home at concentrations of up to 40 times greater than recommended (Miller, 1992). It has been estimated that up to one third of all buildings in the United States suffer from indoor air pollution (Miller, 1992). Selected pollutants found in indoor air include formaldehyde, carbon monoxide, carbon dioxide, nitrous oxides, benzopyrene, and asbestos (Koren, 1991). Some of these are released by the building structure or furnishings. Additional pollutants may be a result of smoking, heating, cooking, household cleaning products, and personal hygiene products. Health effects of these pollutants include nose, throat, and eye irritations as well as respiratory dysfunction, heart disease, damage to the central nervous system (CNS), and cancer (Briasco, 1990; Koren, 1991). Bronchitis, pneumonia, asthma, and acute respiratory infections occur twice as often in children under the age of 2 whose parents smoke, and the more smoking in the home, the higher the prevalence of respiratory symptoms (Murdock, 1991, p. 12).

Cigarette Smoking. Cigarette smoking is an important cause of illnesses and deaths and has received attention at local, state, and national levels. Attention was initially focused on smoking and health as a result of the report *Smoking and Health: Report of the Advisory Committee to the Surgeon General of the Public Health Service* (U.S. Department of Health, Education and Welfare, 1964). In this report, following a review of 7,000 studies, the reviewers concluded that there was a causal relationship between cigarette smoking, lung cancer, and other serious diseases. They also stated that remedial action was needed. Later, the Federal Cigarette Labeling and Advertising Act of 1965 and the Public Health Cigarette Smoking Act of 1969 were passed by Congress.

These laws required health warnings on cigarette packages and banned cigarette advertising on mass media sources. The U.S. Public Health Service established a national clearinghouse for smoking and health in 1964 that has published more than 20 reports on the health consequence of smoking.

Cigarette smoking causes 390,000 deaths in the United States each year and is considered to be the largest preventable cause of illness and premature death in the United Stages. Diseases resulting from cigarette smoking include a variety of cancers (lung, laryngeal, esophageal, and urinary/bladder), coronary artery disease, chronic obstructive lung disease, some forms of cerebrovascular disease, spontaneous abortion, retarded fetal growth, and fetal or neonatal death (Rice, 1991, p. 296). In addition, smoking during pregnancy can lead to stillbirths, miscarriages, premature births, and low-birth-weight infants (U.S. DHHS, 1989, p. 19).

A variety of efforts have been initiated to reduce or eliminate cigarette smoking. Radio and television advertising for cigarettes has been eliminated; programs are available to help smokers stop; literature is available on the effects of smoking and resources to assist with stopping; rights of nonsmokers are stressed; smoking has been eliminated in many restaurants and public buildings, or smoking and nonsmoking areas have been identified; and high taxes have been added to the cost of cigarettes. Cigarette vending machines have been removed from many hospitals and businesses, and many airline flights are now smoke free. Despite resistance from tobacco companies, efforts to reduce smoking have proceeded. Recently, some states have also brought action against tobacco companies to recover money spent for tobacco-related illnesses. In a June 8, 1996, newspaper article ("San Francisco Files Suit," 1996), it was reported than San Francisco sued the tobacco industry to recover millions of dollars that the city and county of San Francisco spends yearly in the treatment of smoking-related illnesses. The suit alleged that six tobacco companies and two trade associations had violated state and federal laws in a 40-year conspiracy to conceal the addictive nature of tobacco. Similar suits have been filed in nine states in the past 2 years. Efforts discussed above to reduce or eliminate smoking demonstrate a multilevel focus on interventions to reduce this community hazard (see the discussion of multilevel intervention models in Chapter 8).

Additional pollutants found in the air are identified in Table 4.2, which includes sources of exposure, routes of entry, systems affected, primary manifestations, and aids to diagnosis. Some of these pollutants are specific to industrial settings.

Air Pollution Education. There are a variety of teaching areas for community health nurses in relation to air pollutants. In terms of primary prevention, the nurse can teach about carpooling to limit pollutants, replacement of asbestos insulation when found in buildings, dangers of space and kerosene heaters and the need for frequent cleaning of heating and cooling filters, airing of homes when the weather permits, and the need to limit outdoor activities when high pollution levels are present. Using the political process, the process of building coalitions, or other interventions to be discussed in Part IV later in this book, community health nurses may advocate legislation for safe standards in home building and heating and for reduced levels of pollutant emissions. The nurse can also teach the signs and symptoms of health reactions to pollutants, the measures to take to reduce reactions, and when and where to seek assistance with symptoms (secondary prevention).

CHEMICALS IN WATER

There are several sources of chemical pollution in water. One is acid rain, which is the precipitation of highly acidic moisture as rain, caused by pollutants from auto exhaust, industry, and other sources. Other sources include dumping, runoff, and seepage from manufacturing industries, mining operations, underground storage of chemicals, septic tanks, salt and de-icing chemicals on highways, landfill waste, fertilizers, herbicides, and pesticides among others. Homeowners add to this pollution by dumping chemicals into sink drains or on the ground. Some chemicals found in water are identified in Table 4.2. Additional chemicals of concern were mentioned earlier under waste disposal.

Health effects of chemicals in water include bladder, colon, and rectal cancers; skin conditions; alopecia; seizures; hepatitis; cirrhosis; infertility; congenital defects; developmental delays; anemia; CNS effects; peripheral neuropathy; renal failure; gastritis; esophagitis; heart disease; and stomach cancer.

Nurses can teach groups at risk about the effects of water pollution, symptoms to observe, and where they can receive care. They can also work with the political process to encourage safe drinking water.

MECHANICAL FACTORS

Mechanical factors are stresses on the body that create health hazards. Mechanical stresses include vibration, repetitive motion, and lifting. Examples of vibration and repetitive motion are pneumonic vibrating tools such as grinding and riveting machines, chipping hammers, and drills. These tools may have a frequency rate of up to 50,000 blows per minute depending on the size. Vasospasm or "white finger" is a result of vibration and repetitive motion and is most often caused by using tools that give less than 4,000 blows per minute with 2,000 to 3,000 being the most dangerous. This condition causes spasmodic contractions of the blood vessels in the fingers, causing them to become numb and white.

Repeated motion may lead to changes in the joints, resulting in tenosynovitis and bursitis. In tenosynovitis, repeated use or sudden strain of a tendon may cause a rupture of the blood vessel into the tendon sheath, resulting in pain on exertion. Bursitis may result from constant abnormal friction on the tendon, usually at the joint. Pain and limitations in movement are the result, due to the fluid in the bursa. Pneumatic drills held against the shoulder may cause bursitis. Carpal tunnel syndrome may also result from repeated motion and is seen in those who type or use computers as well as in meatpackers, garment workers, and many assembly line workers. Tenosynovitis and bursitis may be prevented in some people by the use of rubber pads to prevent constant pressure of tissue against hard surfaces and by periodic changes in position and methods of work. Protective mittens and mechanical devices to hold vibrating tools in place may also be effective in reducing the problems associated with repetitive motion. When spasms are discovered, the work should be discontinued to prevent further complications.

Lifting of loads is another work-related problem that places severe stress on the body. The usual method of lifting a weight, which is incorrect, is to bend at the waist while keeping the legs straight. A better method is to stand close to the object with the feet 8 to 12 inches apart and to bend the knees rather than the back. This puts the pressure on the leg muscles rather than on the back. Correct lifting of a weight should reduce the associated stress to the body.

PSYCHOSOCIAL FACTORS

SOCIETAL VIOLENCE

Pope et al. (1995) list violence, stress, and high-demand/low-control occupations under the category of psychosocial environmental health hazards. Stressors might include noise, overcrowding, lack of social interaction, lack of privacy and space, boredom, crowds, and change. Likewise, societal stresses such as crime, poor economic condition, rising unemployment, and changing mores affect populations in different ways. In addition, although Pope et al. list high-demand/low-control occupations as a separate psychosocial environmental factor, it could easily be listed under the category of stress. Another category of stressors involves natural disasters, such as earthquakes, floods, hurricanes, drought, and volcano eruptions.

Humans react differently to these stressors. Often, an important difference in reactions is related to the attitude of the person facing the stressor. For example, some people might look at overcrowding in a household as a lack of space and privacy and react negatively, whereas another might see this as opportunities for interaction and love. Humans react differently to different stressors and to the same stressor at different times. Many aspects of stress, stressors, and stress management techniques are discussed in a previous book by the author (Helvie, 1991).

Violence is a growing environmental concern. Factors that may trigger violence include poverty, widespread unemployment, proliferation of handguns, lack of child abuse facilities, violence on mass media, hate crimes, and the reluctance of police and the justice system to consider women's abuse as serious.

Hate crimes against racial, ethnic, or religious minorities and against lesbians and gay men are reported often by mass media. For example, Hall and Stevens (1992) reported increased threats, malicious innuendos, and violent crimes against Arab Americans throughout the United States during the U.S.-Iraq war. They also note that women and children are frequent targets of violence because of their relative political powerlessness. In addition, cultural norms of violence are reinforced by male images of male aggressiveness and sexual dominance (Hanmer & Maynard, 1987).

Violence in the home has received increased attention recently. Although this usually takes the form of wife abuse, it may also involve male, child, or elder abuse. According to Gelles and Strauss (1988), 95% of all abusers are male. Wife abuse occurs more often as a result of pregnancy, alcohol use by the abuser, the abuser's having a role model who abused in the family of orientation, social isolation, and a lack of social support for women. According to Barber-Madden, Cohn, and Schloesser (1988) and Grisso et al. (1991), one third of all women are assaulted by husbands or male companions at least one time during a relationship; 30 of every 1,000 women are severely abused, physically, by a male partner each year; and spouse abuse is the leading cause of injury for women. Berrios and Grady (1991) add that domestic violence accounts for 30% to 50% of all police cases.

Certain characteristics are associated with the abusers and victims. First, there is a socioeconomic relationship. Although abuse occurs at all economic levels, families at or below the poverty level are five times more likely to experience it. Education and occupation also seem to be related. Compared with other occupations, abusers are more prevalent among skilled or semiskilled workers. In addition, personality traits of abusers have been identified. They are more often emotionally dependent and very egocentric. Abuser characteristics include poor social skills, an explosive temper, a need for instant gratification, and low tolerance of frustration. A variety of methods are used to exert power over a partner: for example, coercion and threats, intimidation, emotional abuse, isolating the spouse, economic abuse, excusing the behavior as a male privilege, using children as weapons, and minimizing or denying the behavior and blaming the spouse.

The traits of the battered spouse in this dyad include an inability to identify one's own ego needs and a tendency to subordinate one's needs to those of the spouse or children. Most battered spouses are economically and emotionally dependent on the batterer.

There is a cyclic pattern to most domestic violence episodes. Three phases were identified by Walker (1979): (a) the tension-building phase, (b) the battering phase, and (c) the apologetic phase. During the tension-building phase, anger and frustration of the batterer and belittling of the victim increase. At this time, the victim becomes more attentive, nurturing, and self-deprecating in an attempt to reduce the anger and frustration in the batterer. Despite these attempts, the tension continues to increase.

During the battering phase, the batterer vents his or her emotions by physically punishing the victim. Following dissipation of these emotions, the batterer moves to the apologetic phase. Now the abuser is contrite and loving and says the episode will not be repeated. The abuser may bring gifts to the victim and make other efforts to please the victim.

Despite the abuse suffered in these situations several attempts are usually made before the victim can leave the abuser permanently. According to Andresen (1985), 55% of the women at one shelter had returned to their spouse by 2 months after leaving the shelter. Reasons for this behavior included hope that the batterer would reform, feeling that there is no place to go, financial concerns, emotional dependence, fear of reprisals from the batterer, fear of living alone, and the difficulty of leaving with children because of finances or feared difficulty in finding housing.

CHILD ABUSE

Statistics for child abuse are alarming: 25 of every 1,000 children are abused or neglected yearly; homicide is the leading cause of death in children 6 weeks to 2 years of age; and sexual abuse occurs in 1 in 5 to 10 girls and 1 in 10 to 50 boys by adolescence (American Academy of Nursing Expert Panel, 1993; National Center for Child Abuse and Neglect, 1988; "Policy Statement," 1993). An increase of 212% in child abuse and neglect cases has been reported from 1976 to 1986, according to the American Humane Society (Starr, Dubowitz, & Bush, 1990).

Statistics indicate that abusers are likely to show an ongoing abuse or neglect pattern rather than a single episode and to target children who are different, such as children with handicaps, and those who are poor, young, black, and with little education (American Association for Protection of Children, 1990). But other reports question some of these characteristics. In terms of physical and emotional abuse, women are more frequent abusers of children than are men (National Center for Child Abuse and Neglect, 1988).

Abuse may be physical, sexual, or emotional. About 1,400 children died in 1991 as a result of physical abuse (Children's Defense Fund, 1992). Examples of mild to moderate physical abuse include pushing, throwing, or spanking with bare hands; severe abusive behaviors include kicking, biting, spanking with an object, and threatening or using a weapon. Emotional abuse includes words or actions that depreciate the child's self-worth. This is an ongoing process, and constant criticism eventually convinces the child that he or she is worthless, stupid, crazy, unwanted, or unloved. These children have a vacant or frozen affect, are delayed developmentally, have poor personal hygiene and dress, have poor school attendance and performance, do not cry, and avoid or overreact to physical contact.

Sexual abuse includes any behavior in which children are used to meet the sexual needs or desires of adults. Sexual abuse is usually committed by family members but can be committed by others in the community. Conte and Berliner (1981) say that about 90% of all abuse is committed by a family member or acquaintance. These cases often are discovered years after the abuse occurred.

NEGLECT

Neglect is an omission or failure to act, as opposed to abuse in which an act is committed. Neglect can be physical or emotional. Failure to provide for the basic needs of food, clothing, and shelter constitutes physical neglect, whereas failure to provide for the child's needs for love, belonging, and recognition constitute emotional neglect. Neglect is an ongoing pattern and not a single episode. Substance abuse and alcohol abuse in parents have been identified as factors in child abuse.

Primary prevention is an important aspect of nursing with abused children. In this role, the nurse should educate groups about the needs of children for physical care and emotional love, the effects of substance abuse and alcohol on children, signs and symptoms of child abuse, resources available for mental health counseling for at-risk parents, and bonding behaviors. In addition, nurses should educate groups who may observe behaviors indicating abuse or who work with these groups, such as teachers, health personnel, and judges. Nurses may also work with the political or other community subsystems to develop community services such as crisis hotlines, respite care for children, and homemaker education and services.

At the secondary level, nurses should assess groups in schools, clinics, or other community settings for evidence of abuse and refer them to community agencies, if this is appropriate. Identified families should be referred to self-help groups. Nurses should also work with community subsystems to ensure the availability of 24-hour trauma centers and with multidisciplinary committees to review and recommend treatment for identified cases.

Primary preventive interventions are important for spouse abuse also. Teaching of groups should include effective communication between partners, joint decision making, and appropriate and inappropriate behavior in relationships, such as conflict resolution. Other areas of teaching might include the legal rights of women and resources for abusers and victims. This teaching might occur in parenting classes, civic meetings, or the mass media.

NURSING AND THE ENVIRONMENT

Examples of nursing interventions for each category of environmental hazards were identified earlier. These interventions are directed toward decreasing the effects of these hazards on the health of aggregates or to make people more resistant to environmental assaults. This involves intervening before the environment brings the disease- or injury-producing agent together with populations (primary prevention) or identifying these effects at an early stage in the disease- or injury-producing process (secondary prevention). Nursing actions should be directed toward both the population and community subsystems that affect populations. For example, nurses may teach population groups how to avoid exposure to certain chemical or biological hazards in the community and at the same time may work with the political subsystem to encourage laws to prevent industrial dumping of toxic waste in water. When possible, a multilevel model of intervention is most effective (see Chapter 8). A case study by a nursing leader in occupational health nursing at the end of this chapter shows how nurses can use knowledge of the environment to protect workers.

Nursing interventions are based on an assessment. Often, these assessments are carried out jointly with others in the community, including health and nonhealth community members. Assessment always involves the consumer of services (see community assessment). To make a plan specific to a community, the nurse should assess the types and sources of environmental hazards on the basis of data presented earlier in this chapter, what the community believes its environmental problems are, the health effects of the hazards identified, and potential resources to assist with resolving the problems. Interventions may involve primary, secondary, and tertiary levels of intervention.

Pope et al. (1995) say that the environment is a primary determinant of health, that nurses are in a good position to address environmental concerns with individuals and communities, and that there is a need to increase the awareness of all nurses of the relationship of the environment and health. They present a general overview of the field and identify undergraduate and graduate nursing courses in which environmental content could be added with minimal effort. They also identify references for this content. It is my hope that this important area of nursing, identified by Florence Nightingale more than 100 years ago, will again have a proper place in nursing education and practice.

Case Study 2
Detecting the Source of Lead Poisoning

JACQUELINE AGNEW

For centuries, lead has been recognized as a dangerous environmental and occupational toxin. Despite our recognition of the severe health consequences associated with lead exposure, it continues to present a threat in our communities and workplaces. Lead is one example of many potentially harmful exposures that result in highly preventable morbidity and mortality (Landrigan, 1992). It is therefore important for nurses to assume a role in controlling lead exposure and preventing lead poisoning. This case study illustrates many facets of inorganic lead poisoning and the areas, from physiology to policy, that must be understood by nurses who have a responsibility to protect communities from environmental hazards. Although the focus is on a single, serious toxin, the principles discussed here can be applied to many other situations in which preventable exposures are a concern.

A CHILD WITH SYMPTOMS

The school nurse was surprised to hear the first-grader's report that she had bumped her head after being pushed by Tess. She knew Tess to be a

relatively quiet and bashful student, whose only problems in school were related to her absences, which seemed to be more frequent. The nurse had come to know Tess quite well as a result of her trips to the nurse's office to deliver her absence notes from home or to complain about stomach pains that eluded explanation. The mysterious set of circumstances prompted the nurse to request a conference with the teacher, principal, and school psychologist. She soon learned that the same conference had been requested by Tess's teacher.

During the conference, the teacher stated that she had noted several behavioral changes in Tess over the school year. In addition to the absences, these included a decreasing attention span, whereas the other children were showing improved ability to attend to their schoolwork. At times, according to the teacher and principal, Tess acted listless and cranky, to the point of occasional aggressiveness with other children such as the classmate with the bumped head. These changes were seen as unusual by all members of the team, and the teacher asked if any home circumstances of this 6-year-old might be contributing to her problems.

Tess lived in a small row house in a low-income neighborhood with two brothers, aged 3 and 7, and her mother. Tess's uncle, her mother's brother, was living with them temporarily, since finding short-term work as a laborer on a construction job 4 months ago. Although her mother had been out of work since the birth of the youngest boy, Tess's uncle was able to bring some income into the household. The family used food stamps and received medical care at the local city health department health clinic, but there was every indication of conscientious attention to the children's needs. They'd had their preschool physical examinations at the clinic, been immunized, and been screened for blood lead levels before the school year began. The second-grade teacher reported that Tess's brother was a well-behaved, eager student who had not changed noticeably over the school year. The team members concluded that they would hold a conference as soon as possible with Tess's mother.

The school nurse continued to ponder the information exchanged at the interdisciplinary meeting and realized there could be a reasonable explanation for the problems described. Tess often said she was tired and that she ached; she had once been seen at the local emergency room to rule out appendicitis when she complained of stomach pain. Although tests for appendicitis were negative, her mother mentioned that Tess periodically stayed home from school for gastrointestinal symptoms. Although the nurse knew that blood lead levels were evaluated for all children seen at the city health clinic, she noted that she was seeing similarities between students she had known with lead poisoning and Tess.

At the meeting with Tess's mother, school personnel expressed their concerns about Tess and learned that their observations and alarm were shared by her mother. She thought that the gastrointestinal symptoms might be related to a lingering flu-like syndrome, but she had also noticed her daughter's fatigue and irritability as well as alterations in Tess's usual upbeat personality. Her mother described how Tess had once been very excited about helping with household chores, but she no longer enjoyed even her most favorite task of helping her mother with the laundry. The family's adjustment to having their uncle move in had gone smoothly, and Tess loved to go for rides in his car, something her mother did not own.

When the school nurse moved the discussion to the issue of lead level screening, she learned that Tess had been found to have a blood lead level of 9 µg/dl (micrograms per deciliter) before the start of first grade; her brothers' levels were 5 and 7 µg/dl. The nurse agreed that these were below the level at which education and follow-up screening would have been initiated (10 µg/dl). She also knew, however, that lead body burden is cumulative and that additional or continuing sources of lead exposure could cause the lead level to rise beyond the previous documented level. She made a request that Tess's mother take Tess to the clinic for a comprehensive health examination. She also made a phone call to the clinic to express her concerns about the potential for lead poisoning.

SIGNS AND SYMPTOMS OF LEAD TOXICITY

What are the potential consequences of exposure to this odorless and tasteless substance that is very common in our environment, and what were the signals that suggested that lead poisoning might be the problem for this 6-year-old child? Lead is a heavy metal that causes toxicity of many systems at all ages but is especially harmful to the nervous system of children and fetuses. Because the blood-brain barrier is less developed in the fetus and child, lead is able to cross that barrier and reaches the central nervous system more easily. At high levels (PbB $\geq$ 80 µg/dl) in children, it can cause coma, seizures, and death. Lower levels adversely affect the renal, gastrointestinal, and hematologic systems and cause more subtle central nervous system effects, such as hearing impairment, balance dysfunction, and learning problems. A disturbing finding that has spawned much recent debate is that levels as low as 10 µg/dl in children have been associated with decreased intelligence and impaired neurobehavioral development. Symptoms of lead poisoning in children include anorexia, vomiting, abdominal discomfort, constipation, irritability, lethargy, insomnia, and hyperactivity. These symptoms are nonspecific and therefore are frequently mistaken for other illnesses.

Adults also experience lead poisoning. In adults, lead affects the same organ systems, but nervous system effects tend to differ from those seen in children. Adults are more likely to exhibit peripheral nervous system effects of sensory and motor disturbances, although they also can experience the most severe central nervous system effects of seizures, coma, and death at very high blood lead levels ($\geq 100\,\mu g/dl$). Hematologic, renal, and gastrointestinal signs and symptoms include anemia, nephropathy, abdominal pain, vomiting, anorexia, and constipation. Additional potential consequences of lead exposure include difficulty concentrating or behavioral manifestations that are often described by family members or friends as irritability or other "personality changes." Another important outcome of lead toxicity seen in adults is an adverse effect on reproductive health; lead can cause spontaneous abortions and has been implicated in sperm abnormalities.

SCREENING GUIDELINES

Unlike many metals, such as zinc and iron, that are required by various physiologic systems in the human body, lead has no known positive biological function. Once absorbed following inhalation or ingestion, however, it accumulates in many different tissues, particularly in bone. Blood lead levels provide an estimate of lead exposure levels in recent months and also reflect, in part, total lead body burden. The increasing evidence that demonstrates associations between increased lead levels and impaired health in children has brought about, over the years, a downward revision of the blood lead values considered to be unacceptable in children. That blood lead level is now set at $10\,\mu g/dl$ according to screening guidelines published by the Centers for Disease Control and Prevention (CDC, 1991). It is important to note that the CDC is now in the process of preparing an updated publication titled "Guidelines for Screening and Management of Children With Lead Poisoning." Following public review, comments, and editing, the guidelines are expected to be published in 1997. This will be an excellent resource for all nurses who deal with children in the community.

The national strategy for improving the health of the nation, *Healthy People 2000,* established as one objective the elimination of blood lead levels above $25\,\mu g/dl$ in children under the age of 5 (U.S. Department of Health and Human Services [DHHS], 1991). In keeping with this objective, screening programs identify asymptomatic lead-poisoned children and allow early intervention to reduce blood lead levels as quickly as possible. All children should be screened for lead poisoning, but the groups of children aged 6 months to 6 years who should be made priorities for screening are the following:

- Children who live in or frequently visit deteriorated housing built before 1960
- Children who live in housing built before 1960 with recent, ongoing, or planned renovation or remodeling
- Siblings, housemates, or playmates of children with known lead poisoning
- Children whose parents or other household members participate in a lead-related hobby or occupation
- Children who live near active smelters, battery recycling plants, or other industries likely to result in atmospheric lead release

These characteristics form the basis of a questionnaire to evaluate risk of lead exposure (CDC, 1991). A positive answer to any of the questions means that the child is potentially at high risk for high lead exposure.

Current recommendations for screening and follow-up are summarized in a publication by the CDC (1991) and are based on the child's age, risk of lead exposure, and previously measured lead levels. Screening can be done on a capillary blood specimen obtained by a careful technique that minimizes contamination of the sample, but elevated results should be confirmed on a venous blood sample.

RESULTS OF THE CLINIC VISIT

The suspicions of the school nurse were confirmed when the results of Tess's blood lead test were returned. Her venous blood lead level was $28\,\mu g/dl$, a significant increase from $9\,\mu g/dl$ only 6 months before. The elevated value triggered several actions. At the clinic, Tess was given a complete medical evaluation, her brothers were immediately screened for lead levels, and as a state requirement, Tess's elevated lead level was reported to the state environmental health department. (This is not a uniform requirement in all states, but Tess lives in a state with a heavy metal registry where results of $\geq 25\,\mu g/dl$ for adults and $\geq 10\,\mu g/dl$ for children must be reported.)

The pediatric evaluation included a detailed history that covered the presence of symptoms, behavior, nutritional status with an emphasis on iron and calcium intake, family history of lead poisoning, a review of previous lead levels, and occupational histories of adults in the household. The pediatrician learned that Tess had become more fatigued, restless, and irritable since the start of the school year 6 months before. She also heard about the recurring abdominal distress that seemed to be without explanation. The pediatrician knew that Tess's mother spent all of her time with her children after being laid off from her grocery store job. Her mother said she had not noticed any disturbance of the paint in the house, and no remodeling or renovation had been done.

The physical examination included particular attention to the neurologic examination and developmental expectations. No abnormal findings were noted. Iron status was evaluated by measurement of serum ferritin, the most definitive indication of overall iron status. This value was 13 µg/dl, a low but normal result. The pediatrician concluded that Tess was experiencing lead poisoning that had been very recent in onset. Fortunately, neither her symptoms nor her lead level would necessitate chelation treatment at this time, but the source of her poisoning must be identified and immediately eliminated from her environment.

The decision to screen Tess's brothers was very appropriate, but when the results were returned, they were perplexing. Their levels had risen only slightly, from 5 and 7 µg/dl in the fall to 10 and 11 µg/dl in March. These new levels were also reported to the state; fortunately, the boys were asymptomatic. Although all children seemed to have encountered a new source of lead in their environment, there was a strong suggestion that it was most strongly affecting Tess. That source needed to be identified.

RESPONSE TO REPORTS OF ELEVATED LEAD LEVELS

According to the policy of the state environmental health department, a child with a blood lead level above 20 µg/dl would be entered into the lead poisoning prevention program, a collaborative arrangement with local health departments. This meant that a county or city public health nurse would make a home visit to assess the home, educate family members, and further

evaluate the child. Dependent on findings during the home visit, other health department team members could follow up with more detailed paint and dust sampling and testing. What sources of lead might be present in a home, and how might a child be exposed?

SOURCES OF LEAD EXPOSURE

Lead is absorbed by inhalation or ingestion, but generally, there are differences between children and adults in terms of exposure. For example, adults with lead toxicity tend to be exposed to lead in their occupations if they work in jobs such as smelting, cabling, radiator repair, or heavy construction where welding or metal burning takes place. Children usually encounter lead in their environment and engage in behaviors that place them at risk of ingesting or inhaling lead dust. Common behaviors that may promote ingestion of lead include the following:

- Playing on floors and in soil where lead dust may be present
- Placing hands and objects in the mouth
- Pica (ingestion of nonfood items such as dirt)
- Chewing on windows, furniture, or other surfaces coated with lead-based paint.

Paint is especially of concern if it was applied before 1978, the year the Consumer Product Safety Commission banned addition of lead to new residential paint. Additional potential sources of adult and child lead exposure include some foods and water, and some medicinal and cosmetic preparations from foreign cultures are high in lead content.

THE HOME VISIT AND ASSESSMENT

A city health department nurse soon visited the family one day after school. All of the children were home with their mother, but their uncle was still at work. The children followed quietly as their mother showed the nurse their bedrooms and the areas in which they played. The nurse observed that the home was an old row house of a vintage that signaled many coats of interior lead-based paint, but the woodwork was not visibly deteriorating, and there were no signs of chewing or biting on the window sills. The nurse knew that old paint can flake off as a dust, especially when windows are raised and lowered, but the housekeeping was quite good, and window wells were not noticeably dusty. In the kitchen, the mother brought out a few dishes from a very plain set of dishes that were not pottery and that did not appear to be glazed. Questions about use of herbal or imported remedies were all answered negatively. The children took only prescribed medicines. The nurse could not be sure of the level of lead in the family's drinking water, but a quick check of lead poisoning cases in the city had shown none others within a few blocks.

Because the lead toxicity was of unknown origin, the nurse had arrived prepared to draw blood samples from Tess's mother and uncle. After learning that the uncle would be home in 15 minutes, she decided to go on to the education phase of the visit and draw the blood samples before leaving. She first discussed the potential health effects of lead in children and stressed the need for continued follow-up for lead level and health assessment. She explained the relationship between nutrition and lead absorption. She pointed out that because lead is more easily absorbed on an empty stomach, all three meals are important for children. In addition, it is thought that calcium and iron inhibit the absorption of lead and that iron deficiency can enhance lead toxicity. Thus, calcium and iron are essential components in children's diets. She made certain that Tess's mother was armed with a list of resources and phone numbers for future questions and assistance. The final part of the nurse's teaching focused on potential lead sources and how they could be controlled. Although the nurse did not strongly feel that the home's paint was the source of the problem for this family, she did cover methods for cleaning wood surfaces with a damp cloth or mop and a phosphate solution. She explained that an environmental team from the health department would visit at a later date to check lead levels in the paint and to sample for lead dust.

As the nurse completed her teaching, the children's uncle arrived home from work. He was introduced by his sister but could not shake hands because he was so dirty from work. The nurse explained that she would like to draw a sample of his blood, and he joked that she was welcome to do so if she could locate his arm under all of the grime from work. They were soon in a discussion about his new job in the city. The nurse learned that he worked as a laborer, but his specific job at the site was actually one of demolition of an old five-story commercial structure that was being torn down and rebuilt. After the old beams were brought down, he used a torch of very intense temperature to cut the iron into sizes to be hauled away. The nurse began to realize that this man performed a job of potentially high lead exposure and that the source of lead in the home may have been found.

Lead-based paint, because of its anticorrosive properties, is often used in construction to coat metal structures. Activities such as sanding or abrading the surfaces in any way will create lead dust, and high temperatures of welding or burning will generate lead fume. Unventilated or indoor areas increase the concentration of lead in the atmosphere. In addition to the hazard presented to the worker who may inhale or ingest the lead dust or fume, lead particles can be carried away from the job site on clothing, hair, shoes, hands, or articles such as lunch boxes and cars. The hazard to workers increases if there are not good hygiene facilities at the job site and if workers smoke or eat around their work. Workplaces in general industry that pose a potential for lead exposure are subject to the Occupational Safety and Health Administration (OSHA) lead standard, which addresses air-level monitoring, worker education and periodic screening, and control of lead exposure, including measures such as showers and the provision of facilities for a clean change of clothes before going home. There is a separate, much less stringent, federal OSHA standard for the construction industry, but the family in this case study lived in one of the states that has mandated that the OSHA lead standard for general industry be used in the construction industry.

CONCLUSION OF HOME VISIT

The nurse discussed with the two adults the possibility that not only the uncle but other household members could be exposed to lead from the construction job if lead-contaminated dust was coming home on his clothes, shoes, and body.

Tess may have experienced more contact with the dust than her brothers if she frequently helped with his laundry and rode in his car. The uncle said he had not experienced any symptoms, but the nurse drew blood samples from both adults before leaving the home. She also ascertained the name of his employer and the location of the construction job.

Realizing that conditions at the job site sounded harmful and that other workers may also be exposed to lead, the nurse immediately made a referral to the state occupational safety and health agency. (States that do not have a state agency are covered by regional offices of OSHA.) The referral would trigger an inspection of the site to evaluate potential lead exposure to all workers. The possibility of other family exposures would also be considered.

THE ISSUE OF HOME CONTAMINATION FROM WORK EXPOSURES

The problem of home contamination from work exposures has received only limited attention and is often an overlooked pathway by which toxins reach family members. This problem has been called one of "paraoccupational exposure" or "take-home toxins" and refers to cases in which workers inadvertently transport the hazardous material to their homes on their skin, hair, clothes, cars, or other items. Workers who do not have adequate changing facilities at work and who launder their work clothes at home are especially at risk for these incidents, which have caused a wide range of health effects and even death in family members. Substances for which there are published reports of paraoccupational exposures include lead, mercury, asbestos, beryllium, and pesticides (Chisolm, 1978; McDiarmid & Weaver, 1993). A recent review by the National Institute of Occupational Safety and Health (NIOSH) of all literature on this topic (1996) indicated that the problem extends worldwide; incidents from 28 countries and 36 states in the United States have been reported (DHHS, 1995). The Workers' Family Protection Act of 1992 (Public Law 102-522, 29 U.S.C. 671a) directed NIOSH to conduct the review and has established the Workers' Family Protection Task Force to evaluate the need for additional research on this important issue.

FOLLOW-UP AT THE WORKPLACE

The uncle's blood lead level results of 35 µg/dl further suggested a workplace exposure, and an evaluation of that construction site by the state occupational safety and health agency was soon under way. The company contracting the job was not aware of the danger to the workers and had not taken steps to evaluate exposures or provide for appropriate surveillance of workers. Air monitoring demonstrated high air lead levels at locations on the job site that were indoors and therefore poorly ventilated. Five other workers who used torches to cut scrap metal were screened for lead levels and nurses from the health department made visits to their homes to evaluate risks to family members. Although most had children, none were found to have lead values above the level of concern of 10 µg/dl, probably because the children did not have close contact with workers' clothes or cars. All workers had moderately elevated levels similar to Tess's uncle's, but they were asymptomatic. The company was in jeopardy of being fined for failure to protect the health and safety of workers by adhering to the lead standard. The response was to immediately institute the required environmental controls, worker training, air and blood lead monitoring, and hygiene facilities. Successive monitoring showed a progressive decline in workers' blood lead values following cessation of their exposure.

FOLLOW-UP IN THE HOME

An environmental sanitation team visited Tess's home to instruct and assist the family with cleanup procedures for the lead dust decontamination. This included wet mopping all surfaces with a phosphate cleaning solution and vacuuming carpets with a high-efficiency particulate vacuum. The family was instructed to wash all toys and to frequently wash their hands. Nurses and the environmental team continued to follow the family until the children's blood lead levels decreased to less concerning levels (below 10 µg/dl). Tess's mother's lead level, slightly elevated, also returned to a lower level. Throughout the process, feedback was provided to school personnel by Tess's mother and the community health nurse. The nurse was also instrumental in explaining to the entire family that home contamination is a common problem and should not serve as grounds for guilt on the part of the worker who unknowingly transported the contaminant.

SUMMARY

Lead poisoning is one of many examples of environmentally mediated, but highly preventable, adverse health conditions. This case study illustrates the role of nurses in reducing and preventing this threat to the health of individuals and communities. As recommended in the report on "Nursing, Health, and the Environment" by the Committee on Enhancing Environmental Health Content in Nursing Practice, established by the Institute of Medicine (Pope, Snyder, & Mood, 1995), environmental health should receive emphasis in defining the scope of responsibilities for nursing practice. As this example demonstrates, it is important to consider all settings where environmental hazards may be encountered, including the workplace, home, and community. Occupational histories of client populations can be very informative in formulating preventive strategies.

Nurses should be familiar with major environmental hazards and should give particular attention to the types of industries that employ their community populations. Other potential sources of toxic exposures include hazardous waste sites, major transportation routes where crashes and spills can expose neighborhoods, and air, water, and soil with dangerous concentrations of pollutants. Housing conditions also play an important role in exposing residents to lead, radon, and indoor air contaminants such as cigarette smoke and mold.

In addition to excellent knowledge regarding potential hazards and health effects, nurses need a comprehensive understanding of all agencies whose missions are relevant to the prevention of environmental disease. As seen in this case study, a number of agencies at the federal, state, and local levels have responsibilities aimed at controlling environmental hazards through promulgation of standards, development of guidelines, or provision of resources. Close coordination among these organizations and appropriate referrals are imperative. Nurses may also interact with authorities when advocacy roles of nurses demand not collaboration but confrontational strategies to resolve a community's environmental problems (Pope et al., 1995, p. 258).

In summary, environmental issues are becomingly increasingly important in the domain of community health nurses. Nurses have a definite role to play in reducing the morbidity and mortality of this preventable epidemic.

REFERENCES

Centers for Disease Control. (1991). *Preventing lead poisoning in young children: A statement by the Centers for Disease Control* (Publication No. 1991-537-304). Washington, DC: Government Printing Office.

Chisolm, J. J. (1978). Fouling one's own nest. *Pediatrics, 62,* 614-617.

Landrigan, P. J. (1992). Commentary: Environmental disease—A preventable epidemic. *American Journal of Public Health, 82,* 941-943.

McDiarmid, M. A., & Weaver, V. (1993). Fouling one's own nest revisited. *American Journal of Industrial Medicine, 24,* 1-9.

Pope, A., Snyder, M., & Mood, L. (Eds.). (1995). *Nursing, health, and the environment.* Washington, DC: National Academy Press, Institute of Medicine.

U.S. Department of Health and Human Services. (1991). *Healthy people 2000: National health promotion and disease prevention objectives* (DHHS Publication No. 91-50213). Washington, DC: Government Printing Office.

U.S. Department of Health and Human Services, Centers for Disease Control and Prevention, National Institute for Occupational Safety and Health. (1995). *Report to Congress on Workers' Home Contamination Study conducted under the Workers' Family Protection Act* (29 U.S.C. 671a). Cincinnati, OH: Author.

REFERENCES

American Academy of Nursing Expert Panel. (1993). AAN working paper: Violence as a nursing priority: Policy implications. *Nursing Outlook, 41*(2), 83-92.

American Association for Protection of Children. (1990). *Highlights of the official child neglect and abuse report, 1988.* Denver, CO: American Humane Association.

Anderson, K. (1994). *Mosby's medical, nursing, and allied health dictionary.* St. Louis, MO: C. V. Mosby.

Andresen, P. (1985). The prevention and treatment of spouse abuse: A community health perspective. *Journal of Community Health Nursing, 2,* 181-190.

Auerbach, L. (1985). The occupational health and safety act. In D. S. Blumenthal (Ed.), *Introduction to environmental health.* New York: Springer.

Baetjer, A. (1965). Atmospheric pollution. In P. Sartwell (Ed.), *Preventive medicine and public health.* New York: Appleton-Century-Crofts.

Barber-Madden, R., Cohn, A., & Schloesser, P. (1988, Summer). Prevention of child abuse: A public health agenda. *Public Health Policy,* pp. 167-176.

Benenson, A. S. (1990). *Control of communicable diseases in man* (15th ed.). Washington, DC: American Public Health Association.

Berrios, D., & Grady, D. (1991). Domestic violence: Risk factors and outcomes. *Western Journal of Medicine, 166,* 133-136.

Blumenthal, D. S. (Ed.). (1985). *Introduction to environmental health.* New York: Springer.

Blumenthal, H. (1985). The health effects of low-level ionizing radiation. In D. S. Blumenthal (Ed.), *Introduction to environmental health* (pp. 79-116). New York: Springer.

Briasco, M. E. (1990). Indoor air pollution: Are employees sick from their work? *AAOHN Journal, 38,* 375-380.

Carson, R. (1962). *Silent spring.* Burlington, MA: Houghton Mifflin.

Children's Defense Fund. (1992). *The state of America's children.* Washington, DC: Author.

Chiras, D. D. (1994). *Environmental science: Action for a sustainable future.* Redwood City, CA: Benjamin/Cummings.

Committee on Advances in Assessing Human Exposure to Airborne Pollutants. (1991). *Human exposure assessment for airborne pollutants: Advances and opportunities.* Washington, DC: National Academy of Science.

Conte, J., & Berliner, L. (1981). Sexual abuse of children: Implications for the practice social case work. *Journal of Contemporary Social Work, 62,* 601-606.

DiChristina, M. (1990). How can we win the war against garbage. *Popular Science, 231,* 57.

Elmer-Dewitt, P. (1992). How do we patch a hole in the sky that could be as big as Alaska? *Time, 139*(7), 64-65.

Farfel, M., & Chisolm, J. (1990). Health and environmental health outcomes of traditional and modified practices for abatement of residential lead-based paint. *American Journal of Public Health, 80,* 1240-1245.

Gelles, R., & Strauss, M. (1988). *The definitive study of the causes and consequences of abuse in the American family.* New York: Simon & Schuster.

Gibbons, W. (1991). Low-level radiation: Higher long-term risk? *Science News, 139,* 181.

Goldstein, M., Schwartz, B., Friedman, C., Maccarillo, B., Borbi, M., & Tuccillo, R. (1990). Lyme disease in New Jersey outdoor workers: A statewide survey of seroprevalence and tick exposure. *American Journal of Public Health, 80,* 1225-1229.

Grisso, J., Wishner, A., Schwartz, D., Weene, B., Holmes, J., & Sutton, R. (1991). A population-based study of injuries in inner-city women. *American Journal of Epidemiology, 134,* 59-68.

Hall, J., & Stevens, P. (1992). A nursing view of the U.S.-Iraq war: Psychosocial health consequences. *Nursing Outlook, 40,* 113-120.

Hanmer, M., & Maynard, M. (Eds.). (1987). *Women, violence and social control.* Atlantic Highlands, NJ: Humanities.

Helvie, C. (1991). *Community health nursing: Theory and practice.* New York: Springer.

Koren, H. (1991). *Handbook of environmental health: Principles and practices* (Vol. 1, 2nd ed.). Chelsea, MI: Lewis.

Lead paint warnings give buyers, renters a heads up before moving. (1996, December 7). *Virginian Pilot,* p. B1.

Lemonick, M. (1992, February 17). The ozone vanishes. *Time,* pp. 60-63.

McCunney, R. (1992). Occupational exposure to noise. In R. J. Rom (Ed.), *Environmental and occupational medicine* (2nd ed.). Boston: Little Brown.

Miller, G. (1992). *An introduction to environmental science: Living in the environment.* Belmont, CA: Wadsworth.

Moeller, D. (1992). *Environmental health.* Cambridge, MA: Harvard University Press.

Moore, A., Herwaldt, B. L., Craun, G., Calderon, R., Highsmith, A., & Juranek, D. (1993). Surveillance for waterborne disease outbreaks—United States, 1991-1992. *Morbidity and Mortality Weekly Report, 42*(SS-5), 1-22.

Murdock, B. (1991). *Environmental issues in primary care.* Minneapolis, MN: Freshwater Foundation's Health and the Environment Digest.

National Center for Child Abuse and Neglect. (1988). *Study findings: National study of the incidence and severity of child abuse and neglect* (DHHS Publication No. OHDS81-30325). Washington, DC: Government Printing Office.

National Safety Council. (1994). *Accident facts.* Itasca, IL: Author.

Nightingale, F. (1859). *Notes on nursing.* London: Harrison & Sons.

Policy statement: Domestic violence. (1993). *American Journal of Public Health, 83,* 458-462.

Pope, A., Snyder, M., & Mood, L. (Eds.). (1995). *Nursing, health and environment.* Washington, DC: National Academy Press.

Rice, D. (1991). Health status and national health priorities. *Western Journal of Medicine, 154,* 294-303.

Salazar, M. (1987). Noise is a pollutant, too. *The Washington Nurse, 17*(5), 17.

San Francisco files suit against tobacco industry. (1996, June 8). *Virginian Pilot,* p. A5.

Spradley, B., & Allender, J. (1996). *Community health nursing: Concepts and practice.* Philadelphia: J. B. Lippincott.

Starr, R., Dubowitz, H., & Bush, B. (1990). The epidemiology of child maltreatment. In R. Ammerman & M. Hersen (Eds.), *Children at risk: An evaluation of factors contributing to child abuse and neglect.* New York: Plenum.

Turk, J., & Turk, A. (1988). *Environmental science.* Philadelphia: W. B. Saunders.

U.S. Department of Health, Education and Welfare. (1964). *Smoking and health: Report of the Advisory Committee to the Surgeon General of the Public Health Service.* Washington, DC: Government Printing Office.

U.S. Department of Health and Human Services. (1989). *The surgeon general's 1989 report on reducing the health consequences of smoking: 25 years of progress.* Washington, DC: Government Printing Office.

U.S. Department of Health and Human Services. (1991). *Healthy people 2000: The surgeon general's report on health promotion and disease prevention* (DHHS Publication No. 91-50212). Washington, DC: Government Printing Office.

U.S. Department of Health and Human Services. (1993). *Progress Report for environmental health.* Washington, DC: Government Printing Office.

U.S. Environmental Protection Agency. (1990). *National air quality and emission trends report, 1988* (EPA-450/4-90-002). Washington, DC: Author.

Walker, L. (1979). *The battered woman.* New York: Harper & Row.

Zuk, G., & White, S. (1990). Six pressing environmental problems: An interview with Lester Brown. *National Forum, 70*(1), 8-11.

CHAPTER 5

SOCIAL AND CULTURAL FORCES INFLUENCING COMMUNITY HEALTH

OBJECTIVES

1. Define culture.

2. Discuss social and cultural diversity in the United States.

3. Compare health- and illness-related values, beliefs, and practices and patterns of the dominant cultural groups with those of groups from culturally diverse backgrounds.

4. Discuss health and illness patterns and values among various social groups.

5. Discuss cultural assessment, cultural sensitivity, and transcultural nursing.

6. Discuss the health and health concerns of special lower socioeconomic groups (migrant workers and homeless people).

THEORETICAL FRAMEWORK

The health status of the community population depends on its interactions (exchanges) with the internal and external environments. Chapter 2 presented a theoretical framework for this book that discussed exchanges such as those of food, housing, and social and recreational services that influence health. This framework also described the interaction of subsystems, such as health, education, recreation, and transportation that influence the health of the community. In addition, the concept of aggregates that are at risk of illnesses because of demographics was introduced. Some aggregates are more susceptible to illnesses because of the interactions of community subsystems and other factors. Some of these factors were discussed in Chapters 3 and 4. For example, in Chapter 3, the lack of health care was identified as problematic for individuals and families of lower socioeconomic status. In Chapter 4, lead was presented as one health concern of families living in older low-cost housing.

In addition, interactions with the environment are a result of people's knowledge, beliefs, values, and attitudes, all of which will influence the health of certain social cultural groups (aggregates). This chapter explores some of these concepts and relates them to health.

Nurses also carry a sociocultural heritage into the community. They must, therefore, be aware of the differences between their background and that of clients to be effective. An understanding of the nursing process, the theory of nursing, and health problems, beliefs, values, and practices of community aggregates will assist in ensuring the best nursing care.

HEALTHY PEOPLE 2000 OBJECTIVES

Healthy People 2000 (U.S. Department of Health and Human Services [DHHS], 1991) identified 114 objectives related to ethnic and other minority groups. This emphasis was a result of finding differences in the health statistics of different ethnic and economic groups in previous reports. Objectives related to areas such as growth retardation in low-income children; smoking patterns in different cultural groups; alcohol-related accidents, suicides, and cirrhosis among Native Americans; homicide among cultural groups; infant mortality in cultural groups; and diabetes, hepatitis, and HIV/AIDS among these groups were identified. A goal was presented in relation to each objective. For example, the goal for reducing growth retardation in low-income children under 1 year of age was to decrease it to less than 10%; the goal for infant mortality was a reduction to 11 per 1,000 live births among African Americans, 8.5 per 1,000 live births among Native Americans, and 8 per 1,000 live births among Puerto Ricans; and the goal for diabetes was a reduction to no more than 62 cases per 1,000 Native Americans, 49 per 1,000 Puerto Ricans and Mexican Americans, and 32 per 1,000 African Americans and Cuban Americans.

CULTURE AND TRANSCULTURAL NURSING DEFINED

Culture is the way of life of individuals or groups. It involves behaviors, ideas, and values that are learned from families and others and that assist in adapting to a changing environment. Because these learned behaviors are culturally based, they vary from culture to culture. Statistics show that they also influence health and illness patterns.

By other definitions, culture is a major construct that describes the beliefs, behaviors, sanctions, values, and goals identifying the way of life of people (Tuck, 1986); the social heritage and the way of acting and doing things that is passed from generation to generation through teaching and demonstrating (Gordon, 1964); and the learned, shared, and transmitted values, beliefs, and norms of a group that are patterned and that guide thinking, decision making, and actions (Leninger, 1978).

A second important concept is transcultural nursing. This was defined by Leninger (1981) as a formal area of study that focuses on the comparative analysis of diverse health-illness caring beliefs, values, and practices of cultures and subcultures for the purpose of generating scientific culture-specific or culture-universal therapeutic nursing care practices.

CULTURAL DIVERSITY IN THE UNITED STATES

Diverse cultural groups are increasing rapidly in the United States. The U.S. Department of Commerce (1993) estimates that the non-Latino white population will constitute only 52% of the total population by 2050 compared with about 75% in 1992 and 83.2% in 1980 (U.S. Department of Commerce, 1980). With this increase in diversity, it is important that community health nurses have a good understanding of cultural groups.

POPULATION STATISTICS AND COMPOSITION

In the 1990 census (U.S. Department of Commerce, 1993), there were almost 30 million African Americans, constituting just over 12% of the U.S. population. In this census, there were also 22 million Latinos, making up 9% of the population; 3.5 million Asian Americans, constituting 2.9% of the population; and 1.9 million Native Americans, constituting 0.8% of the population. The Latino category consisted of people from Cuba, Chile, the Dominican Republic, El Salvador, Guatemala, Mexico, Nicaragua, and Puerto Rico. The Asian group included Chinese, Filipinos, Japanese, Koreans, Vietnamese, Hawaiians, Samoans, and Guamanians. The Native American group included Indians, Eskimos, and Aleutians.

GROWTH STATISTICS

In 1980, African Americans made up 11.7% of the population (26,488,218 people), compared with 12% in 1990, and were projected to make up about 15% in 2050. Latinos made up 6.4% of the population (14,605,283 people) in 1980 and 9% in 1990, with a projected population percentage of slightly above 18% in 2050, and are considered to be the fastest-growing population. Native Americans made up 0.6% of the population (1,481,195 people) in 1980, 0.8% in 1990, and a projected percentage of 1.2% in 2050. Asians made up 1.5% of the population (3,500,636 people) in 1980, 2.9% in 1990, and a projected 10% in 2050. Whites (non-Latino) made up 83.2% of the population (226,504,825 people) in 1980, 75.4% in 1990, and a projected 62.1% of the population in 2025. The percentages for whites had decreased from 87.5% of the population in 1970 (U.S. Bureau of the Census, 1993; U.S. Department of Commerce, 1980, 1993).

HEALTH AND ILLNESS STATISTICS FOR CULTURAL GROUPS

AFRICAN AMERICANS

Health and illness statistics vary among cultural groups. African Americans have higher mortality rates than do whites and a life expectancy of 69.1 years compared with 75.6 years for whites. African Americans have an excess in death rates at all ages until age 75, and there is an extremely high death rate during the first year of life. Of the leading causes of death in the United States (cardiovascular, malignant neoplasms, accidents, and influenza and pneumonia), the adjusted rates are higher for blacks than for whites. For example, the adjusted rate for cancer is 159 per 100,000 for blacks and 127 per 100,000 for whites. The maternal death rate is also four times higher than for whites.

Other causes of mortality among African Americans include stroke, diabetes mellitus, cirrhosis, homicide, and malnutrition. Mortality rates for communicable diseases, especially HIV/AIDS, are higher in blacks than in whites. One third of all reported cases of AIDS are among African Americans, and African American men make up 80% of these cases (National Center for Health Statistics, 1993). Of women of childbearing age with AIDS, 57.6% are black; of children under 15 with AIDS, 54.5% are black; and of teenagers with AIDS, 40.2% are black (Knox, 1990).

Some factors accounting for this disparity have been identified. Stress, low incomes, discrimination, poor education, poor housing, and inadequate or no health insurance have been reported. Increased numbers of single-parent households run by women, a high rate of unmarried teen pregnancies, and a lack of male role models have added to these concerns (Friedman, 1990).

HISPANIC AMERICANS

The life expectancy for Hispanic Americans is slightly longer than that of the general population, but most of this time may be spent in ill health (U.S. DHHS, 1993a). Among Hispanic Americans, tuberculosis is very common, especially in the age group under 35. Rates for tuberculosis are five times those of the general population ("Prevention and Control of Tuberculosis," 1992). Obesity, hypertension, and diabetes are also prevalent. A report from the Texas Special Committee on Diabetes Services, states that the incidence of diabetes in Mexican Americans is five times the national average, and complications are more frequent (Reinert, 1986). However, despite lower socioeconomic status and higher rates of diabetes and obesity, Mexican Americans have lower rates of cardiovascular disease than do whites (U.S. DHHS, 1986). Among communicable diseases, rates of HIV/AIDS, pneumonia, and other diseases identified below are high. The rate for AIDS in the United States is proportionately higher in the Hispanic American population; 13.25% of people with AIDS are Hispanic, whereas only 7.5% of the population is Hispanic. The frequency of AIDS is also higher in women of childbearing age, children under the age of 15, and teenagers (Knox, 1990). Of the health problems common to Mexican Americans, 85% are communicable diseases and include respiratory infections, diarrhea, skin disorders, parasitic diseases, and nutritional problems that occur often during the first year of life (Anthony-Tkach, 1981). Other health concerns include malnutrition, alcohol and drug abuse, gastroenteritis, parasitic infections, violence, and accidents. Refugees from Central and South America also experience posttraumatic stress disorders (Magar, 1990).

ASIAN AMERICANS

Asian Americans have a higher death rate than does the white population, and tuberculosis is a serious problem in this group. Tuberculosis mortality is almost 10 times higher among Asians than among the white population in the United States ("Prevention and Control of Tuberculosis," 1992). Other diseases prevalent in the Asian American population include cancer, mental illness, respiratory diseases, arthritis, parasitic diseases, and malnutrition. Those who have fled their countries under adverse situations often experience high suicide rates and stress-related illnesses. Among Vietnamese, the following diseases are prevalent: tuberculosis, intestinal parasites, malnutrition, anemia, skin diseases, hepatitis, malaria, and dental problems. Among the Japanese, the following diseases are prevalent: cancer (esophagus, liver, stomach), hypertension and vascular lesions of the central nervous system, and stress-related diseases (ulcers, colitis, psoriasis). On the other hand, the Japanese have a lower prevalence of multiple sclerosis, cardiovascular and renal disease, and certain cancers, such as colon, lung, breast, and prostate cancers.

NATIVE AMERICANS

Until recently, Native Americans had the highest infant mortality rate in the United States. Now it is comparable to that of the general population. However, birth trauma and asphyxia rates are double, fetal alcohol rates are 6 times, and postnatal death rates are more than 2 times the rates for the general population (Hanley, 1991). They also have the shortest life expectancy of all groups in the United States (National Indian Health Board, 1984). Leading causes of death include heart diseases, accidents, malignant neoplasms, cirrhosis and other chronic liver diseases, cerebrovascular diseases, homicides, suicide, diabetes, and alcoholism (Lamarme, 1989). The mortality rate for heart disease is 393 per 100,000, which makes it the leading cause of death (U.S. DHHS, 1993a). Diabetes occurs three to four times more often among Native Americans than in the general population, and it is estimated that more than 10% of Navajos on reservations are affected (Hanley, 1991). According to Spector (1991), many of the chronic diseases are related to alcohol abuse, which is "the most widespread and severe problem in the Native American community" (p. 244). A closely related problem is domestic violence.

Infectious diseases are also problematic among Native Americans, and mortality from them is twice that for the general population. Meningitis, sexually transmitted diseases, and hepatitis are major problems (Rhodes, Hammond, Welty, Handler, & Amler, 1987), and there is also increased mortality from parasitic infections, pneumonia, and kidney infections (Becker, Wiggins, Peck, Key, & Samet, 1990). Death rates from tuberculosis are also very much higher in some parts of the United States among Native Americans. In addition, tuberculosis morbidity is more than four times that of the white population ("Prevention and Control of Tuberculosis," 1992).

POVERTY AND CULTURE IN DISEASE

According to the Centers for Disease Control (CDC; 1993), poverty has a greater influence on health and illness than does race. Without adequate incomes, these groups are unable to provide for the basic necessities of food, shelter, and clothing. In addition, the governmental system of health care often excludes them from free health care (see Chapter 3), and they are often unable to pay for health care because their money must be used for more immediate necessities. Likewise, preventive services are often not used (see health beliefs and practices in this chapter). Additional stressors related to low incomes that affect the health of these groups include limited occupational and educational opportunities, unsafe neighborhoods, and substandard and hazardous housing (Haan, Kaplan, & Camacho, 1987).

HEALTH VALUES, BELIEFS, AND PRACTICES OF CULTURAL GROUPS

Health values and beliefs of cultural groups influence health practices, which in turn influence health statistics. In addition, changes can be made only within a cultural belief context. For example, Hispanic Americans believe that certain foods or conditions are "hot" and others are "cold." They believe one cannot eat a hot food after a hot experience but, rather, must eat a cold food to restore balance. Thus, after delivering a child (a hot experience) a woman could not eat a hot food (see Table 5.1) but should eat a cold food to restore balance. Likewise, during pregnancy (a hot experience) she should not take prenatal vitamins (a hot food). However, if she took the prenatal vitamins with fruit juice, they would be cooled and that would be acceptable. Without this knowledge, the nurse might continue to encourage prenatal vitamins without an understanding of why the vitamins were refused and what could be done to change the behavior. Health beliefs can also determine what people will do when ill and who they will turn to for help. Thus, it is important for nurses to have an understanding of cultural values and beliefs of health as a basis for working with cultural groups.

Benjamin Paul (1955), in his classic *Health, Culture and Community,* discusses many situations in which health workers tried to intervene in communities to improve health. Some of these were successful and others were unsuccessful depending on whether or not health workers tried to bring about change within the belief system of the recipients of care. For example, workers who tried to improve the diet of malnourished South African Zulus by adding milk needed to consider that cattle were intimately connected with beliefs about ancestors and valued norms of behavior. Only by introducing milk in powdered form were they successful in using it to improve nutrition. Another case, involving Western medicine in rural Rajasthan in India, revealed a profound difference between Western and indigenous health beliefs:

> To the western doctor complaints of physical weakness signifies malnutrition and anemia and called for the prescription of iron tonics and vitamin concentrates. . . . But according to the cultural system of the patient, symptoms of physical disability were connected to moral weakness by a chain of convictions involving nutrition, blood, semen, and transgression of the ethical code. Ideal remedies therefore included pilgrimages and ritual baths to wash away one's sins—atonement rather than tonics. (Paul, 1955, p. 107)

Table 5.1 lists some cultural beliefs about health and illness, types of health care providers used, folk healers used, and preventive and treatment efforts for four major cultural groups in the United States: African American,

text continues on page 137

TABLE 5.1 Cultural Variations in Beliefs Concerning Health and Illness

Concepts	African Americans	Hispanic Americans	Asian Americans	Native Americans
Health	Total harmony with nature	Result of good luck Reward for good behavior	Harmony with nature (spiritual and physical) Balance of yin and yang	Harmony between human beings and the universe
Illness	Punishment for wrongdoing caused by magic or worry Disharmony Illness can be natural or unnatural due to environment, divine punishment, or impaired social relations	Imbalance of hot and cold (see specific illness section later) Illness of 2 types: natural—caused by imbalance with nature and God; unnatural—caused by satanic forces	Imbalance of Yin and Yang (Yin—negative, female, dark, cold, empty; Yang—positive, male, light, warmth) Soul loss—spirit possession	Disharmony with environment, such as violation of natural laws, storms, lightning, witchcraft, spirits Price paid for past or future deeds caused by evil spirits
Time orientation	Present	Present	Past (tradition)	Present
Family authority	Joint decision	Male Joint decision	Male	Female All family members
Source of health care	Traditional for serious problems Folk medicine for common problems	Traditional—naturally caused illnesses Folk medicine—unnaturally caused illnesses	Traditional—physician Folk medicine	Traditional—deals with symptoms Folk medicine—deals with underlying causes
Type of folk healer used	Born healer—cures all illnesses Spiritualist—acquires power from spiritual experience (used for financial, spiritual, natural problems)	Family member (for minor illness) Herbalist—yerbero	Acupuncturist—restores balance of Yin and Yang Herbalist	Family member Medicine man—practices magic for supernatural illnesses

TABLE 5.1 Continued

Concepts	African Americans	Hispanic Americans	Asian Americans	Native Americans
	Old woman practitioner—learns healing from others (used for simple conditions caused by natural forces)	*Curandero*—holistic healer by birth, calling, or apprenticeship (treats all illnesses)	Female shaman—prescribes after ecstatic trances from dancing, prophesy	Herbalist
	Voodoo priest—cures magical illnesses	Spiritualist—analyzes dreams and predicts future (protects against or treats magical illnesses)		Seer or prophet
		Massager—*sabador* (treats traditional and nontraditional illnesses)		
		Witch—*brujo* (uses magic to cause, prevent, or treat illnesses)		
Prevention	Proper diet—3 nutritious meals	Proper diet to prevent imbalance. Balance of hot and cold foods and avoidance of excess rice, apples, bananas, coffee, fried foods	Herbal tea to prevent illness	Herbal tea to prevent illness
	Rest	Work, prayer, herbs to prevent illness	Ginseng—restores frail children	Isolation to prevent communicable diseases
	Clean environment	Avoid overheating—prevent nosebleed	Meditation	Charms worn to prevent evil and disease
	Laxatives	Avoid cold food/drink if hot (prevent chill)	Amulets to ward off evil spirits	Avoid cutting hair to maintain strength
	Asafetida—rotten flesh worn around neck to prevent communicable diseases[a]	Avoid drafts—cover head outside (prevent illness)		Carry medicine bundle to ensure blessing
	Cod liver oil	Keep windows closed at night		
	Periodic purge—keeps system open	Wear religious medals or amulets		
	Avoid red meat—prevents "high blood"	Purge to prevent *empacho* (see section on "Specific illnesses and treatments")		
	Sulfur and molasses rub in springtime			
	Charms around neck and copper and silver bracelets—protect from evil and illness			
	Physician not routinely consulted			

General treatments	Voodoo—with oil, candles Prayer—most common Laying on of hands Magical rituals Self-medication Sugar and turpentine for worms Poultices (infections) Goldenrod for fever Sassafras tea for colds Bluestone mineral for colds Salt and porkcloth for cuts Clay wrap for spirits Garlic for evil spirits Herbal tea for pain, fever, colds Lemon and honey for colds	Application of opposite of disease—hot illness, cold treatment (see next section for hot and cold foods) Herbs—most popular Offering money, penance, confession or candle lighting, making promises, visiting shrines Laying on of hands Massage Cleansing by passing unbroken egg or tied bunch of herbs over body of sick person	Body massage Poultices Exercise Acupuncture for pain Herbs Ginseng as a sedative and to improve digestion Quicksilver—external treatment for VD Seahorse for gout Turtle shell for gallstones and weak kidney Rhinoceros horns for snakebites and boils Deer antlers for impotence and to strengthen bones Cold Rx for hot disease Hot RX for cold disease Single dose of medication adequate for cure	Sweat baths Massage Herbs Pinongum on wound for cuts Cliff rose for clean wound Sand Sagebrush to bring a boil to a head Sunflower water for spider bite Bladder pot for snake bite Fleabane for headache Blue gilia tea for indigestion Thistle flower for worms Yucca plant stem for laxative Juniper ash for poultice to reduce edema Zuni tea or Goldenrod for colds, sore throat
Specific illnesses and treatments	High blood—excessive blood from rich food, especially red meat. Rx: Lemon, vinegar, epsom salts, astringents to sweat out excess blood	Susto—from fright and loss of soul, restlessness in sleep, listlessness, anorexia, depression, loss of strength. Rx: Curandero soul; back massage	Excessive yin—frequent colds, nervousness, gastric problems, cancer, diarrhea. Rx: Moxibustion—heated pulverized wormwood applied to skin over certain meridian points.	

TABLE 5.1 Continued

Concepts	African Americans	Hispanic Americans	Asian Americans	Native Americans
	Low blood—too little blood; anemia due to overtreatment of high blood. Rx: decrease astringents, increase red meat or something the color of blood such as wine or beets	*Empacho*—food ball on stomach wall causes vomiting, pain, diarrhea, and cramps from excessive food. Rx: rubbing and pinching spine during prayer, massage, increase fluids, ingest "cold medicine" (quicksilver) followed by "hot laxative" (castor oil)	Excessive Yang—fever, dehydration, irritability, tenseness, elevated blood pressure, sore throat (cold weather affects lungs)	
	Thin blood—increased susceptibility to diseases. Rx: dress warmly; in cold weather, stay inside	*Malojo*—Excessive admiration from another: causes severe headache, sleepiness, high fever, crying, diarrhea, restlessness, irritability, weight loss. Rx: care given by admiring person. Mix hen's egg with water, place under head of bed	Yang (hot)—most meats, sweets, coffee, spicy condiment (garlic), chicken broth, ginger, rice, port, chicken, eggs, peanuts	
	Bad blood—VD	*Malpuesto*—magical conditions from social problems (e.g., lovers' quarrel) causes convulsion or emotional liability. Rx: magical interventions by *curandero*	Yin (cold)—most fruit, vegetables, fish, duck, and things from water	
	Poison blood—illness due to witch-craft (rashes). Rx: catnip tea, sulfur and molasses or castor oil to purge the system of impurities	*Envida*—illness from envy	Dermabrasive techniques—for headache, sinusitis, colds, sore throat, cough, diarrhea, fever	
		Hot and cold—includes food, beverage, animals, people, conditions	Pinching—causes bruises and welts	
		Food: hot—beef, chili peppers, oils, hard liquor, acidic and spicy foods, mustard; cold—beans, rice, wheat, pork, peaches	Cupping—hot cup placed on skin to remove toxins and excess energy as it cools	
		Conditions: Hot—menstruation or delivery (avoid hot foods)	Rubbing—rubbing body with lubricated spoon to bring toxins to body surface	
			Burning—cigarette to abdomen to compensate for heat loss in diarrhea	

a. See Spector (1991), p. 146).

Asian American, Hispanic American, and Native American. These patterns have been summarized from a variety of sources, including Andrews and Boyle (1995), Galanti (1991), Giger and Davidhizar (1991), and Spector (1991).

The reader should consider this table as only a beginning guide to beliefs and practices among various cultural groups because these groups are heterogeneous. For example, Asian Americans include Chinese, Japanese, Filipino, Koreans, Laotians, and Vietnamese; and Latinos come from Cuba, Chile, the Dominican Republic, El Salvador, Guatemala, Mexico, Nicaragua, and Puerto Rico. Each of these groups will have some beliefs that are different. In addition, within a group, such as the Japanese, not all will subscribe to the same beliefs. For example, Giger and Davidhizar (1991) say that one should not generalize about Native Americans because the beliefs and practices will vary among the 300 plus federally recognized groups in the United States. However, there are commonalities among the groups. Table 5.1 can provide initial information, but further assessment of specific groups is necessary.

CULTURAL ASSESSMENT AND CULTURAL SENSITIVITY

Many cultural assessment tools address the cultural values and beliefs of individuals and families (Helvie, 1991; Leninger, 1978; Orque, Block, & Monroy, 1983). This book focuses on the community, and any assessment tool included should have that focus. Two books with assessment tools directed toward aggregates are by Brownbee (1978) and Smith and Maurer (1995). The reader is referred to these sources for further information. In addition, Tuck and Harris (1988) list assessment factors for cultural groups, such as racial and ethnic background, reasons for migration, reception by receiving host, level of involvement in community, demographics, length of time in the country, common stereotypes regarding the group, major health problems, major source of health and illness care, health beliefs and practices, dietary and language requirements, religion, and socioeconomic issues.

Cultural sensitivity is an important aspect of nursing and facilitates communication and the effective use of nursing process with all aggregates. Bennett (1986) says that the learner progresses from ethnocentrism (tendency to believe one's ways are best and to act superior in relation to other ways as a result) to increased cultural sensitivity in a stepwise fashion. Steps in this process include the following:

1. *Denial:* There is no recognition of cultural differences, there is cultural blindness and ethnocentricism, and different behavior is labeled deviant.

2. *Defense:* Cultural differences are recognized, but one's own beliefs are defended as superior or correct.

3. *Minimization:* Cultural differences are recognized, but the differences are minimized (e.g., a nurse teaches the basic four food groups to a Mexican family who is receiving adequate nutrition but using a diet that may not completely fit the basic four categories).

4. *Acceptance:* The learner recognizes and values different cultural beliefs and practices, such as using alternative therapies in nursing.

5. *Adaptation:* The learner adapts to another culture and stereotypes are minimized (this stage is believed to occur rarely).

6. *Integration:* Learners move comfortably between cultures but at the same time recognize differences in cultural practices (this stage is believed to be very rare).

TRANSCULTURAL NURSING

A definition of transcultural nursing was provided earlier. According to Leninger (1988), who developed this area of nursing, "Care is the essence of nursing and the central, dominant, and unifying feature of nursing" (p. 152). Care is an important component of recovery from illness, and unfavorable life situations and will vary from culture to culture. For example, culture mainly determines the perception of health and illness and the concepts of appropriate treatment and prevention for groups and thus may provide the framework for appropriate cultural care. In addition, individuals may modify or internalize various aspects of cultural patterns, so an individual framework must also be used. Leninger's focus is on developing a scientific and humanistic body of knowledge to provide culture-specific and culture-universal care. The theory consists of a set of interrelated cross-cultural concepts and hypotheses that consider individual and group caring behaviors, values, and beliefs based on culture.

The theory of cultural diversity and universality is presented in the "sunrise model," which shows a cognitive map of components, including technological, religious, kinship, political/legal, economic, educational, and cultural values that influence the care patterns and well-being of individuals, families, communities, and institutions. Three major modalities guide nursing decisions and actions:

1. *Cultural care preservations and/or maintenance:* actions or decisions that assist, support, or enable clients of any culture to preserve or maintain a state of health, recover from illness, or face death

2. *Cultural care accommodations and/or negotiations:* actions or decisions that assist clients to adapt to or negotiate a beneficial health status

3. *Cultural care repatterning or restructuring:* actions or decisions that assist clients "[to change their] lifeways for new or different patterns that are culturally meaningful and satisfying or that support beneficial and healthy life patterns" (Leninger, 1988).

The theory is used mainly to generate data about care meanings, patterns, experiences, and other aspects of care of diverse populations so that both universal care features and differences can be identified.

SOCIOECONOMIC GROUP CONCEPTS

If nurses study the health statistics of populations by demographic variables, they will also find an unequal distribution of diseases among socioeconomic groups. For example, Najman (1993) reports a direct link between low income and early death, and others (Andersen, Chen, Aday, & Cornelius, 1987; Halfon & Newacheck, 1993; Martin, 1992; National Center for Health Statistics, 1981) have found more anemia, arthritis, asthma, diabetes, hearing problems, influenza and pneumonia, tuberculosis, and eye abnormalities among lower- than among middle- and upper-income individuals.

In the April 1996 issue of the *American Journal of Public Health,* several articles document the association between sociodemographic factors and health. Link and Phelan (1996), in an editorial in that issue, say there are associations between "socioeconomic status and life expectancy, infant mortality, and the consumption of fruits and vegetables to name a few" (p. 471) and that in research reported in the journal 25 or 50 years ago one finds similar results. Thus, it is important to have information on health patterns, health beliefs, and needs among social groups.

CONCEPT OF SOCIAL CLASS

Social classes are often distinguished in terms of income, occupation, education, lifestyle, and access to services. Hollingshead (1957) developed a two-factor index consisting of the occupation and education of the head of the household from which to arrive at a social class standing. Other authors have added income to these two factors, and still others add additional variables. Goode (1977) ranks people in social groups by education, income, occupation, and prestige, or a combination of these. According to Murray and Zentner (1993), determinants of social class include race, occupation, education, lifestyle, financial status, and language.

Regardless of the indicators used, there has been an attempt to differentiate social classes in the community. Some authors have identified three classes (lower, middle, and upper), whereas others have identified additional categories, such as lower middle and upper middle. Each class has its own health problems, beliefs, values, and advantages or disadvantages regarding health care services.

There is no overall agreement about where a certain income or other criteria fit within a specific social class—for example, into which social class a $10,000 income would fit. The one exception is the poverty index established by the government. It is obtained by multiplying the cost of food for a minimum diet (Economic Food Plan) by a cost factor of 3 to obtain a standard basis subsistence amount. Adjustments may be made for family size, rural or urban residence, and age of family members (Schultz, 1985). This is commonly used as a measure of poverty. However, it has been criticized for several reasons. The major one is that it has remained stable since the mid-1970s despite inflation.

Despite some disagreement, social class rankings based on occupation and income seems to correlate well with social and health patterns and have been used often in research. According to Green and Anderson (1986, p. 35), level of education is the best predictor of health behavior of social class variables. Modifying behavior, such as smoking cessation, exercise, weight control, immunizations, and dental care, is more common among people with higher educational levels. In addition, this group tends to respond better to the suggestions of health professionals and, in general, to be healthier.

SOCIAL CLASS AGGREGATES IN THE COMMUNITY

At any point in time, the community is made up of different social class group proportions that may change over time. When neighborhoods age, the middle- and upper-class aggregates often move out and lower-class groups move in. The social class of the particular group has relevance for the community health nurse because the knowledge, attitudes, beliefs, and behaviors of groups vary. Groups are often classified by upper, middle, and lower social class, which may help determine their educational level for teaching purposes, their lifestyle and habits, and customs and exposures influencing health. Some generalizations may serve as a starting point for viewing these groups. However, nurses should assess group beliefs, habits, and behaviors as a basis for interventions with a specific group.

People of the middle and upper classes usually enjoy better health, are more self-sufficient regarding health matters, avail themselves of the best medical and health care, and respond better to appeals to modify behavior in a positive health-related way. For example, they are the most likely to modify diet as needed, to quit smoking, to control their weight, and to obtain immunizations and dental care. The lower class usually have the worst outcomes and are the most difficult to persuade to obtain treatment and preventive services. Poor health outcomes are partly a result of the income level, which may lead to poor housing, inadequate diets, crowded conditions, and other factors that reduce their resistance to disease agents. Lack of access to health care may also be a factor (see access to health care in Chapter 3).

Noack (1988) says mortality rates are the best indicator of ill health and these are inversely related to occupational class, socioeconomic group, level of education, and income. The incidence of nearly all diseases has a social class difference. In addition, morbidity rates also show an inverse relationship with social class. For example, Neal (1995) says that the "death rates for poor are approximately twice the rate of persons above the poverty level" (p. 239).

STUDIES OF CLASS BEHAVIOR

Hogelin (1988) says Americans recognize that developing nine of the leading causes of premature death (e.g., heart diseases, lung cancer) are a result of adult health behavior. He also calculates the years lost in life and the associated behaviors leading to the premature death for the listed causes. For example, in 1983, 1,559,000 years of life were lost from diseases of the heart before age 65. Associated behaviors leading to this premature death included cigarette smoking, diet (obesity), failure to follow hypertension treatment, and sedentary lifestyle.

Although a literature review uncovers few current studies on class and health behavior, past studies on class values, attitudes, and behaviors are valuable as a starting point for community health nurses working with community aggregates. Watts (1967) compared some characteristics of lower- and middle-class people and found that lower-class people are more oriented to the present than to the future: They take advantage of what is immediately available rather than plan for a future they cannot visualize. This attention to the present is often a necessity because they must continually be aware of meeting basic needs. Middle-class groups are more future oriented and more able to plan ahead and save for a desired goal. There are therefore more likely to take advantage of preventive services than are lower-class groups.

In his classic *The Health of Regionville,* Koos (1954) categorized his study population into social classes and asked each group if the following symptoms were significant and if they required the attention of a doctor: loss of appetite, persistent backache, continued coughing, persistent joint and muscle pain, blood in the stools, blood in the urine, excessive vaginal bleeding, swelling of the ankles, loss of weight, bleeding gums, chronic fatigue, shortness of breath, persistent headache, fainting spells, pain in the chest, lump in the breast, and lump in the abdomen. He found that the highest social class was consistent in recognizing the symptoms as important, the skilled workers were less concerned, and the lowest class was indifferent to the symptoms. He concluded that there were obvious differences between the social classes concerning their attitudes toward symptoms and thus toward seeking treatment. For example, one lower-class housewife told the interviewer she would be "hooted out of town" if she consulted a doctor about a backache. Some symptoms were given more importance if they occurred in a young person but were disregarded if they occurred in a middle-aged or elderly member of the family. In addition, cost was often a deterrent to seeking care, especially when it was an unknown factor and the family's income was low.

Research has confirmed that when symptoms are considered normal, no action for seeking health care follows. In addition to social class, other factors may also influence health behavior. Koos (1954) found that people afraid of surgery, where indicated, would ignore the most pressing symptoms to avoid going under the knife.

The results of this research suggest the following implications for community health nurses:

- Before individuals will take health action they must recognize that they have a problem (lower-class aggregates are less likely to recognize this; different people have different concepts and values in health).

- For health action to occur, sometimes the fear of treatment must be less than the fear of the consequences of not having treatment.

- In some instances, especially among lower-class aggregates, the cost of care is a crucial factor in seeking treatment.

- Health action is tied closely to people's overall belief systems.

Community health nurses help population aggregates by working within each aggregate's concept of health, by explaining treatments and the consequence of not receiving treatment, by explaining the cost of care and financial assistance available, by determining the belief system of the group and working within it, and by connecting new ideas of care with old ideas of the particular group.

Rosenstock's (1966) research on motivation in health action also has important implications for nursing work within community aggregates. He found that before people will take health action they must believe (a) that the problem does or could affect them, (b) that the problem will not subside on its own, (c) that medical help will make a difference because there is knowledge about and treatment for the condition, and (d) that the treatment is less threatening than the consequence of no treatment. Thus, if a nurse is working to reduce hypertension among black men (the group at highest risk for this condition), he or she must tell them that they are more likely to have or to develop hypertension, that the condition may lead to severe heart disease or stroke and will not subside on its own, that medical care does make a difference and that it is known that controlling hypertension has decreased mortality from stroke and heart disease (U.S. DHHS, 1990), and that treatment consists of taking daily medication with infrequent side effects and very little effect on daily activities as opposed to the consequences of heart disease and stroke, which can affect activities for the rest of a person's life. Other teaching models for mass education are discussed in Chapter 10.

Another study that found socioeconomic group differences in beliefs and attitudes toward health and health practices and the use of health personnel in the treatment of diseases was carried out by the National Opinion Research Center and sponsored by the Health Information Center (King, 1962). The 2,379 adults studied were a representative sample of the American public. Variables of age, sex, region of country, size of community, occupation, education, income, and family structure were obtained, and because of sampling techniques the results can be generalized.

In relation to the expectations of illness, each respondent was asked to agree or disagree with certain statements regarding health, such as the following:

- No matter how careful a person is, he has to expect a lot of illness during his lifetime.
- Aches and pains are not important—you just get used to them.
- People understand their own health better than most doctors do.
- You shouldn't go to the hospital unless there is no other way to get care.

Results showed that people with low education and income had the highest agreement rate with the statement that people should expect a lot of illness and that one should get used to aches and pains. These rates were in marked contrast to those of respondents with high income and education.

Knowledge about diseases also varies with social class. Dunnell and Cartwright (1972) found that the proportion of people giving four or five correct answers to questions about whether diabetes, anemia, bronchitis, tuberculosis, and polio were "catching" fell from 82% for people in Social Class I (highest class) to 53% in Social Class V. These results confirmed earlier results by King (1962).

According to Mechanic (1982), lower-class groups have less information and knowledge about diseases and are more likely to hold irrational ideas about illnesses. They also rely more on folk medicine and fringe practitioners, and they delay seeking medical treatment more than do middle- and upper-class groups. Some of the reasons for delaying treatment from physicians or for seeking help outside the organized care system (folk medicine) were discussed earlier.

Noack (1988) says that from surveys over the past 20 years it is clear that people in the lower class smoke more cigarettes, eat more unhealthy foods, report fewer leisure time activities, and have more risk behaviors than do middle- and upper-class groups. The Alameda study (see Haan et al., 1987) also reported more positive health practices among the middle and upper classes than among the lower classes.

SPECIAL LOWER-CLASS GROUPS

Two groups of lower-class clients have special health concerns and are discussed next: migrant workers and the homeless population.

MIGRANT WORKERS

There are about 4.2 million migrant workers and dependents in the United States (CDC, 1992, p. 2) and about 2.5 million hired farmworkers (Martin & Martin, 1994). These workers move from place to place, have unique health risks, and often receive infrequent health care. In addition, state and federal laws often do not include or protect them. Most migrant workers are excluded from provisions of the Fair Labor Standards Act (PL85-231) such as minimum wage/maximum hours and child labor laws (Goldfarb, 1981). In addition, they are excluded from collecting the unemployment and workmen's compensation guaranteed in state laws, and they may be discriminated against regarding the Social Security Act (PL85-109) (Moses, 1989, p. 115). They are partially or completely excluded from joining unions and participating in collective bargaining (National Labor Relations Act, PL85-791), and they lack the guarantee of health and safety in the workplace (Occupational Health and Safety Act of 1970, PL95-251).

DEMOGRAPHICS

Of migrant workers, 80% are male, 70% are the under the age of 34, and 2% are between 14 and 17 years old (median age is 26 years). Seventy-eight percent are white; 14% are Hispanic; and 8% are black. Median age of whites is 24 years; of Hispanics, 29 years; and of blacks, 30 years. In terms of education, 23% have under 8 years of schooling, and 50% have 12 years or more. Salary for the group in 1987 was $3,400 for 112 days of farm work and $3,300 for nonfarm work, for a total of $6,700 for the year (Martin & Martin, 1994).

Migrant workers are poor and usually unskilled. They travel with their families from one harvest site to another along certain routes. It is estimated that between 800,000 and 900,000 people follow the harvest site routes each year (Martin & Martin, 1994, p. 5). They earn small amounts of money and live in substandard temporary housing that is crowded and has primitive cooking facilities (Watkins, Larson, Harlan, & Young, 1990, p. 567). About 2 million farmworkers make about $5,000 annually for 6 months of work (Martin & Martin, 1994). It is estimated that 42% of their farm housing is substandard

(Goldfarb, 1981, p. 42). Consequently, meals are often unbalanced and workers are malnourished. In addition, children are often required to work in the fields or are left unsupervised. Because of frequent moves, these groups do not have continuous routine health care or preventive services. Their income is usually inadequate to pay for health services, and according to Goldfarb (1981) 90% do not have health insurance. In addition, most are unaware of free or low-cost health services available to them.

HEALTH PROBLEMS

Many health problems of this group are reflected in the statistics. The life expectancy of the migrant worker is 49 years (Goldfarb, 1981, p. 34). When compared with the national life expectancy of 75 years, this shows a decreased life expectancy of 26 years. The National Migrant Resource Program (1990) found comparable figures in 1990. The death rate for agricultural workers is high, with only miners exceeding that rate (CDC, April 27, 1984). In addition, there are high numbers of deaths and disabilities from chemicals. According to Goldfarb (1981), at least 800 farmworkers die each year and 800,000 are injured from the use of pesticides. Immediate effects of these exposures are skin rashes, upper respiratory tract irritability, and eye irritations; chronic long-term effects include cancer, blindness, infertility and sterility, chronic liver damage, and Parkinson's disease. Although there may be legislation to reduce problems related to pesticides, the workers may fail to understand the warnings if these are written in an unknown language or if they enter the fields too soon after spraying.

In addition, "Migrant farm workers' infant mortality rate is 25% greater than the national average; . . . the rate of parasitic infection among some sets of farm workers approximates 50 times that of the total population" (National Migrant Resource Program, 1990, p. 4). When compared with the general population, migrant workers have higher rates of tuberculosis, parasitic infections, communicable diseases, diabetes, hypertension, malnutrition, infant mortality, and high-risk pregnancies (CDC, June 5, 1992). They also have a high incidence of digestive diseases and inadequate diets, high rates of hospitalizations and chronic illnesses among children, and low rates of childhood immunizations (Watkins et al., 1990, p. 568).

In a 1992 article in *Morbidity and Mortality Weekly Report* by the Advisory Council for the Elimination of Tuberculosis, the problem of tuberculosis among migrant farmworkers was elaborated on. The council reported that tuberculosis is 6 times more likely to occur in this population than in the general adult working population. To reduce this problem, they suggest detection and diagnosis of those with active tuberculosis, treatment and monitoring, contact investigation and appropriate preventive measures for exposed persons, screening and preventive therapy for infected workers who are asymptomatic, and widespread tuberculin testing.

MIGRANT HEALTH ACT

The Migrant Health Act funds more than 100 migrant health projects in the United States, including 400 actual clinic sites in 43 states and Puerto Rico

(Martin & Martin, 1994) that serve more than 500,000 farmworkers and their families. However, surveys show that only about 12% to 15% of the eligible migrant families use these services (Decker & Knight, 1990; Galarneau, 1993; Helsinki Commission, 1993; U.S. DHHS, 1993b). Factors that account for poor attendance at the clinics include (a) lack of money for minimal care, (b) lack of knowledge of resources for care, (c) lack of state and federal support for marginal-income families, (d) lack of transportation and time to go to distant sites, (e) lack of child care facilities, (f) clinic hours while workers are in the fields, (g) fragmented care resulting from inadequate histories on records that remain stationary as workers move from place to place, and (h) discrimination against workers and families.

In addition to health care centers for migrant workers, the government provides Head Start programs for 11,700 children and a job training program for migrant and seasonal farmworkers. There is also a high school equivalency program (HEP) and the College Assistance Migrant Program (CAMP) to help migrant workers complete secondary school and 1 year of college. Other programs that may be available for low-income families but not specifically for migrant workers include the food stamp program and the supplemental food program for women, infants and children (WIC). Because of limited funds, none of these programs is able to accommodate all people who are in need.

COMMUNITY NURSING AND THE MIGRANT

Community nurses work with this population to assess health problems and to identify barriers to care. Any of the interventions discussed in Part IV of this book would be appropriate to introduce change related to the assessment. For example, the nurse might use political action or coalition building to remove barriers (to provide child care, services in the evening, mobile unit services at the migrant site, etc.). The nurse might also obtain funding to provide immunizations at the site if low immunization levels were assessed. Part of this process would include an evaluation of the possible effect of the planned change on the health of the population (see the discussion of interaction of subsystems in Chapter 2).

HOMELESS POPULATION

DEFINING THE HOMELESS

Various definitions of *homeless* have been used in the literature. A simple definition of homelessness is the absence of a stable residence in which to sleep and receive mail (Robertson, Roper, & Boyer, 1984). A similar definition is that a person is homeless if he or she does not have a stable, reliable source of housing (Raeburn & Buss, 1986). According to Levin (1983), homelessness relates to lack of adequate shelter, resources, and community ties. The Community Service Society of New York (Hopper & Baxter, 1981) added to this concept finding shelter in well-hidden sites that were known only to the homeless person. The U.S. General Accounting Office (1985) uses elements of the above definitions to define the homeless as "those persons who lack resources and community ties necessary to provide their own adequate shelter" (p. 2). The Ohio Department of Mental Health (1985) offered a more comprehensive definition of homelessness: "Those living in extremely substandard housing such as flop houses or single room occupancy hotels are homeless if they only have sufficient resources to reside in these places less than 45 days and consider themselves homeless" (p. 3). This group also includes those who are forced to move in with relatives and friends on a temporary basis (45 days or less) because they have become homeless.

Homeless people may also be defined as those without a permanent resident who seek security, rest, and protection from the elements. They often live in areas that are not meant to be shelters, such as parks, bus terminals, and cars; occupy structures without permission as squatters; or are provided temporary shelter by private or public agencies. Some definitions also include people living in single-room occupancy hotels and motels or those residing in social and health care facilities on a short-term basis without permanent housing.

The U.S. Department of Housing and Urban Development (1984) defined the homeless this way:

> (a) [those] in public or private emergency shelters which take a variety of forms—armories, schools, church basements, government buildings, former fire-houses and, where temporary vouchers are provided by private or public agencies, even hotels, apartments, or boarding houses; or (b) [those] in the streets, parks, subways, bus terminals, railroad stations, airports, under bridges or aqueducts, abandoned buildings without utilities, cars, trucks, or any other public or private space that is not designated for shelter. (p. 2)

Because of differing definitions, different numbers of homeless people have been offered. Two aspects of the definitions seem to account for this variation—namely, time and place. For example, some researchers consider only those sleeping in emergency shelters or places not usually used for shelter, such as parks and cars. Others include these places in their definition but also add all people living with friends or living in hotels. In relation to time, some researchers consider those who are sleeping in unconventional places for a short time to be homeless, whereas others consider only those with chronic long-term disrupted housing as homeless.

NUMBERS OF HOMELESS

In my own course on homelessness, I ask students to select the correct number of homeless people in America from the following: (a) 250,000 to 500,000, (b) 500,000 to 1 million, (c) 2 million, and (d) more than 3 million. Usually, some students select each category, and I tell them they are all right depending on which author they quote, which definition of homelessness was used, and what method was used for counting. For example, the Community for Creative Non-Violence (Hombs & Snyder, 1982) in Washington, D.C., used information from more than 100 agencies in 25 cities and states as a basis for their numbers and concluded that in 1980, 2.2 million people nationally lacked shelter and that the number could reach 3 million by 1983.

In another study by the U.S. Department of Housing and Urban Development (HUD; 1984) approaches used for counting the homeless included use of published local statistics, interviews with local observers in 60 metropolitan areas, interviews with a national sample of shelter managers, and a combined shelter and street count. HUD evaluated 100 local and national studies and carried out more than 500 interviews with local observers in the 60 cities. They also made site visits to 10 areas, carried out a national survey of shelter operators, and surveyed 50 states regarding their activities with the homeless. From the data, they concluded that on an average night (December 1983 to January 1984), there were between 195,000 and 586,000 homeless, with the most reliable figure being 250,000 to 350,000.

Another figure, determined by the National Coalition for the Homeless (Ito, 1988), is 2.5 million in 1985, up from half a million in 1982. According to the U.S. Conference of Mayors (1986a, 1986b), there has been an annual increase of 20% in numbers of the homeless seeking emergency shelter.

Numbers in this study showed differences regionally. The West had the highest numbers, with 31% of the homeless but only 19% of the population. All other regions had a similar proportion of the homeless, ranging from 22% in the north central United States to 24% in the South and Northeast. The homeless population also varied by the size of the city. The larger cities had more homeless, with 13 per 10,000 population compared with 12 per 10,000 population in medium-sized communities and 6.5 per 10,000 population in small communities. This variation is probably related to the increased numbers of emergency shelters, social service benefits, and job opportunities in large urban areas.

DEMOGRAPHICS OF THE HOMELESS

There are more homeless men than women. The percentage of homeless women ranges from 14% to 30%, with most studies finding about 22% of the population being women. However, in the past, women made up only 5% of the homeless. The mean age from studies has ranged from 34 to 37 years of age, with the population being younger than previously. Currently, 65% of the homeless are in their late 20s to mid 30s. Children are the fastest-growing population of the homeless (U.S. Conference of Mayors, 1989). Children and members of their families make up about 38% of the estimated 3 million homeless people in the United States (Cuomo, 1983). Between 1984 and 1988, the number of homeless families in shelters more than quadrupled to more than 60,000 people (Kosof, 1988).

According to the HUD study (1984), the majority of homeless are white but minorities are overrepresented: 44% of the shelter population was black, Hispanic, or Native American. More recent figures show an equal percentage of whites and minorities among the homeless. Twenty years ago, at least 90% of the homeless were white. Blacks are found more often in cities in the East and Midwest, whereas Hispanics are more often found in California and the Southwest.

Although the majority of homeless adults have not been married, many have been. Single rates among the homeless range from 54% to 60%. Thus, up to 46% have been married. Of those who have been married, the majority are separated or divorced. The proportion of high school graduates among the homeless is comparable to that of the general population, but fewer homeless people have attended college (Rossi, Fisher, & Willis, 1986).

From 20% to 25% of the homeless are working, and others are looking for work. According to Rossi et al. (1986), the average monthly income of homeless people in Chicago is about $168. Thus, it is necessary for many to rely on public assistance or help from charities.

PRIMARY GROUPS OF HOMELESS PEOPLE

The homeless population is not homogeneous. Nine major groups who make up the homeless population have been identified: (a) the traditional single, older transient male; (b) runaway youth; (c) deinstitutionalized mentally ill; (d) evicted families; (e) low-income persons with mental or physical disabilities; (f) abused or battered women with or without children; (g) illegal immigrants; (h) alcoholics; and (i) refugees of disasters (Erickson & Wilhelm, 1986, p. xxvii).

CAUSES OF HOMELESSNESS

Six reasons for the increased numbers of homeless in America have been identified: inflation, a shortage of affordable housing, Reaganomics, poor planning for deinstitutionalization, unemployment, and the breakdown of traditions (Hopper & Hamburg, 1984). Marginal- or fixed-income families, when faced with inflation, were unable to continue to meet their needs without additional support services. A decrease in affordable low-income housing has led to homelessness for marginal families with minimal marketable skills. Many of the single-room-occupancy hotels have been torn down, and at the same time the government has decreased the numbers of subsidized homes built. During the Reagan administration, many federally funded programs, such as food stamps, welfare, school lunches, unemployment assistance, and housing subsidies, were decreased, which also contributed to homelessness. The proportion of the homeless who are mentally ill and who were put out of mental institutions when emptied found a lack of aftercare programs to assist with their mental health needs. In the early 1980s when the homeless problem increased, the United States was experiencing an economic recession, with higher rates of unemployment and massive layoffs. Last, there has been a breakdown in the traditional relationships and responsibilities in the United States. In the past, the unemployed were taken in by families, but that is not the typical pattern today. Thus, a combination of factors has led to increased numbers of homeless people.

POTENTIAL SOLUTIONS

According to Erickson and Wilhelm (1986), there are four program options for solving the problems of the homeless. First, there must be efforts to prevent homelessness by expanding low-income housing nationally and expanding the number of residential community mental health programs such as halfway houses for alcoholics and drug users. Next, there should be emergency short-term shelters for people who are homeless while their needs for jobs, long-term housing, social, and health and mental health services are evaluated.

Third, there should be adequate long-term residences for the homeless while they locate jobs, housing, and whatever other services they need. Last, there should be provisions for permanent subsidized housing or specialized facilities.

In my own experiences with the homeless, follow-up case management is useful for improving the outcomes of families with children after leaving a homeless shelter. Helvie and Alexy (1992b) found that by providing case management services to families for 1 year after leaving the shelter, all of those discharged were able to remain independent for more than a year. This was in contrast to the 50% returning to the shelter or becoming homeless within 1 year who had not received case management services. Services offered included locating resources, serving as a resource link, assisting with completing applications, providing transportation, and being an advocate or support person.

HEALTH PROBLEMS

Some health problems are more specific to the homeless and relate to their activities, whereas others are seen in the general public as well as in the homeless. Two major problems that are more specific to the homeless are scabies and lice. Although these are not life threatening, the complications from secondary infections, such as internal abscesses, pyogenic pneumonia, septicemia, and secondary impetigo with acute glomerulonephritis, can be serious. These are transmitted by exchanging clothing, picking up clothing on the streets, lying next to an infected person, and exchanging headgear or combs. Symptoms include a rash, itching, and a low-grade fever in some instances. Treatment may be difficult because contacts may not be treated simultaneously and reinfection can occur.

Thermoregulatory disorders are also common because of the exposure of homeless people to sun, wind, rain, and snow. Cold-related illnesses include hypothermia (core body temperatures of less than 95 °F), frostbite, and trench foot; heat-related illnesses include heat stroke, heat exhaustion, and heat cramps. Some of these are life threatening and were discussed in Chapter 4. In addition to problems related to the weather extremes, drugs may also influence thermoregulatory disorders. Prescribed psychiatric drugs or street drugs, including alcohol and nicotine, may alter the individual's ability to correctly perceive environmental conditions or impair body circulation and make the individual more susceptible to environmental conditions.

Trauma is a significant cause of death and disability among the homeless (Jackson & McSwane, 1992), and according to Brickner, Scharer, Conanan, Elvy, and Savarese (1985), it is one of the leading causes of death and disability. Major trauma such as stabbing, shooting, head trauma, fractures, or suicide attempts require immediate emergency treatment and follow-up care that is often not obtained. Postoperative complications such as hemorrhage, shock, sepsis, myocardial infarction, respiratory failure, and death are common (Greenfield, 1984).

Minor traumas such as burns, bites, sexual assaults, sprains, eye injuries, cellulitis, or concussions, although not life threatening, may cause permanent disability. These also require treatment and follow-up care.

Cardiovascular and respiratory diseases are also common among the homeless. Diseases in these categories include hypertension, peripheral vascular disease, pneumonia, tuberculosis, and chronic obstructive pulmonary diseases (COPD). Hypertension is problematic because of the high-sodium diet, the consumption of alcohol, and the stress of living on the streets. Peripheral vascular diseases and cellulitis are common because the homeless have little opportunity to put their feet up during the day or at night. Pneumonia and tuberculosis are also common because of crowded conditions, stress, poor diet, lack of proper rest in shelters, and so forth. The homeless also frequently use tobacco and other substances that contribute to COPD (Brickner et al., 1985; Jackson & McSwane, 1992).

AIDS has also increased among the homeless. HIV infection among the homeless is estimated to be twice that of the general population. Sexual assaults and intravenous drug use have added to the risks of exposure. When infectious diseases occur among this group, they may be a more virulent form requiring longer hospitalization, and the homeless are less likely to continue long-term treatment (Fetter & Larson, 1990; Jackson & McSwane, 1992).

In addition to physical illnesses among the homeless, there are also mental illnesses. It has been estimated that 30% of the homeless have major mental illnesses, including schizophrenia.

STRESS, COPING, AND SOCIAL SUPPORT

Helvie (Helvie, 1994b; Helvie & Alexy, 1992a, 1993) looked at coping, stress, social support, and illness among homeless populations. A study of 50 homeless men between the ages of 22 and 55 (Helvie, 1994b) obtained data on perceived stress, social support, and illnesses by means of standardized tests. This study showed a direct relationship between perceived stress and psychological illness. In addition, the study showed an inverse relationship between perceived stress and physical illness, meaning that the higher the score of perceived stress, the lower the likelihood of reporting physical illness, although the relationship was not significant at the 0.05 level.

No relationship was found (a) between demographic variables and perceived stress, (b) between demographic variables and physical or psychological illness, or (c) between perceived stress, social support, and illness as measured by correlation statistics.

In another study, 50 women were given tests on family coping and social support at admission and 3 months after discharge from a shelter for the homeless (Helvie & Alexy, 1992b). Results showed no relationship between length of homelessness before admission and coping and social support on admission but did show a relationship between (a) family type and coping (more stress [coping] in broken families); (b) coping and social support (a higher number of social supports among women with high stress [coping]); (c) coping and age (higher distress in older women); and (d) admission variables and number of children, family type, and coping (there were more preadmission evictions, domestic violence, and unemployment among women with larger families, women who had broken homes, and women who had high distress levels on coping). There was also a slight nonsignificant change in the mean coping scores of the group between admission and 3 months after discharge from the shelter. An interesting finding was the significant change in social support be-

tween admission and 3 months after discharge (fewer people in the social network after discharge). This finding may be related to the case management
follow-up (Helvie & Alexy, 1992b), in which the case manager tries to help
families become self-sufficient.

In another study (Helvie & Alexy, 1993), 50 mothers newly admitted to a
homeless shelter were given a standardized test that measures hassles on a scale
related to work, family, friends, the environment, practical considerations, and
chance occurrences. This study showed that stress was higher in young mothers,
mothers with less education, single mothers who had never been married, and
African American mothers.

WELLNESS AMONG THE HOMELESS

Very little has been written about wellness and health promotion among
homeless populations. Helvie (1995) examined the wellness behavior of two
homeless populations. Data were collected on 64 homeless men and 41 homeless mothers living in homeless shelters. Study questions included the following: (a) How do homeless men and homeless mothers rank on individual
categories and overall ratings of wellness behavior? (b) Is there a significant
difference in wellness behaviors of the two groups? (c) Do these groups rank
above or below national norms? and (d) Do demographic variables (age, race,
education, working status, length of homelessness) influence wellness? Wellness behaviors were measured on the Wellness Inventory, a 100-item tool of the
National Wellness Institute (1993). This tool has 10 questions in each of the
following categories: physical fitness and nutrition, medical self-care, safety,
environmental wellness, social awareness, sexuality and emotional awareness,
emotional management, intellectual wellness, and spirituality and values. Each
question was rated from 1 (*almost never*) to 5 (*almost always*), giving a score
for each category from 10 to 50 and for the total tool of 100 to 500. A score of
425 to 500 on this tool was considered high-level wellness by the makers of the
tool; 350 to 424 meant both positive and negative aspects of health; and under
349 meant the person's lifestyle could be adversely affecting his or her health
status and future quality of life.

The sample of men ranged in age from 18 to 59, with a mean age of 36.
The sample was 70% Caucasian, 28% black, and 2% other. Twenty percent of
the men had some high school, 30% were high school graduates, 34% had some
college, and 16% were college graduates. More than half (59%) were working
full-time, 14% were working part-time, and 25% were not working. A majority
(55%) had been homeless for less than 3 months. The sample of women ranged
in age from 17 to 47, with a mean age of 28. Thirty-seven percent were Cauca-
sians, 54% were black, and 9% were other. Thirty-one percent had less than a
high school education, 49% were high school graduates, 20% had some college,
and there were no college graduates. Twenty-nine percent were working full-
time, 39% were working part-time, and 29% were not working. A majority
(64%) had been homeless less than 3 months.

Table 5.2 shows the mean total scores and the mean scores for each category of the Wellness Inventory (National Wellness Institute, 1993) for homeless
men and homeless women. Table 5.3 shows the *t* and *p* values for differences

TABLE 5.2 Mean Scores of Homeless Men and Women on the Wellness Inventory Categories

Category	Mean Score	
	Homeless Men (n = 64)	Homeless Women (n = 41)
Physical fitness and nutrition	29.640	30.341
Medical self-care	28.344	27.390
Safety	38.250	36.756
Environmental wellness	31.045	26.073
Social awareness	37.000	33.610
Sexuality and emotional awareness	37.672	30.829
Emotional management	38.891	31.900
Intellectual wellness	37.297	28.560
Occupational wellness	38.234	18.049
Spirituality and values	36.859	34.049
Total score	354.625	297.390

TABLE 5.3 Difference Between Homeless Men and Women on the Wellness Inventory

Category	t	p
Physical/nutrition		n.s.
Medical self-care		n.s.
Safety		n.s.
Environmental	3.15	.002
Social awareness	2.28	.025
Sexuality/emotional awareness	3.83	.000
Emotional management	4.50	.000
Intellectual wellness	5.32	.000
Occupational wellness	7.73	.000
Spirituality		n.s.
Total score	4.48	.000

between men and women on each category. Table 5.4 shows the percentages of men and women within the three levels of health established by the National Wellness Institute. Table 5.5 gives the probability values for men and women for relationships between demographic variables and total wellness scores.

The results showed that men ranked higher than women on the total wellness score, a difference significant at the .005 level. Men also ranked higher on the following categories on the wellness tool: environmental, sexuality/ emotional awareness, emotional management, intellectual wellness, and occupational wellness, all of which were significant at the .005 level. Women did not rank higher than men in any category. When placed in the National Wellness Institute categories, 23% of the men ranked high on the total wellness score and 36% ranked satisfactory, for a total of 59%. No woman ranked high on the total wellness score and 10% ranked satisfactory.

TABLE 5.4 Percentages of Homeless Men and Women Within the Three Levels of Health Established by the National Wellness Institute

Wellness Level	Men (n = 64)	Women (n = 41)
High-level wellness (425-500)	23	0
Satisfactory-level wellness (350-424)	36	10
Adverse lifestyle for health (< 349)	41	90

TABLE 5.5 Relation of Demographic Variables to Total Wellness Scores Among Homeless Men and Women

Variable	Men	Women
Ethnicity	n.s.	n.s.
Length of homelessness	marginal ($p = .057$)	marginal ($p = .078$)
Work status	$p = .027$	$p = .005$
Education	$p = .017$	$p =$ n.s.
Age	n.s.	n.s.

When demographic variables were correlated with the wellness scores, the results showed that the higher the education of the men, but not of the women, the higher the wellness score; for both men and women, working was associated with higher wellness scores; and for both men and women, the longer the period of homelessness, the higher the wellness score.

OTHER HEALTH STUDIES

Some other studies on the health of homeless populations have been carried out. In one study by the National Health Care Program for the Homeless reported by Wright (1990), data were included from 19 cities and almost 100,000 homeless clients seen in clinics almost 300,000 times. The most common acute condition in this group was respiratory infections (33%), followed by traumas (25%), which included lacerations, wounds, sprains, bruises, and fractures in the order of frequency, and minor skin conditions (15%). When compared with the rates of health conditions of a random sample of clients seen in an ambulatory setting, the rates for the homeless were 3 to 6 times more prevalent. Nutritional disorders (primarily malnutrition and vitamin deficiencies) were also seen in about 2% of the sample compared with fewer than 0.1% in the comparison sample. About two thirds of the health concerns seen in the clinic arose from acute conditions, and one third arose from chronic conditions.

The major chronic illnesses seen in the homeless population were hypertension, arthritis and other musculoskeletal disorders, dentition problems, gastrointestinal problems, peripheral vascular disease, neurological disorders, eye disorders, genitourinary problems, musculoskeletal concerns, ear disorders, and COPD. The rates for these diseases usually exceeded the control sample by a significant amount.

In a New York City study, Wright and Webster (1987) again found trauma, upper respiratory infections, chronic lung disease, skin conditions, peripheral vascular disease, and hypertension to be common problems. They also found that these disorders were considerably higher in the homeless population than in a nonhomeless group. Similar results were found by Brickner et al. (1985), Crystal and Goldstein (1984), the Institute of Medicine (1988), Marwick (1985), and the U.S. Conference of Mayors (1985).

SPECIAL HEALTH NEEDS

Dietary restrictions are a part of the treatment of several diseases, but these are almost impossible for the homeless to comply with. The homeless usually lack both the provisions for cooking and the funds for purchasing appropriate foods. Often, the homeless will patronize fast food restaurants or soup kitchens or eat from trash bins or from handouts that do not provide for special dietary needs. Foods available from these sources are usually high in carbohydrates and fat, with few vegetables and fresh fruits.

Taking prescribed medications also presents problems for the homeless. According to surveys, many of the homeless have mental illnesses, and their confusion works against complying with medical regimes. The lack of a routine also creates problems in taking medications. In addition, lack of money to purchase clocks or watches to schedule medications works against compliance. Storage of medications may also be a problem for the homeless, who must move from shelter to shelter without provisions for securing property. Freezing of liquid medications may be a problem in cold weather, and overheating may be a problem in warm weather for those medications that require a certain range of temperature. Insulin for diabetics would be an example. Finding a place to give insulin or a place to store needles and syringes may also be a problem. In my own experience with the homeless, often a practical approach based on an assessment of the situation may make the difference between compliance and failure to comply. For example, recently I saw a man at the shelter who had a muscle strain and needed heat applications. An assessment indicated a lack of electricity in the trailer where he slept. Thus, a heating pad would not work. However, because hot water was available, a hot water bottle solved the problem, and the patient complied with the request for heat to the strain.

Only about 50% of homeless patients kept their clinic appointments; only 59% kept their emergency referrals; and 14% refused to be admitted for severe illnesses (Brickner et al., 1985). This lack of adequate care and follow-up increases the special health needs of the homeless.

NURSING AND THE HOMELESS

Nursing can make a difference with the homeless population. Educators have discovered that this is a good population for student nurses to learn about a variety of health concerns. I have attended the homeless shelter dinner hour for several years and usually take students with me. In that setting, students can learn about the homeless and their concerns as well as screen for a variety of health conditions. Students have identified areas of concern and then intervened. For example, one student saw several people with sore feet and obtained donations of soap and body lotion from local businesses. She then prepared a class on foot care and also passed out the soap and lotion. Students have presented a variety of wellness classes as part of their community health nursing experience. One group of students planned and carried out a health fair for a homeless population based on an assessed need for screening for diabetes and hypertension and for teaching about breast and testicular self-examinations, diet, and community resources (Helvie, 1994a). Another group, as part of their community health nursing course, identified a need for homeless people to have access to resource manuals and developed and placed these in strategic places throughout the community. As part of this project, students obtained donations for printing the brochures and obtained media coverage on local television to advertise the project (Helvie, 1996).

In addition, primary care is being provided to homeless populations in a variety of settings. In my own community of Virginia Beach, the homeless have access to a free clinic run by a nurse practitioner. Both acute and chronic health care are provided. In addition, the Division of Nursing at Health and Human Services has been active in encouraging and financially supporting the start-up of nurse-managed clinics. Several of these have been located in homeless shelters, making care readily accessible. The shelter experience discussed above led to the request for and funding of a grant from the Division of Nursing for a nursing center in the local homeless shelter. This growing population will continue to need the services provided by nurses for many years.

The advanced practice nurse is involved in assessing health patterns among various community aggregates and the patterns and practices that influence these patterns as a basis for planning community care. The reader is referred to Chapters 6 and 7 on community assessment and community analysis. The nurse is also involved in planning for the best ways to intervene to reduce illness, death, and disability among these groups (see Chapters 8 and 9 on planning). Selected interventions appropriate to the advanced practice nurse are identified in Chapters 10, 11, 12, and 13.

REFERENCES

Advisory Council for the Elimination of Tuberculosis. (1992). Prevention and control of tuberculosis in migrant farm workers. *Morbidity and Mortality Weekly Report, 44*(RR-10), 1-13.

Andersen, R., Chen, M., Aday, L., & Cornelius, L. (1987). Health status and medical care utilization. *Health Affairs, 6*(1), 136-156.

Andrews, M., & Boyle, J. (1995). *Transcultural concepts in nursing care.* Philadelphia: J. B. Lippincott.

Anthony-Tkach, C. (1981). Care of the Mexican American patient. *Nursing and Health Care, 2,* 424-427.

Becker, T., Wiggins, C., Peck, C., Key, C., & Samet, J. (1990). Mortality from infectious diseases among New Mexico's American Indians, Hispanic whites, and other whites. *American Journal of Public Health, 80,* 320-322.

Brickner, P., Scharer, L., Conanan, B., Elvy, A., & Savarese, M. (1985). *Health care of homeless people.* New York: Springer.

Brownbee, A. T. (1978). *Community, culture, and care.* St. Louis, MO: C. V. Mosby.

Centers for Disease Control. (1984, April 24). Leading work-related diseases and injuries—U.S. Severe occupational traumatic injuries. *Morbidity and Mortality Weekly Report, 33,* 213-215.

Centers for Disease Control. (1992, June 5). Prevention and control of tuberculosis in migrant farm workers. *Morbidity and Mortality Weekly Report, 41,* 1-15.

Centers for Disease Control. (1993). Use of race and ethnicity in public health surveillance. *Morbidity and Mortality Weekly Report, 42*(RR-10), 1-17.

Crystal, S., & Goldstein, M. (1984). *Correlates of shelter utilization: One-day study.* New York: Human Resources Administration.

Cuomo, M. (1983). *1933-1983. Never again: A report to the National Governor's Association Task Force on the Homeless,* Albany, NY: Governor's Office.

Decker, S., & Knight, L. (1990). Functional health assessment: A seasonal migrant farm worker community. *Journal of Community Health Nursing, 7*(3), 141-151.

Dunnell, K., & Cartwright, A. (1972). *Medicine takers, prescribers and hoarders.* London: Routledge & Kegan Paul.

Erickson, J., & Wilhelm, C. (1986). *Housing the homeless.* New Brunswick, NJ: Rutgers University, Center for Urban Policy Research.

Fetter, M., & Larson, E. (1990). Preventing and treating human immunodeficiency virus infection in the homeless. *Archives in Psychiatric Nursing, 4,* 379-383.

Friedman, M. (1990). Transcultural family nursing: Application to Latino and black families. *Journal of Pediatric Nursing, 5,* 214-222.

Galanti, G. (1991). *Caring for patients from different cultures: Case studies from American hospitals.* Philadelphia: University of Pennsylvania Press.

Galarneau, C. (Ed.). (1993). *Under the weather: Farm worker health.* Austin, TX: National Advisory Council on Migrant Health, Bureau of Primary Health Care, & U.S. Department of Health and Human Services.

Giger, J., & Davidhizar, R. (1991). *Transcultural nursing: Assessment and intervention.* St. Louis, MO: Mosby Year Book.

Goldfarb, R. (1981). *A caste of despair.* Ames: Iowa University Press.

Goode, W. (1977). *Principles of sociology.* New York: McGraw-Hill.

Gordon, W. (1964). *Assimilation in American life: The role of race, religion, and national origin.* New York: Oxford University Press.

Green, L., & Anderson, C. (1986). *Community health.* St. Louis, MO: Times Mirror/Mosby.

Greenfield, L. J. (1984). *Complications in surgery and trauma.* Philadelphia: J. B. Lippincott.

Haan, M., Kaplan, G., & Camacho, T. (1987). Poverty and health: Prospective evidence from the Alameda County study. *American Journal of Epidemiology, 125,* 989-998.

Halfon, N., & Newacheck, P. (1993). Childhood asthma and poverty: Differential impact and utilization of health services. *Pediatrics, 9*(1), 55-61.

Hanley, C. E. (1991). Navaho Indians. In J. N. Giger & R. E. Davidhizar (Eds.), *Transcultural nursing* (pp. 240-259). St. Louis, MO: Mosby Year Book.

Helsinki Commission. (1993). *Migrant farm workers in the United States: Briefing of the Commission on Security and Cooperation in Europe.* Washington, DC: Government Printing Office.

Helvie, C. O. (1991). *Community health nursing: Theory and practice.* New York: Springer.

Helvie, C. (1994a, November). *Community project for the homeless.* Paper presented at the annual meeting of the American Public Health Association, Washington, DC.

Helvie, C. (1994b, November). *Stress, social support and illness among homeless men.* Paper presented at the annual meeting of the American Public Health Association, Washington, DC.

Helvie, C. (1995, October). *Wellness among the homeless.* Paper presented at the annual meeting of the American Public Health Association, San Diego.

Helvie, C. (1996). Students implement community project for the homeless. *Journal of Nursing Education, 36*(8), 13-15.

Helvie, C., & Alexy, B. (1992a, November). *Family coping and social support at admission to and following discharge from a homeless shelter.* Paper presented at the annual meeting of the American Public Health Association, Washington, DC.

Helvie, C., & Alexy, B. (1992b). Using after-shelter case management to improve outcome for families with children. *Public Health Reports, 107,* 585-588.

Helvie, C., & Alexy, B. (1993, October). *Stress among mothers newly admitted to homeless shelters.* Paper presented at the annual meeting of the American Public Health Association, San Francisco.

Hogelin, G. (1988). The behavioral risk factor survey in the United States, 1981-1983. In R. Anderson (Ed.), *Health behavior, research and health promotion.* New York: Oxford University Press.

Hollingshead, A. B. (1957). *Two factor index of social position.* New Haven, CT: August B. Hollingshead.

Hombs, M., & Snyder, M. (1982). *Homeless in America: A forced march to nowhere.* Washington, DC: Community for Creative Non-Violence.

Hopper, K., & Baxter, E. (1981). *Private lives/public space: Homeless adults on the streets of New York City.* New York: Community Service Society.

Hopper, K., & Hamburg, J. (1984). *The making of America's homeless: From skid row to new poor.* New York: Community Service Society.

Institute of Medicine. (1988). *Homelessness, health and human needs.* Washington, DC: National Academy Press.

Ito, S. (1988, March 17). Plans to house homeless on VA property dropped. *Los Angeles Times.*

Jackson, M. P., & McSwane, D. A. (1992). Homelessness as a determinant of health. *Public Health Nurse, 9* 185-192.

King, S. (1962). *Perceptions of illness and medical practice.* New York: Russell Sage.

Knox, R. A. (1990, June 17). Most favor bigger role in U.S. AIDS fight. *Boston Sunday Globe,* p. 22.

Koos, E. (1954). *The health of Regionville.* New York: Columbia.

Kosof, A. (1988). *Homelessness in America.* New York: Franklin Watts.

Lamarme, R. (1989). The dilemma of Native American health. *Health Education, 20*(5), 15.

Leninger, M. (1978). *Transcultural nursing: Concepts, theories, and practices.* New York: John Wiley.

Leninger, M. (1981). Transcultural nursing: Its progress and its future. *Nursing and Health Care, 2*(7), 365-371.

Leninger, M. (1988). Leninger's theory of nursing: Cultural care diversity and universality. *Nursing Science Quarterly, 1*(4), 152-160.

Levin, I. (1983, August). *Homelessness: Its implications for mental health policy and practice.* Paper presented at the annual meeting of the American Psychological Association, Anaheim, CA.

Link, B. G., & Phelan, J. C. (1996). Understanding sociodemographic differences in health: The role of fundamental social causes, *American Journal of Public Health, 86,* 471-472.

Magar, V. (1990). Health care needs of Central American refugees. *Nursing Outlook, 38,* 239-242.

Martin, D. A. (1992). Children in peril: A mandate for change in health care policies for low-income children. *Family and Child Health, 15*(1), 75-90.

Martin, P., & Martin, D. (1994). *The endless quest.* San Francisco: Westview.

Marwick, C. (1985). The "sizable" homeless population: A growing challenge for medicine. *Journal of the American Medical Association, 253,* 3217-3225.

Mechanic, D. (1982). *Symptoms, illness behavior, and help seeking.* New York: Prodist.

Moses, M. (1989). Pesticide related health problems and farm workers, *AAORN, 37*(1), 115-180.

Murray, R., & Zentner, J. (1993). *Nursing assessment and health promotion strategies through the life span* (5th ed.). Norwalk, CT: Appleton-Lange.

Najman, J. M. (1993). Health and poverty: Past, present and prospects for the future. *Social Science and Medicine, 35,* 157-166.

National Center for Health Statistics. (1981). *Eye conditions and related need for medical care among persons 1-74 years of age: Health, United States, 1971-72* (DHHS Publication No. 83-1678). Washington, DC: Government Printing Office.

National Center for Health Statistics. (1993). *Health, United States, 1992.* Hyattsville, MD: U.S. Public Health Service.

National Indian Health Board. (1984). *National Indian Health Board Reporter, 3*(12), 4.

National Migrant Resource Program, Inc. (1990). *Migrant and seasonal farm worker health objectives for the year 2000.* Austin, TX: Author.

National Wellness Institute. (1993). *Wellness inventory.* Stevens Point: University of Wisconsin, National Wellness Center.

Neal, M. (1995). Epidemiology: Unraveling the mysteries of disease and health. In C. Smith & F. Maurer (Eds.), *Community health nursing.* Philadelphia: W. B. Saunders.

Noack, H. (1988). The role of social-structural factors in health behavior. In R. Anderson (Ed.), *Health behavior, research and health promotion* (pp. 53-68). New York: Oxford University Press.

Ohio Department of Mental Health. (1985). *Homelessness in Ohio: A study of people in need.* Columbus: Author.

Orque, M., Block. B., & Monroy, L. (1983). *Ethnic nursing care.* St. Louis, MO: C. V. Mosby.

Paul, B. (1955). *Health, culture and community.* New York: Russell Sage.

Prevention and control of tuberculosis in U.S. communities with at-risk minority populations. (1992). *Morbidity and Mortality Weekly Report, 41*(RR-5), 1-11.

Raeburn, F. S., & Buss, T. (1986). *Responding to America's homeless: Public policy alternatives.* New York: Praeger.

Reinert, B. (1986). The health care beliefs and values of Mexican-Americans. *Home Healthcare Nurse, 4*(5), 23-27, 29-31.

Rhodes, E. R., Hammond, J., Welty, T. K, Handler, A. O., & Amler, R. W. (1987). The Indian burden of illness and future health interventions. *Public Health Reports, 102,* 361-368.

Robertson, M., Roper, R., & Boyer, R. (1984). *Emergency shelter for the homeless in Los Angeles County.* Los Angeles, University of California at Los Angeles, Basic Research Project, Document No. 2, School of Public Health.

Rosenstock, I. M. (1966, July). Why people use health services. *Milbank Memorial Fund Quarterly,* pp. 94-127.

Rossi, P., Fisher, A., & Willis, G. (1986). *The condition of the homeless of Chicago.* Amherst: University of Massachusetts, Social and Demographic Research Institute.

Schultz, J. H. (1985). *The economics of aging* (3rd ed.). Belmont, CA: Wadsworth.

Smith, C., & Maurer, F. A. (1995). *Community health nursing* (pp. 149-151). Philadelphia: W. B. Saunders.

Spector, R. E. (1991). *Cultural diversity in health and illness.* Norwalk, CT: Appleton-Lange.

Tuck, I. (1986). Transcultural nursing: From theory to practice. In *Proceedings of the First Annual Transcultural Nursing Conference.* Nashville, TN: University of Tennessee, Virgin Islands Nursing Association and the School of Nursing.

Tuck, I., & Harris, L. (1988). Teaching students transcultural concepts. *Nurse Educator, 13*(3), 36-39.

U.S. Bureau of the Census. (1993). Population profiles of the U.S., 1993. *Current Population Reports* (Series p-23, No. 185). Washington, DC: Government Printing Office.

U.S. Conference of Mayors. (1985). *Health care for the homeless: A forty-city review.* Washington, DC: Author.

U.S. Conference of Mayors. (1986a). *The continuing growth of hunger, homeless and poverty in American cities: 1986.* Washington, DC: Author.

U.S. Conference of Mayors. (1986b). The growth of hunger, homelessness and poverty in America's cities: A 25 city survey. In *Hunger among the homeless: Hearings before the Select Committee on Hunger* (Serial No. 99-13, U.S. Congress, House 99th Congress, 2nd Sess., pp. 103-140). Washington, DC: Government Printing Office.

U.S. Conference of Mayors. (1989). *A status report on hunger and homelessness in American cities: 1989. A 27-city survey.* Washington, DC: Author.

U.S. Department of Commerce. (1980). *Statistical abstracts of the United States, 1980.* Washington, DC: Government Printing Office.

U.S. Department of Commerce. (1993). *Statistical abstracts of the United States, 1993.* Washington, DC: Government Printing Office.

U.S. Department of Health and Human Services. (1986). *Report of the Secretary's Task Force on black and minority health: Vol. 8. Hispanic health issues.* Washington, DC: Author.

U.S. Department of Health and Human Services. (1990). *Prevention 89/90: Federal programs and progress.* Washington, DC: Government Printing Office.

U.S. Department of Health and Human Services. (1991). *Healthy people 2000: National health promotion and disease prevention objectives.* Washington, DC: Author.

U.S. Department of Health and Human Services. (1993a). *Health United States, 1992, and Healthy People 2000 review.* Washington, DC: Government Printing Office.

U.S. Department of Health and Human Services. (1993b). *1993 recommendations of the national advisory council on migrant health.* Austin, TX: National Advisory Council on Migrant Health, National Migrant Resource Program.

U.S. Department of Housing and Urban Development. (1984). *A report to the Secretary on the homeless and emergency shelters.* Washington, DC: Author.

U.S. General Accounting Office. (1985). *Homelessness: A complex problem and the federal response* (GAO/HRD 85-40). Washington, DC: Author.

Watkins, E. L., Larson, K., Harlan, C., & Young, S. (1990). A model program for providing health services for migrant farmworker mothers and children, *Public Health Reports, 105,* 567-576.

Watts, W. (1967). Social class, ethnic background and patient care. *Nurse Forum, 6,* 155-162.

Wright, J. (1990). The health of homeless people: Evidence from the National Health Care for the Homeless Program. In P. W. Brickner, L. Scharer, B. Conanan, M. Savarese, & B. Scanlan (Eds.), *Under the safety net: The health and social welfare of the homeless in the United States* (pp. 15-31). New York: Norton.

Wright, J. D., & Webster, E. (1987). *Homelessness and health.* New York: McGraw-Hill.

CHAPTER 6

COMMUNITY ASSESSMENT
Methods, Approaches, Models, and Process

OBJECTIVES

1. Discuss methods for assessing communities.
2. Identify approaches used in community assessment.
3. Discuss different nursing and health models useful in community assessment.
4. Use the Helvie energy theory in community assessment.

The first step in helping a community improve its health is to assess the health problems. A total community assessment is rarely carried out, and when it is, a team of community professionals is usually involved. A review of *Healthy People 2000* (U.S. Department of Health and Human Services [DHHS], 1991) will show just how complex an assessment of health concerns can be. It is more usual to carry out a more limited assessment. A community assessment should be based on a theoretical framework and should include an evaluation of internal and external community factors influencing health. More specifically, the community assessment involves the collection of information, facts, concerns, and opinions about the demographics, health, and environmental problems of a community. In addition, the sociocultural, economic, and environmental factors that influence community health should be assessed. Health trends should also be evaluated as a basis for setting priorities. In this chapter, the assessment process using the Helvie energy theory will be discussed and applied in two examples. The first application involves a fictitious urban community called Rudyville. The second case study, written by a nursing leader, involves data from an actual rural community.

THEORETICAL FRAMEWORK

The Helvie energy theory of community was presented in Chapter 2 and underlies community assessment in this chapter. In addition, other nursing models useful as assessment tools will be discussed briefly. A community assessment tool based on the Helvie energy theory can be found in the appendix and provides the format for presenting assessment data in this chapter.

COMMUNITY FOCUS

Concepts of community were discussed in Chapter 2. However, it needs to be reemphasized that a community focus for community assessment requires a readjustment in thinking. Unlike an assessment of an individual patient's health, which involves taking vital signs and checking other indicators of patient health, a community assessment requires an understanding of statistical measures and rates. Instead of assessing a pregnant woman or a cancer patient, the nurse must look at statistics regarding pregnancy or cancer and determine whether the rates have gone up or down as a basis for planning.

TOOLS FOR A COMMUNITY FOCUS

Demography assists in maintaining a community focus by providing data on populations and methods for calculating population rates. The demographic information sources discussed throughout this chapter provide the nurse with important community, state, and national data on factors such as birth rates; age, race, and sex composition of the population; socioeconomic status; housing conditions; mortality rates; and other factors discussed as secondary data and used in the case studies.

Demographic measures commonly used in community assessment include incidence and prevalence rates. The *incidence rate* is the number of people developing the condition or illness over an interval of time divided by the population at risk times a constant such as 100,000 population. The *prevalence* rate is the number of people (all cases) with a condition or illness at a point in time divided by the population at risk times the constant. An increase in the prevalence of a disease or condition (all cases) does not differentiate whether cases are living longer or more new cases have accounted for the increase. The incidence rate would help to differentiate.

METHODS AND APPROACHES FOR COMMUNITY ASSESSMENT

METHODS

There are various methods for collecting community assessment data. These are discussed below.

WINDSHIELD SURVEY

In a windshield survey, the community nurse rides a bus or drives through the community and identifies multiple dimensions of the community, the environment, and the lifestyles of its inhabitants. The following characteristics lend themselves to this method of observation:

1. Quality of housing—age, style, and construction materials; presence of single- or multiple-family dwellings; size of lots; presence of vacant houses; condition of houses (well kept, deteriorating); and signs of heating and cooling units in housing
2. Neighborhood hangouts—where, frequented by whom and at what times, and whether open or closed to strangers
3. Schools—elementary, secondary, trade, professional, or universities
4. Vacant lots—how many, private or public ownership, in well-kept condition or a trash heap
5. Neighborhood decay—for example, abandoned cars, trash, abandoned houses, and multiple real estate signs
6. Geographical boundaries—for example, rivers, highways, and mountains
7. Racial and social class composition
8. Transportation system—major highways, extent and quality of public transportation, condition of roads
9. Presence of shops, food stores, and malls
10. Open spaces
11. Churches indicating religious preference
12. Availability of protective services such as police and fire stations

SECONDARY DATA

A second method of data collection is the secondary data assessment and surveys. In this method, the community nurse uses data published previously, which may include (a) statistical data, (b) published documents, (c) meeting minutes, (d) health survey results, and (e) health records. These data are collected from multiple sources on specific assessment forms that vary depending on the theoretical framework and models used. In the past, most of this information was published in written form, but it is now increasingly available on computers.

Some sources for obtaining secondary data are listed in Table 6.1. The sequence of data presented follows the theoretical framework of this book (Chapter 2) and is reflected in the community assessment tool in the appendix. This sequence will also be used to present the steps in community assessment in this chapter.

Selected National Sources of Secondary Data. Several sources of national data might be useful to the community health nurse carrying out a community assessment:

■ The *American Medical Association* maintains a file of all physicians in the United States.

TABLE 6.1 Sources of Secondary Data for Community Assessment

Data	Source	Importance
A. Geography		
Topography	Almanac	Influences types of health problems
Climate	Chamber of Commerce	and access to care
B. History of the study area	Chamber of Commerce	Identifies trends in development,
	History society	health problems and resources,
	Library	political support, etc.
C. Economic subsystem of community		
Employment level	Almanac	Influences nature of health problems,
Types of work	Census data	access to care, use of community
Income level	Chamber of Commerce	resources (welfare, free medical
Governmental budget by category	Employment commission	care)
D. Education subsystem		
Number of educational facilities	Census data	Influences social class and illness
Educational level of population	Interviews with school principals	patterns, access to care, and
Health personnel	School district	understanding of health and
	Telephone directory	related information
E. Communications subsystems		
Newspapers	Chamber of Commerce	Identifies types and quality of health
Radio stations	Local libraries	information, resources for mass
Television stations	Newspaper managers	media presentations, concerns of
Health coverage	Telephone directory	community aggregates
Speakers bureau	Television managers	
F. Political subsystems		
Parties and leaders	Local election boards	Reflects community values, citizen
Major issues and actions implemented	Local party organization	involvement and concerns, and a
	Local representatives	mechanism for political action by
	Newspapers	the nurse and others
G. Recreation subsystem		
Numbers	Newspapers	Identifies resources available for
Locations	Parks and recreation staff members	community, concern for leisure
Type	and documents	time and quality of life
Age group	Telephone directory	
Leadership		

continued

TABLE 6.1 Continued

Data	Source	Importance
H. Religious subsystem		
Religious distribution	Chamber of Commerce	Reflects values in community, involvement of members, and resources for spiritual needs
Key leaders	Newspapers	
Values, beliefs	Telephone directory	
	Windshield survey	
	Personal interviews	
I. Populations subsystem		
Characteristics	Census of population and housing	Identifies health problems, trends types, services needed, including community health nursing, priorities, and resources
Numbers	Chamber of Commerce	
Density	Health facilities	
Changes	Local and state health departments	
Age distribution	Local mental health centers	
Sex and race	Local hot lines	
Vital statistics	Libraries	
Social problems	National Center for Health Statistics	
Health problems	National vital statistics reports	
Immunizations	State Department of Health	
Leading cause of death		
Chronic disease		
J. Health subsystem		
Hospital services	Annual reports	Identifies resources available and client satisfaction
Nursing homes	Chamber of Commerce	
Ambulance services	Community service directory	
Occupational health services	Health professional organizations	
School health services	Local and state health and health planning agencies	
Health department services	Personal interviews	
Health manager	Planning boards	
Services in homes and types	Telephone directory	
Clinic services		
School services		
K. Protection (services)		
Fire	Chamber of Commerce	Identifies resources available and protective service adequacy
Police	Local fire, police, health, transportation departments, social service department, hospitals, schools, Local Red Cross	
Health		
	Telephone directory	

Data	Source	Importance
Environment	United Way directory	
Transportation		
Social		
Community nursing		
Ambulance		
Hospitals		
Education		
Disaster		
L. Housing		
Condition	Housing and urban development director	Influences health statistics and quality of life
Types		
Complaints		
M. Sanitation		
Air	Local and state health departments	Influences health statistics and quality of life
Water	Newspapers	
Sewage		
Vector control		
Food and milk		
N. External community		
Threats	State and national health statistics	Influences community health statistics
Resources		
Statistics		

NOTE: Sequence of data follows the theoretical framework reflected in the community assessment (see the appendix).

- The *American Hospital Association* carries out annual surveys on a variety of hospital functions, including characteristics of clients, services provided, number of beds, and length of stay.

- The *Bureau of the Census* of the Department of Commerce completes census data of the United States every 10 years and also estimates the monthly employment and unemployment rates and other characteristics of the workforce, the total population, and selected subgroups.

- The *Bureau of Health Professions* within the Health Resources and Services Administration determines the current and future supply of health care personnel.

- The *Centers for Disease Control and Prevention* include the following centers and programs:

  1. The *Center for Chronic Disease Prevention and Health Promotion* provides data on abortions in all states.

2. The *Center for Infectious Diseases* collects and maintains morbidity data nationally on conditions such as aseptic meningitis, AIDS, diphtheria, encephalitis, food-borne outbreaks, rabies, and tetanus and publishes other public health statistics in *Morbidity and Mortality Weekly Report (MMWR),* as well as making them available at most local health departments.

3. The *Center for Preventive Services* conducts national immunization surveys to determine immunization levels.

4. The *Epidemiological Program Office* (EPO) in conjunction with the *Council of State and Territorial Epidemiologists* operates the *National Notification Disease Surveillance System,* which provides weekly information on disease occurrences.

■ The *Department of Health and Human Services, National Center for Health Statistics* (NCHS) has several valuable sources of secondary data:

1. The *National Health Interview Survey* (NHIS) collects continuing data, such as personal and demographic characteristics, illnesses, injuries, disabilities, chronic conditions, and health resources from a national sample.

2. The *National Health and Nutrition Examination Survey* obtains data from physical examinations and clinical, laboratory, and related tests on a continuing national sample. Data have been collected on arthritis, diabetes, allergies, speech pathology, cardiovascular and respiratory conditions, kidney and liver functions, hearing conditions, and nutritional status of the American people.

3. The *National Survey of Family Growth* conducts surveys and provides data on the social and demographic factors related to adoption, childbearing, and maternal and child health. Data include cohabitation, marital status, sexual activity, contraception and sterilization, infertility, breast-feeding, pregnancy loss, low-birth-weight infants, and use of medical care for family planning, infertility, and prenatal care.

4. The *National Vital Statistics System* collects and publishes national information on births, deaths, divorces, and marriages. Data from the NCHS are published annually in *Health, United States* with the appropriate year added to the title.

■ The *Environmental Protection Agency* is responsible for national environmental protection and collects data on environmental pollutants.

■ The *National Cancer Center of the National Institute of Health* maintains 11 population-based cancer registries and provides data on all residents diagnosed with cancer during the year.

■ The *National Institute of Occupational Safety and Health* (NIOSH) collects periodic data on employee exposure to various environmental factors.

Although some of the most important national sources of secondary data have been identified here, several others are identified in the *Health, United States* series (see, e.g., NCHS, 1992). One book that assists in using census data is *Using the 1990 U.S. Census for Research* (Barnett, 1994). This book includes a section on using the computer (CD-ROM) as a source of secondary data.

SURVEY DATA

Survey data from a community sample are useful but less efficient and economical than windshield or secondary data because they require time and money to obtain. However, it may be necessary to conduct one's own survey when data cannot be obtained by other methods. For example, secondary data may be available for the total community but not for particular high-risk aggregates.

Surveys may be used to collect demographic data, to establish a need for a program or service, to identify use patterns of services and facilities, or to identify strengths or problems in aggregates or the total community. Surveys may be written or verbal. Low return rates and the cost of postage have been identified as disadvantages of written and mailed surveys. Interviews may provide additional information but are time consuming.

The extent of the sample will vary by the size of the community. If there is a small community population, the entire aggregate or community may be surveyed. In large communities, the cost, time, and difficulty in reaching people may require the use of a random sample (Polit & Hungler, 1993). This approach allows the results to be generalized to the total aggregate or community. A further discussion of surveys and sample instruments appears in Chapter 7.

KEY INFORMANT INTERVIEWS

Interviews with key informants are another source of community data. Key informants are people with positions in a community that give them insights into community problems and needs. They may also be able to identify the basis for resistance to health programs—and how to reduce resistance—or know contact persons to assist with beneficial community programs. Some key informants might be public officials, school personnel, health care professionals, prominent business or religious leaders, local politicians, directors of housing projects, and unofficial community spokespersons.

PARTICIPANT OBSERVATION

In this approach, the nurse participates in community life or the life of an aggregate group and makes observations about its health and health needs. For example, the nurse interested in data on alcoholism might attend open Alcoholics Anonymous meetings and detox centers, and the nurse interested in a homeless population might attend free health clinics, soup kitchens, libraries, or other hangouts of the group.

Community nurses might also attend and observe at significant community events, such as social gatherings, religious ceremonies, political meetings, and community health activities. This allows nurses to learn about individual and group behavior, practices, and similarities and differences. For example, the nurse can identify community leaders who can be used as key informants and learn about who attends what meetings, who makes decisions, who has health concerns, what attitudes are expressed about access to and adequacy of health services, and who does or does not support community health and community health nursing.

COMMUNITY FORUM

A community forum allows community members to provide information and opinions about health and community needs, services, or other topics of concern. Forums may be open to total communities or aggregates of the community, depending on the focus of information needed. This is a relatively cost-efficient and effective way to obtain opinions from the community.

COMMUNITY ASSESSMENT APPROACHES

Although there are multiple methods for collecting community data, there are only two basic approaches. These approaches are called *data gathering* and *data generating*. Data gathering involves collecting existing, often published, data that are readily available and have been collected by others. Usually, these are statistical data; they were called *secondary data* above. The data gathered may concern demographics, vital statistics, health care staffing, and community organizations and services.

Generated data are more difficult to obtain and are usually costly and time consuming to collect. Data generation involves interacting with community members and collecting data from them firsthand. Data collected may concern knowledge, beliefs, and values of members of the community or aggregates; their goals and perceived needs for health; community norms and problem-solving processes; or community power and influence structures. Data are qualitative and are collected by observation or interview (see methods of community assessment above).

Both approaches are valuable for obtaining a comprehensive picture of the community. In addition, several methods within each approach may be necessary to collect the needed data. The scope and complexity of data collection depend on several factors:

1. If nurses are assessing a community's or an aggregate's health status, data collection will be more extensive than if they are collecting additional data about a known problem.
2. Time available will influence the complexity of the community assessment: Less time will mean a less complex assessment.
3. Population size will also influence the community assessment: A smaller population may be assessed as a total in more depth, whereas a larger population may require a less in-depth assessment of a community sample.
4. The relationship between cost and perceived benefit may also limit the scope of a community assessment.
5. The expertise of the nurse or other data collector will also affect the process.

USING AN ASSESSMENT TOOL BASED ON THEORY OR MODELS

Although the assessment tool for this book is based on the Helvie energy theory (Chapter 2) and is discussed later in this chapter, some additional tools are available in the literature. Some community health nursing authors have developed assessment tools based on a theory or nursing model (Anderson & McFarlane, 1996; Berentson, 1985; Clark, 1996; Cookfair, 1996; Finnegan & Ervin, 1989; Hanchett, 1988; Helvie, 1991; Krieger & Harton, 1992; Smith & Maurer, 1995), whereas others do not include assessment tools or base tools on a theory or model (Clemen-Stone, Eigsti, & McGuire, 1995; Martin, 1988; Spradley & Allender, 1996; Stanhope & Lancaster, 1996; Turner, 1991).

An assessment model is important because it provides a format for data collection. This ensures that the data are collected in a systematic way. The models presented below direct the nurse in collecting data specific to the model.

EPIDEMIOLOGICAL MODEL OF COMMUNITY ASSESSMENT

Finnegan and Ervin (1989) use an epidemiological model for community assessment. In this model, a classification of human, disease agent, and environmental factors (see Helvie, 1991, for enlargement on this conceptual framework) is used as the organizer for the data collection tool. Data on human factors, such as social, economic, cultural, demographic, and attitudinal factors, answer the "who" of epidemiology. Data on variables such as age, race, sex, ethnicity, income, cultural norms and values, occupational and educational levels, and health status of the community would be included under this category.

Data on the disease agent factors answer the "why" and "how" questions of epidemiology. When infectious diseases were prevalent, the disease agent was separated from environmental factors in the triad. Because the focus has shifted to other diseases and conditions, epidemiologists now often consider the agent an integral part of the environment. Use of the framework involves assessing agent, host, and environmental factors that have created an imbalance at a point in time. These then form the basis of nursing diagnoses and interventions in the community.

Data on the environmental factors answer the "where" (place) and "when" (time) questions of epidemiology. Place factors include data on the physical, biological, and social environments; time factors include time of day or year and trends over time.

PATTERNS MODEL OF COMMUNITY ASSESSMENT

Krieger and Harton (1992) use Gordon and Kucharski's (1987) 11 functional health patterns as a model for community assessment. They developed an assessment typology based on these health patterns and then created the Community Health Assessment Tool (CHAT). CHAT is not meant to be all-inclusive but, rather, to provide a structure that allows nurses to be as comprehensive as they wish.

The authors adapted Gordon and Kucharski's 11 individual functional health patterns to the purposes of assessment with a community focus: (a) The "health perception/health management pattern" now concerned the adequacy of the community's health and safety efforts; (b) the "nutritional/metabolic pattern" became the adequacy of the community's nutrition efforts, including nutritional education; (c) the "elimination pattern" became waste management in the community; (d) the "activity/exercises pattern" became an assessment of community transportation and recreation; (e) the "sleep/rest pattern" became community rhythms and cycles; (f) the "cognitive/perceptual pattern" became community decision-making processes; (g) the "self-perception/self-concept pattern" became the community's view of itself; (h) the "role/relationship pattern" became the community definitions for both formal and informal roles; (i) the "sexuality/reproductive pattern" became the community's resources for reproductive functions and family structure; (j) the "coping/stress tolerance pattern" became community support services; and (k) the "value/belief pattern" became the community's response to spiritual, cultural, and ethical needs.

Categories of community assessment were then developed for each of these 11 functions. The health perception/health management pattern has three subcategories: protective services, morbidity and mortality statistics, and health resources. Protective services include police, fire, and disaster response; morbidity and mortality statistics include rates for reportable and other specific diseases and crude and cause-specific death rates for the top 10 (and other) causes of death; and health resources include those involving health promotion, ambulatory care, and long-term care.

Elimination pattern has two subcategories: (a) sanitation, which includes water, sewage, trash and garbage removal, rodent and vermin control, and (b) ecological concerns, which include air and noise pollution, hazardous waste, and recycling programs. Other areas of assessment for each of the 11 patterns can be found in the original article.

NEUMAN'S MODEL OF COMMUNITY ASSESSMENT

Several nurse authors have referred to Neuman's model (1989) as it relates to community, and some have used it as a basis for community assessment (Anderson & McFarlane, 1996; Cookfair, 1989). This model begins with a wheel that has at its center the people in the community. Assessment data related to the population in this core include demographics such as age, race, and sex, as well as the history, values, and beliefs of the population. Around this population at the center are the spokes of the wheel, eight subsystems of the community that affect and are affected by the population: recreation, physical environment, education, safety and transportation, politics and government, health and social services, communication, and economics.

NORMAL AND FLEXIBLE LINE OF DEFENSE

Surrounding the community in the wheel model is a solid line (the wheel's circumference) representing the community's normal line of defense. This represents the community's usual coping mechanisms and the community's level of health at a point in time resulting from the usual coping methods. Usual coping may involve responses such as the usual response of the fire department to an alarm, police to a burglary call, city council to a request for zoning changes, or the health department to unimmunized children. Results of these coping actions will be reflected in the level of health of the community, as indicated by characteristics such as low infant mortality and high immunization levels based on statistics.

Beyond the normal line of defense in the model is the flexible line of defense, a "dynamic level of health resulting from a temporary response to stressors. This temporary response may be a neighborhood mobilizing against an environmental stressor such as flooding or a social stressor such as an unwanted 'adult' bookstore" (Anderson & McFarlane, 1996, p. 169). In my own community a few years ago, a riot was handled at the flexible-line-of-defense level by calling in the National Guard and state police for assistance and by setting up temporary prisons and judicial hearing stations. This resulted in the maintenance of law and order. Because it was anticipated that riots might become an annual occurrence at that particular time of year, a further system of parking permits, police checks, and other measures was established to prevent the occurrence and to maintain order in subsequent years.

The model also shows interaction between the eight subsystems as depicted by the broken lines between them. These show that each subsystem influences and is influenced by the others.

Communities have lines of resistance or internal mechanisms that defend against stressors. These might include, for example, "an evening recreation program for young people . . . to decrease vandalism and a freestanding, no-fee health clinic to diagnose and treat sexually transmitted diseases" (Anderson & McFarlane, 1996, p. 172). Internal and external stressors or both penetrate the normal or flexible line of defense and may cause community disequilibrium. The reaction to the stressors may be reflected in health and other community statistics.

Community assessment is based on an evaluation of all of these factors. The nurse assesses the population, the subsystems, the lines of defense, the community's resistance, the stressors, and the reaction to stressors.

OREM'S SELF-CARE COMMUNITY ASSESSMENT MODEL

Berentson (1985) applies the Orem Model (1980) to community assessment. This model features seven concepts: (a) universal self-care requisites, (b) developmental self-care requisites, (c) health deviation self-care requisites, (d) therapeutic self-care demands, (e) self-care agency, (f) self-care deficit, and (g) adequate self-care actions. The first four of these concepts can be used for assessing the community's ability to perform the functions necessary to maintain its current level of functioning or to move to a higher level (self-care agency). Requisites are those necessary ingredients for a community to engage in self-care. The three universal self-care requisites are common to all communities and must be provided.

SELF-CARE REQUISITES

Universal self-care requisites are (a) living space and shelter, (b) goods and services, (c) safety and order, (d) education and enculturation, (e) communication, (f) rules and standards of behavior, and (g) opportunity for interaction. *Developmental self-care requisites* are related to the universal self-care requisites and are the needs created by change and development in the community. Thus, the community must provide ways to meet the needs associated with each universal self-care requisite as a result of change and development. For example, a rise in crime in a community (change) must be met with a mechanism to maintain the universal requisite of safety and order. This could be accomplished, by increasing the number of police, jail cells, and judges and other responses. If it is accomplished, the community has provided the mechanism for maintaining safety and order in the light of changing crime patterns. For example, my own city has a resort area along the beach, and many people come into town for vacation each spring and summer (change). At that time, motels open that have been closed for the winter and provide living space for the increased population; restaurants and stores open to meet the needs for necessary goods and services; police officers are moved to the resort area from other areas of the city, and some new temporary police are employed to maintain law and order. Other changes occur as well to accommodate the influx of people. Thus, the community is able to meet the needs of the population created by the increased numbers (change) each summer. Provision of developmental self-care requisites is similar to Neuman's normal line of defense and to Roy's (1984) automatic community responses, discussed later in this chapter.

The third type of self-care requisite, the health deviation self-care requisites, refers to the needs that evolve when there is community dysfunction created by a threat to the community. Examples might include a natural disaster, environmental pollution, crime, poverty, or a communicable disease epidemic. At these times, the community must recognize the threat and seek and implement solutions to reverse it. Provision of health deviation self-care requisites is similar to Neuman's flexible line of defense and Roy's cognitive response.

SELF-CARE DEMANDS

Self-care demands refers to the actions a community must take to meet its self-care requisites. Demands related to the universal self-care requisite of living space and shelter include land planning and zoning, areas for housing and parks, and areas for industry and agriculture. Community self-care demands related to necessary goods and services include accessible goods and services, adequate economic base, health services and personnel, professionals and service people, and public assistance. Other self-care requisites related to the universal self-care demands can be found in Berentson (1985).

There are also developmental self-care demands for each developmental self-care requisite. These include community members who strive toward common goals, emotional commitment to established goals, articulation of community goals, determined procedures to meet goals, attention to the need for change, and attention to sociocultural, demographic, and ecological features of the community.

Finally, there are self-care demands related to the health deviation self-care requisites. These include ways to monitor community functioning, ways to detect threats to the community, community problem-solving mechanisms, ways to access external resources, and community resources to implement plans to alleviate the threat.

These four areas of assessment will determine how well the community is functioning and whether it has self-care deficits. Community self-care deficits will form the basis of nursing diagnoses.

ROY'S MODEL OF COMMUNITY ASSESSMENT

Although some authors have adapted Roy's model (1984) for use in the community, these presentations are more theoretical than practical because specific areas of data collection are missing. The interested reader is referred to Hanchett (1988, 1989).

HELVIE'S ENERGY THEORY FOR COMMUNITY ASSESSMENT

SUMMARY OF THEORY

The Helvie framework for assessment follows the theory presented in Chapter 2 and is reflected in the assessment tool located in the appendix. This theory identifies three types of energy in the community: bound, kinetic, and potential. These are the organizations and community members (including the population and aggregates) along with the dynamic roles, services, knowledge, attitudes, and beliefs that make up part of the internal environment of the community and influence health. The theory continues on to discuss the environment as energy (internal and external) and the exchanges of the population with these environments. The internal environment is identified as community subsystems, including the population. The concepts of energy types and internal energy are similar to Neuman's concepts core and subsystems. The external environment relates to other communities, the state, and nation, and these exchanges may also stress the community and require adaptation. They also provide resources (money, personnel) and serve as a standard against which the community can compare itself.

The community continually attempts to adapt to the internal and external exchanges, and the balance established at any point in time forms the basis for a community assessment. Attempts at adaptation on the part of the community in the Helvie energy theory is similar to the normal and flexible line of defense in Neuman's model, responses to self-care requisites of Orem's model, and the automatic and cognitive community responses of Roy's model. The balance resulting from the adaptation may move the community toward or away from a healthy focus and can be assessed. For example, health statistics show the result of the community's adaptation to internal and external factors. Thus, nurses assess this balance and develop plans to maintain it or to move the community toward a more healthy level.

Because community energy needs vary by time and situation, nurses must look at trends in assessment data and also compare community data with data for other communities, the state, and the nation to determine how well the health of the community is being cared for.

Concepts from this theory are combined with the nursing process in a model presented in Figure 2.3. A case study using the assessment tool and based on this theory is presented next.

COMMUNITY ASSESSMENT APPLICATION—RUDYVILLE

The community assessment was carried out in Rudyville, Virginia, in 1996. Although most of the state and national data are authentic, Rudyville is a fictitious community, and data for the application are drawn from a variety of real and fictitious sources for the purpose of demonstrating the concepts. The case study application following this section is a real community, but the name has been changed.

INTERNAL CHARACTERISTICS

Internal characteristics in the Helvie energy theory include the topography and climate, boundaries, history, and subsystems of the community under study. These are discussed below. External characteristics are included here for comparison only.

TOPOGRAPHY AND CLIMATE

According to the Department of Economic Development, the climate in Rudyville is moderate, with an average of 45 inches of rain and 1.8 inches of snow each year. Annual mean temperature is 59.5 °F, with an August high of 85.7 and a January low of 31.7. Rudyville is a coastal city and is promoted by the Chamber of Commerce as a resort area. As a result, an estimated 2.5 million people visit the city annually, generating $30 million in city tax revenue.

As a coastal city, Rudyville is threatened yearly between June and November by the possibility of hurricanes. For many years, there were no hurricanes along the Atlantic coast, but starting 6 years ago, they have been increasing (2 in 1990, 3 in 1991, 3 in 1992, 6 in 1993, 6 in 1994, and 11 in 1995), and although the forecast is for fewer in 1996 there are predictions of a continuing trend of more hurricanes in the future. Damage from hurricanes has occurred in Texas, Louisiana, Florida, South Carolina, North Carolina, New York, and New England. Because Rudyville is at sea level, flooding is a possibility in addition to more severe damage from hurricanes. Financing of the Disaster Planning Office is shared by the health department and the city. This office reported that if there was a hurricane warning in the area, only 25% of the population would be able to be evacuated before the hurricane because of the number of people, the limited number of roads out of the area, and the limited time between the warning and the event. Warnings have been announced in the past with minimal information about preparation when hurricanes were considered a possible threat. This information was presented by the weather channel on the radio and television.

In addition, being at sea level poses problems for garbage and trash disposal. Currently, trash is placed on top of the ground and periodically covered with soil. One such covered trash heap has become a playground and is aptly called Mount Trashworth. Being at sea level also means that the terrain is flat with the exception of the trash mountains. The flat terrain improves visibility and makes it easier to move from place to place on bicycles or in automobiles.

Because Rudyville is a southern community on the ocean, there is limited snow during the winter months, and the temperature remains moderate. Thus, transportation mobility is good year round.

HISTORY OF RUDYVILLE

The history of Rudyville began when British colonists landed at Cape Henry in 1607 before moving to Jamestown. Wilf County, which surrounds Rudyville, was established in 1691. In 1791, Cape Henry was built as the first federally funded lighthouse. It is symbolic of Rudyville and is used as part of the city seal. In 1906, Rudyville was a town with a population of 642. The health department was established after World War II. The local hospital, Rudyville General, was established during the influenza epidemic in 1918. On January 1, 1963, Rudyville was chartered as a municipal corporation by the General Assembly of Virginia. On that date also, Rudyville annexed adjacent Wilf County and became a city of 125,000 people. The 1990 census shows that 393,069 people live in Rudyville. According to Rudyville's department of economic development, by the year 2000, the population is projected to reach 500,000. Rudyville is the most populous city in Virginia.

Rudyville became a major military base in 1941 and has retained a large naval fleet since that time. Having a large navy population affects the median age of the population, buffers the economy during downward cycles, and in general is a positive factor.

There was an epidemic of the flu in 1918 and a polio epidemic in 1948. Laws regarding compulsory vaccinations and immunizations prior to school enrollment were passed in 1949. Ash Wednesday in 1943 brought a northeastern storm that flooded the coast and surrounding neighborhoods with up to 4 feet of water covering cars, houses, streets, and sidewalks. Flood insurance was a requirement for financing homes following this storm.

BOUNDARIES

Specific boundaries of Rudyville include the cities of Trier and Kuntztown to the west; the Ontario Bay and Buzzard County to the north; the Atlantic Ocean and international waters to the east with 38 miles of shoreline; and Charlestown and South Carolina to the south. There are 66 census tracts in Rudyville, covering a land area of 258.7 square miles. Because Rudyville is at sea level, there are many lakes within the city, covering a total of 51.3 square miles.

TABLE 6.2 Employment Distribution, 1990, for Persons Aged 16 and Over, by Number and Percentage

Category	Rudyville	Virginia	United States
Total population	293,496	4,843,182	191,829,271
Employed	225,245	3, 338,989	125,182,378
Percentage employed	76.8	68.9	65.3
Manufacturing	14,700	457,632	20,461,000
Percentage of total	5.01	9.45	10.67
Wholesale	6,709	101,910	5,011,026
Percentage of total	2.29	2.20	2.61
Retail	36,633	487,016	19,485,666
Percentage of total	12.48	10.06	10.16
Local government	15,287	223,882	8,244,000
Percentage of total	5.21	4.62	4.30
State government	4,157	142,952	5,381,000
Percentage of total	1.42	2.95	2.81
Federal government	17,789	274,832	3,941,000
Percentage of total	6.06	5.67	2.05
Unemployed	8,691	142,048	7,792,248
Percentage of total	2.96	2.93	4.06
Not in labor force	68,224	1,504,193	66,646,893
Percentage of total	23.25	31.06	34.74
Armed forces	38,395	168,579	1,708,928
Percentage of total	13.08	3.48	0.89

SOURCE: 1990 census data.

ECONOMIC SUBSYSTEM

Labor Force. In 1990, the labor force in Rudyville included 225,245 persons, who represented 76.8% of the population of 293,469 people over the age of 16. Table 6.2 shows the total employment numbers and percentages of this population by category of employment for Rudyville, the state, and the nation.

Unemployment Rate. The unemployment rate was 5.9% in 1992, representing an increase from 1990 (2.90%) and from 1987 (3.4%). As Table 6.2 shows, in 1990 it was about the same as that for the state and lower than the rate for the nation as whole. For all years between 1987 and 1991, the rate in Rudyville was lower than that of the state and the nation.

Income Sources. The major sources of income for Rudyville are the tourist/convention business, the military, and defense systems technology. About 2.5 million people visited the resort city in 1991 and spent more than $500 million on hotels, meals, souvenirs, and other services. This generated about $30 million in taxes for the city, and in 1990, conventions produced about $43.7

TABLE 6.3 Family Income Levels, by Percentages, 1990

Category	Rudyville	Virginia	United States
Under $5,000	2	3.1	4
$5,000 to $9,999	2	4.5	5.6
$10,000+	96	92	90.4
Median income	$39,112	$33,328	$35,225

SOURCE: 1990 census data.

TABLE 6.4 Percentage of the Population Under Poverty Levels, by Age and Type of Family, 1990

Category	Rudyville	Virginia	United States
Age			
Under 5 years	8.5	14.5	20.1
5 to 17	7.1	12.4	17
Under 18 years	7.6	13	17.9
Over 18	5.1	9.2	11.3
Over 65 years	8	14.1	12.8
Family type			
All families	4.6	8.3	10.2
Female household heads			
Families with children	20.2	26.7	31.1
Under age 5	40.2	50.3	57.4
Under age 18	26.5	36.4	42.3

million in gross revenue. The four military bases employ 34,233 military and civilian employees and have a combined annual payroll of $715 million. Much of this money is spent in Rudyville.

In addition, agriculture and construction projects contribute to the economy of Rudyville. Data from Rudyville's department of economic development state that there are 165 farms in Rudyville with about 239 acres each. Approximately 39,358 acres of land are under cultivation. Fresh fruit and vegetables are available at the farmer's market, and people are allowed to pick in the fields in season. Agriculture contributes about $75.7 million to the economy annually, and construction and real estate add $364,313,097.

Family Income and Poverty. Family income levels for residents of Rudyville and for the state and nation are shown in Table 6.3. Percentages of the population under poverty levels are given in Table 6.4. State and national figures data were obtained from the 1990 census (U.S. Bureau of the Census, 1990) and are for 1989. The poverty level decreased in Rudyville from 7.7% in 1979 to 4.6% of families in 1989. A similar change was seen at the state and national levels. The percentage of the families under poverty levels in Virginia was 9.2% for families in 1979 and 8.3% in 1989 and in the United States was 9.6% in 1979 and 10.0% in 1989.

In addition, large numbers of people are at or near poverty levels. In Rudyville, a "near-poor" person is one with an annual income less than 200% of the federal poverty level ($13,620 for one person). A person identified as poor is at 100% of the federal poverty level ($6,810 for one person annually). Census data indicate that there were 393,000 people in Rudyville in 1990, with 12,000 poor and 13,000 near-poor. Many of these did not have access to health care.

Health Insurance. In 1991, the Commission on Health Care for All Virginians studied the issues of accessibility and affordability of primary health care for the citizens of Virginia. The 1991 Virginia General Assembly adopted Senate Joint Resolution 179, which directed all district health directors throughout Virginia to assess the primary care needs of their constituency and develop a public-private partnership to provide services to those in need. The assessment was completed and plans were developed for providing health care to the medically indigent. Twenty thousand persons were found to be poor or near-poor and to be without health insurance.

In addition, a 1990 survey conducted by the health department concluded that 29,000 additional doctor visits were needed annually to adequately cover the health care needs of the medically indigent. In 1995, the health department received a new director who provided a new focus for services. At the same time, Medicaid requirements changed at the state level. Thus, the health department closed the adult medical clinic for the medically indigent, which had cared for 3,000 people. This left one free source of care, the Rudyville Free Clinic, which was staffed by volunteers and which has always had a long waiting list. Thus, services for this population are inadequate.

Governmental Budget. Responsibilities of the local government include developing the annual budget, establishing community needs, determining the opinion of community members, and evaluating funding available. The city manager (see "Political Subsystem" below) presents the budget to the city council for the following year at least 90 days prior to the end of the fiscal year. Workshops are initiated to discuss funding levels, and public hearings are scheduled to allow for public comments about the budget before it is adopted. The capital improvement program (CIP) is included in the budget and encompasses the major construction requirements of the city for the following 5 to 10 years. Construction includes schools, municipal buildings, roads, water and sewage systems, and recreation facilities.

The comprehensive plan is the city's official guide for physical development in future years to keep growth in harmony with funding. The plan is adopted by the city council and is supplemented by zoning, capital improvement program funding, and other resources and mechanisms. This plan is reviewed every 5 years.

The city council delegates responsibility to selected appointees. The city attorney has authority for legal matters involving the city. The city clerk maintains the city's official seal and records, prepares the agenda, takes minutes at meetings, and provides a weekly summary. The real estate assessor appraises all properties, including those that are tax exempt, and submits real estate assessments to property owners.

The city budget is approved annually following the process discussed above. Table 6.5 shows the amounts and percentage of the total for local expenditures by category of service for 2 recent years. Local communities surrounding Rudyville have different percentages for certain items in the budget: For example, Trier and Kuntztown, which are comparable in size, show the following allocations: public works, 4.2% and 4.0%, respectively (compared with Rudyville's 6.54%); health, 3.1% and 2.8% (compared with Rudyville's 0.29%); and parks and recreation, 2.8% and 3.2% (compared with Rudyville's 1.83%).

EDUCATION SUBSYSTEM

Rudyville has numerous educational facilities. There are 74 public schools and 15 private schools for kindergarten through Grade 12 and more than 77,000 school students. Of the public schools, 52 are elementary, 13 are junior high, and 9 are senior high. There are also special schools, including a literacy center, an adult learning center, a vocational-technical school, and a center for the gifted and talented. There are four colleges in Rudyville, including three religious colleges and a state community college. In 1992, these schools had 20,259 full- and part-time students enrolled. There are also seven additional private and state colleges and universities within 25 miles of Rudyville. In addition to preparing undergraduates in all areas of study, these schools prepare professionals at most graduate levels, including medicine, nursing, and allied health. There is one medical school, three nursing schools, a physical therapy school, a social work school, and a dental hygiene school within 20 miles of Rudyville. The medical school graduates 65 physicians yearly, and 50% of these are women. It graduates students in all medical specialties. The three nursing schools graduate 550 baccalaureate-prepared nurses (including RN to baccalaureate graduates) annually, 150 master's-prepared nurses with specialties in all clinical areas, and 4 doctoral-prepared nurses. The social work school graduates 65 master's-prepared social workers and 10 doctoral-prepared social workers annually, and the physical therapy school graduates 65 master's-prepared physical therapists annually. The nearest dental school is 100 miles away.

*Educational Level.*The educational level of the population in Rudyville and in Virginia is shown in Table 6.6. This shows that for the population 25 years and older, the following percentages achieved various levels of education: 4.0% achieved less than ninth grade; 37.8 were high school graduates; 34.8% had some college; and 23.4% were college graduates.

Almost 50% of the Rudyville budget is allocated to schools (see "Education" and "Debt: school" in Table 6.5). Schools have lower student-teacher ratios than do those in surrounding communities. They also feature computer stations, driver training courses, and many extras. Despite the size of the budget, school officials overspent the budget by $20 million in 1994-1995 and by $10 million in 1995-1996. Following a grand jury investigation, some school officials and board members were fired or charged with mismanagement.

TABLE 6.5 Rudyville, Virginia, Budget, Summary of Expenditure, by Department from 1991 to 1994 (Amounts and Selected Percentages)

Department	1991-92 Amount ($)	1992-93 Amount($)	1993-94 Amount ($)
Legislative	687,700	637,700	623,300
Executive	1,614,600	1,169,700	1,168,000
Law	1,475,300	1,549,900	1,546,000
Finance	11,458,700	11,145,100	11,134,700
Human resources	2,331,900	2,295,600	2,269,300
Judicial	15,422,100	15,347,700	15,956,500
Health	2,252,400	2,151,500	2,103,900
Social services	15,252,200	18,242,600	15,568,700
Police	39,221,200	41,251,200	42,459,100
Public works	39,405,300	43,737,600	46,684,400
Parks and recreation	13,063,300	14,479,000	13,071,800
Library	7,527,400	7,460,800	7,521,600
Planning	1,564,000	2,566,400	2,517,300
Agriculture	225,100	703,200	656,300
Economic development	1,091,500	1,177,300	1,176,300
General services	16,887,000	16,774,365	19,918,800
Bds. and commiss.	2,032,900	2,231,600	2,248,750
Fire	18,914,200	17,963,000	18,357,200
Public utilities	30,608,800	35,005,500	36,100,900
Mental health	10,903,795	12,134,100	12,250,700
Emergency medical services	1,110,400	1,189,400	1,681,900
Museums	1,751,700	1,713,800	1,735,940
Management and budget	774,100	1,379,500	1,367,092
Conventions and Tourism	6,398,000	6,900,700	6,805,400
Housing and neighborhoods	2,664,300	4,447,100	4,540,300
Education	280,153,300	312,800,200	323,510,300
Debt: school	19,963,470	22,082,700	24,910,100
Debt: other	49,656,300	56,439,300	56,516,400
Nondepartmental	2,321,100	2,158,600	3,005,000
Cont. reserv.	0	3,408,100	8,031,000
Capital projects	16,100,800	11,432,600	23,794,700
Total budget	617,698,800	671,972,600	714,254,700

COMMUNICATIONS SUBSYSTEM

There are two major daily papers in Rudyville, and daily circulation for the two is 201,800 (Rudyville Opinion Survey). A weekly paper in Rudyville has a circulation of 82,655 customers (Rudyville Opinion Survey).

TABLE 6.6 Educational Levels for Population Over Age 25 in Rudyville, Virginia, and the United States

Category	Rudyville	Virginia	United States
Under 9 years	7,133 (4.0%)	443,668 (15.6%)	16,505,211 (13.3%)
High school graduate	67,265 (37.8%)	1,059,199 (37.1%)	47,642,763 (38.2%)
Some college	61,851 (34.8%)	736,007 (25.8%)	29,779,777 (23.9%)
College graduate	41,541 (23.4%)	12,679 (21.5%)	30,624,492 (24.6%)
Total	177,790 (100.0%)	2,851,553 (100.0%)	124,549,240 (100.0%)

TABLE 6.7 Rudyville Media Stations

Name	Address	Audience
Television		
Rudyville ABS	22 W. Hanover Lane	Middle-class white
Rudyville CBS	33 Lake George St.	Lower-class, white, black
Rudyville NBS	45 Lake George St.	All classes, ages, races
Rudyville Prot.	21 Anchor Way	Religious groups
Radio		
Rudyville WQXZ	412 Briton St.	All races, ages, classes
Wellwood University station WXRX	235 Minton St., Norton, VA	Middle- and upper-class, adults

Radio and Television. There are 18 AM and 26 FM radio stations received in Rudyville from surrounding areas. These offer a variety of music as well as reports on news, weather, sports, and road conditions. There is one local radio station and one university-affiliated radio station in a neighboring community 25 miles away. One cable service company went bankrupt recently, but there is one remaining. Three television stations and one religious station present a wide range of programs (see Table 6.7).

Speakers Bureau. There is a speakers bureau that includes health information in Rudyville and also one at the university 25 miles away. Speakers from the university's speakers bureau are available to organizations in Rudyville. Information is offered by nursing and other health faculty members on a variety of topics. In addition, the health director and staff members of the local health department are available and frequently used on mass media channels and by organizations. There is also an on-line service with automated recorded messages on many health-related topics. Rudyville also has a City-Line for citizen information that offers hundreds of recorded messages on city services by telephone.

Influential Community Leaders. Several community leaders influence communication in Rudyville. These are the owners of the major communication systems and are listed in Table 6.8. It should be noted that many of these owners are related to the family who established Rudyville.

TABLE 6.8 Community Leaders in Mass Communication

Name	Affiliation	Telephone
John Rudy	*Rudyville Pilot*	422-4896
Jay Rudy	*Rudyville Times*	428-5127
Jan Elder	*Weekly Beekly*	428-5508
Wilf Mann	Rudyville ABS	428-0908
Carl Rudy	Rudyville CBS	422-0802
Jane Love	Rudyville NBS	428-0222
Jason Pacon	Rudyville WQXZ	421-0009
Mary Rhodes	Wellwood WXRX	683-5555

Mass Media Health Coverage. Health coverage by mass media is inadequate, according to survey data from radio, television, and the public. There is adequate, high-quality information on various disease processes and family care for sick members. However, there is almost no public information on prevention and wellness. This lack of wellness coverage is true of all newspapers and of the radio and television stations.

Health Information in Schools. The health information in schools is presented by nurses from the health department and by physical education teachers. Because the health department nurses have many additional functions in clinics and the community, they spend a limited amount of time in schools weekly. This usually consists of about a half-day a week for small schools and a day a week for larger schools. This time is usually spent in teacher-nurse conferences, preparing for physical exams in selected grades, and record keeping. There is minimal teaching by nurses for the first aid and triage duties that teachers assume and little emphasis on health promotion, prevention, and wellness. In addition, minimal attention is given to health concerns related to developmental stages, such as sex education and AIDS.

The limited information that is currently provided to students consists of classes on personal hygiene, including cleanliness, tooth care, grooming, and toilet care for Grades 1 through 6; classes on nutrition and care for the sick at home for Grades 7 through 9; and classes on auto safety, sports safety, and sexual development for Grades 10 through 12. Periodic blood pressure screening and vision, hearing, and scoliosis screening are required by law.

Physical education teachers have a minor role that is usually confined to ensuring that students participating in athletics have obtained the necessary examinations. In addition, there is some emphasis on treatment and prevention of athletic injuries.

POLITICAL SUBSYSTEM

City Governance. According to the Rudyville Public Information Office, the local government in Rudyville was chartered as a municipal corporation by the General Assembly of Virginia on January 1, 1963. This system of government operates under a city manager, a planning commission, a comprehensive zoning ordinance, and an 11-member city council that is elected in even-numbered years for 4-year terms. Each member, including the mayor, has one vote on issues brought before the council. The city of Rudyville is independent from a county and has one local governing and taxing authority.

Although seven of the city council members run in specific districts of the city, they are voted on by the total city at elections. Four members run at large, including the mayor, who is also elected for a 4-year term. Although the mayor was previously selected by the council members from among its members, for 8 years this person has been elected by the public. In the future, voters will decide whether to vote for candidates for city council from within a district or citywide.

Party Lines. Although the council members do not divide into parties, there is a division between those who are progrowth and business oriented and those who are for slower growth and are resident oriented. This emphasis shifts from time to time, and currently the progrowth faction is in power. Some of this emphasis is seen in the budget (presented in Table 6.5) and plans for the city. Plans include beautification of the oceanfront resort area, heavy advertising of the oceanfront along the northeastern U.S. corridor, and plans for a corridor of indoor and outdoor shops near the oceanfront, a new mall and shopping center near the oceanfront, a sports stadium, an amphitheatre, and additional golf courses.

The influence of the slow-growth faction of the city council can be seen in the population data below. This shows a decrease in the percentage of growth from 104% between 1960 and 1970 to 50% between 1980 and 1990. This resulted from the development of a comprehensive plan for growth and was necessitated by a desire to retain farmland in the southern area of the city, to maintain an adequate water supply, and to coordinate roads, schools, and other necessities with population growth. At times, this plan has been challenged legally, and growth has gotten out of control.

Other Appointed and Elected Officials. Voters also elect constitutional officers for the city who protect the interests of the commonwealth. These include the commonwealth's attorney, the commissioner of revenue, the clerk of circuit court, the city treasurer, and the sheriff.

School and Public Health. The superintendent of schools is appointed by the school board and in the past the board was appointed by the city council. In 1992, this was changed, and the voters now elect the school board. These positions are for 3 years. The budget for the schools is prepared and administered by the school administration and approved by the city council.

The public health activities of Rudyville are directed by the Rudyville health director, the administrator, the nurse manager, and the environmental health manager, all of whom are state employees. Although part of their budget is received from Rudyville, they are also accountable to the state.

Issues Influencing Health. Several issues that influence health have been addressed in Rudyville over the last 5 years. The first involves access to health care. The state legislature mandated an assessment of health care access and plans to solve the problem, if appropriate. This assessment was completed, but access to health care remains a problem. A potential solution was proposed that allowed nurse practitioners greater leeway in providing primary care in Rudyville, but this has not been resolved. Consequently, many people are without health care, as was discussed earlier.

A second issue affecting health involves the local water supply. Water is currently purchased from a neighboring community and is in short supply. Consequently, residents have been on restrictions for 4 years. The city council proposed piping water from a distant source, but lawsuits from a variety of groups have delayed this project. The council continually returns to this plan as the least costly solution to the problem. Considerable tax dollars have been spent on legal battles.

A third area affecting health is a law passed that requires parental notification when minors request treatment for sexually transmitted diseases. It is believed by some that this law will delay treatment and increase the spread of those diseases.

Another issue, passed recently, that will affect health is Chapter 28.5 of the Code of Rudyville regarding smoking in public buildings and restaurants. This law forbids smoking in public buildings and requires separate rooms in restaurants for smoking and nonsmoking patrons.

Another issue passed 2 years ago by the city council that affects health is the provision to allow in-line skating on the same walkway that is used by pedestrians at the oceanfront. This has resulted in injury to pedestrians. Another law passed recently forbids the throwing of balls and other objects at the oceanfront. This law was passed following injuries to some tourists.

RECREATION SUBSYSTEM

One source of recreation is swimming and water sports. Rudyville has 38 miles of shoreline, 28 miles of public beaches, and 79 miles of scenic waterways.

There are 51 miles of bike trails throughout Rudyville. These run parallel to some highways and to the walkway along the oceanfront. Unfortunately, some bicyclists prefer to ride on the walkway with pedestrians, and some have been injured. Law enforcement looks the other way when these laws are broken. In addition, some areas of the city do not have bike trails, and bicyclists ride in the roads, presenting potential hazards.

In-line skating and skateboarding are other sources of recreation for the younger crowd. In-line skates can be rented and are allowed on the walkway by the ocean along with pedestrians. This has also resulted in some pedestrian injuries. Skateboards are not allowed at the oceanfront, and neither skateboards nor in-line skates are allowed on any other city street. Again, the police force usually does not enforce this law. Ball playing at the oceanfront is another form of recreation that was recently prohibited by law. However, this law is not enforced by the police.

The city has the following parks for walking or riding: 2 state parks, 1 regional park, 3 national wildlife refuges, 7 district parks, 5 community parks, and 161 neighborhood parks. These are located throughout the community. There are also six recreation centers in the city with swimming pools, ball courts, and activity rooms. These centers charge a fee and thus are not available to all community members. Likewise, the centers are inaccessible to those without cars. In addition, the city offers 210 tennis courts throughout the area and

10 golf ranges. Large city parks and all recreation centers have personnel available during activity hours. The city also has a series of waterways for the boating enthusiast. These wind throughout the city.

The city has a parks and recreation plan that has identified current and future planned waterways, bike trails, nature walks, and parks. This plan is widely publicized.

RELIGIOUS SUBSYSTEM

Rudyville has 16 Protestant churches (92%), 10 Catholic churches (5.5%), and 4 Jewish synagogues (2.5%). The Protestant religion is very strong, and the Rudyville Protestant Complex houses a church, a religious-oriented university, and a television station. Two other religious churches incorporate schools within their complex. These include a progressive church called "On the Rock" and another run by the Quakers.

Some churches have also become involved in local, state, and national politics by supporting selected candidates and organizing members into voting blocks locally and nationally. Thus, they hold a position of power.

The major religious leaders in the local community are Father Day at the Catholic Church of Divinity (422-2234), Rabbi George at the Beth Shalom Synagogue (422-0002), Reverend Kunstmann at the Lutheran Church (422-4223), Reverend Patrice at the Rudyville Protestant Complex, Reverend Shone at the "On the Rock" Church (422-2314), and Reverend Otto at the Rudyville United Methodist Church (422-4786).

TRANSPORTATION SUBSYSTEM

The international airport is less than 1 mile from the city line and services seven major airline carriers to all parts of the United States with connections to Europe. Short- and long-term parking is available at this facility.

Bus transportation is available for local and long-distance travel. One station near the oceanfront is available for long-distance bus travel out of the area. The local bus service, Rudyville Transit Services, is limited primarily to the northern, heavily populated part of the city. The southern area of the city, which has farmland and some residences, has fewer bus services. For those in the northern section of Rudyville, bus transportation is adequate and passes the hospitals, the health and welfare center, and the oceanfront, although buses run infrequently except during rush hours. They do not pass many of the recreation centers.

Of the residents in Rudyville, 90% use private transportation, and there has been a large increase in traffic on the highways. Between 1982 and 1988, there was an increase of 57,350 cars on the local highways. Many people work in adjacent communities and travel alone to work and back. Road building has not kept pace with population increases. Consequently, the limited roads are packed to capacity during rush hours. The city and state established high-occupancy vehicle (HOV) lanes for autos with two or more passengers during rush hours, but these lanes are usually not crowded. This was an attempt to get individuals to double up for commuting, but it has been largely unsuccessful. In 1990, 82% of the commuters traveled alone. An increase in traffic accidents has occurred with the increase in traffic.

TABLE 6.9 Population Numbers and Percentage of Increase: Rudyville, Virginia, and United States

Population Unit	1986	1991	Percentage of Increase
Rudyville	336,500	406,100	20
Virginia	5,795,000	6,286,000	8
United States	241,096,000	252,177,000	4
Population Unit	1986	1995 (Projected)	Percentage of Increase (Projected)
Rudyville	336,500	439,427	30.6
Virginia	5,795,000	6,551,559	13
United States	241,096,000	261,478,000	08.4

WELFARE SUBSYSTEM

The agency responsible for welfare is the Rudyville Social Services Department, located adjacent to the Rudyville Health Department at 21 James Street in the central part of the city. It is accessible by public transportation. It serves all of the city and offers the following programs: Aid to Families With Dependent Children, food stamps, medical assistance, short-term general relief, fuel assistance, and employment interviews. Interviews for various programs are conducted from Monday to Friday mornings on a first-come, first-served basis.

The social services programs are state supervised, locally administered, and funded by federal, state, and local funds. Section 63.1-43 of the Commonwealth of Virginia Code empowers the director of social services to carry out the functions of social services. The Rudyville code requires social services to have an advisory board consisting of five members appointed by the city council. This board acts in an advisory capacity to the director of social services.

In addition, many churches have food pantries that supply food to needy families and thrift stores that offer free clothing to the needy. The Rudyville homeless shelter offers a free meal daily, clothes-washing, and showering facilities. Addresses for these facilities can be found in a publication titled *Resources for Low Income and Homeless Individuals and Families*.

Welfare Needs. Identified shortages in Rudyville include housing and medical care. For every homeless family accepted in the local homeless shelters, three are turned away. Some of these sleep in cars and in the woods within the city. It is estimated that about 1,000 people are without shelter. In addition, many are without health insurance, as discussed earlier.

POPULATION SUBSYSTEM

Population Numbers and Changes. Population numbers for Rudyville, the state, and the nation for 1986 and 1991 and percentage increases are shown in Table 6.9. In addition, projected numbers and percentage increases for 1995 are included.

TABLE 6.10 Rudyville Population's Age Distribution in 1980 and 1990, Numbers and Percentage of Change

Age	1980 Number	1990 Number	Percentage of Change
Under 5	20,316	34,801	+71.1
5 to 14	45,123	59,807	+32.5
15 to 19	26,434	27,553	+04.2
20 to 34	110,584	126,279	+14.2
35 to 49	48,830	83,620	+71.2
50 to 64	28,449	37,825	+32.9
65 to 79	9,685	19,104	+97.2
80+	2,229	4,110	+84.4

SOURCE: Data from the census bureau.

TABLE 6.11 Virginia Population's Age Distribution in 1980 and 1990, Numbers and Percentage of Change

Age	1980 Number	1990 Number	Percentage of Change
Under 5	360,686	443,155	+22.0
5 to 14	818,575	822,892	+00.5
15 to 19	505,674	438,556	−13.3
20 to 34	1,458,832	1,660,554	+13.8
35 to 49	1,300,555	1,363,753	+04.9
50 to 64	763,302	793,978	+04.0
65 to 79	409,776	525,920	+28.3
80+	95,532	138,550	+45.0

SOURCE: Data from census bureau.

On January 1, 1993, the population in Rudyville was 410,607, showing an increase of 12,307 in 2 years. These figures would seem to be within the projected range in Table 6.9 of 439,427 for 1995. The projected population in Rudyville for the year 2000 is 500,000 people. A summary of the population numbers and increases for Rudyville by 10-year increments follows: 84,215 for 1960, 172,106 for 1970, 262,199 for 1980, and 393,069 for 1990. Increases for each 10 years are 87,891 (104%) for 1960 to 1970, 90,093 (52.35%) for 1970 to 1980, and 130,870 (50%) for 1980 to 1990.

Population Density. The population density was 1,565 people per square mile in 1992, based on a population of 404,822 people and 258.7 square miles of land. This could be contrasted with population densities of 156 per square mile in Virginia, 79 per square mile in Lise County, which is 40 miles away, and 1,410 for the total metropolitan area surrounding Rudyville.

Age Distribution of Population. The age distribution of the Rudyville population in 1980 and 1990 compared with the state of Virginia is shown in Tables 6.10 and 6.11. The median age in Rudyville in 1990 was 28.9, compared

TABLE 6.12 Age Distribution of Population for Rudyville and Virginia, 1990

Age	Rudyville		Virginia	
	Number	Percentage of Total	Number	Percentage of Total
Under 5	34,801	08.8%	443,155	07.1
5-14	59,807	14.7	822,892	13.3
15-19	27,553	07.0	438,556	07.0
20-34	126,279	32.1	1,660,554	26.8
35-49	83,620	21.3	1,363,753	22.0
50-64	37,825	09.6	793,978	12.8
65-79	9,685	02.5	525,920	08.5
80+	4,110	01.0	138,550	02.2

with that for the state (32.6) and for two areas adjacent to Rudyville, Lise County (33.6) and Devon (33.8).

The percentages of the population in each age group in Rudyville in 1980 and in the state in 1990 are presented in Table 6.12.

Sex and Race Distribution of Population. The population distribution by race for 1980 and 1990 is presented in Table 6.13. The population distribution by race and sex for 1990 is presented in Table 6.14 for 1990.

Vital Statistics. The following are some of Rudyville's vital statistics, along with state and/or national comparisons.

Birth rate: In 1990, there were 7,260 live births (18.5 live births per 1,000 population) in Rudyville and 96,777 live births (15.6 live births per 1,000 population) in Virginia.

Infant mortality rate: Rudyville's infant mortality rate per 1,000 live births (all races, urban and rural) was as follows: 13.4 in 1988, 11 in 1989, 9.4 in 1990, and 12.8 in 1991. Virginia's infant mortality rate was 10.1 in 1988, 10.2 in 1990, 10 in 1991. The U.S. infant mortality rate was 8.9 in 1991. These rates are all above the *Healthy People 2000* goal of no more than 7 deaths per 1,000 live births (U.S. DHHS, 1991, p. 368).

Infant, neonatal, and fetal mortality rates by race: In Rudyville, mortality rates for whites in 1980 were infant, 14; neonatal, 11; and fetal, 13.5. In 1990, the rates were infant, 10.5; neonatal, 9.9; and fetal, 8.8. Because Rudyville is primarily an urban area, these rates are compared with the urban rates for Virginia, which for whites in 1980 were infant, 11.9; neonatal, 8.4; and fetal, 11.4. In 1990, these had decreased to infant, 8.3; neonatal, 5.5; and fetal, 7.3. The U.S. rates for 1980 for whites were infant, 11.5; neonatal, 7.9; and fetal, 8.2. For 1990, these rates were infant, 7.7; neonatal, 4.9; and fetal, 6.3.

The Virginia rates for blacks in 1980 were infant, 20.9; neonatal, 15.2; and fetal, 16.1. In 1990, these rates has been combined with rates all other nonwhite races for rates of infant, 18.4; neonatal, 13.7; and fetal, 17.1. Rates for all others in 1980 were infant, 19.6; neonatal, 14; and fetal, 15.2.

TABLE 6.13 Population Distribution by Race for Rudyville and Virginia, 1980 and 1990

	1980			
	Rudyville		Virginia	
Category	Number	Percentage	Number	Percentage
White	226,788	85.5	4,229,798	78.4
Black	26,291	09.9	1,008,668	18.7
Hispanic	5,160	1.9	79,868	1.5
Asian	6,570	2.5	66,209	1.2
Other	633	0.2	9,454	0.2
Total	265,442	100.0	5,393,997	100.0
	1990			
White	316,408	78.1	4,791,739	75.5
Black	54,671	13.5	1,162,994	18.3
Hispanic	12,137	3.0	160,288	2.5
Asian	17,025	4.2	159,053	2.5
Other	4,965	1.2	73,572	1.2
Total	405,206	100.0	6,347,646	100.0

TABLE 6.14 Population Distribution for Rudyville, by Race and Sex

Category	Number	Percentage of Total
White male	161,502	39.9
White female	154,906	38.2
Black male	29,253	7.2
Black female	25,418	6.3
Asian male	7,893	1.9
Asian female	9,132	2.3
Hispanic male	2,462	0.6
Hispanic female	9,675	2.4
Other male	2,506	0.6
Other female	2,459	0.6
Total	405,206	100.0

The U.S. rates for blacks in 1980 were infant, 18.2; neonatal, 11.7; and fetal, 13. In 1990, these rates were combined with all others to make infant rates of 19.4; neonatal, 12.8; and fetal, 13.1. All other rates in 1980 were infant, 14.9; neonatal, 9.4; and fetal, 12.4.

Births of low-birth-weight infants: Low-birth-weight infants in Rudyville for 1991 numbered 521 and made up 7.2% of the live births. This is more than

TABLE 6.15 Suicide Rates (per 100,000 Population) in Virginia, 1975 and 1986, by Selected Ages

Age	1975	1986
15-24	13.6	13
25-34	16.3	17.9
35-44	19.8	16.8
45-54	30.8	16
55-64	25.6	20.3
65-74	25.6	22.6
Total[a]	15.3	14

a. Compare with total suicide rates for Rudyville: 18 per 100,000 in 1975 and 25 per 100,000 in 1986.

TABLE 6.16 Suicide Rates (per 100,000 Population) in Virginia, by Year and Race

Year	White	Nonwhite	All
1950	13.1	4.2	11.1
1960	14.0	5.1	12.2
1970	13.9	5.9	12.4
1980	15.3	6.4	13.4
1986	25.0	6.9	14.0

the state or national percentages. It is also higher that the *Healthy People 2000* goal of no more than 5% of live births.

Legal abortion rates: For Rudyville for 1985 and 1991, respectively, there were 35.4 and 34.4 legal abortions per 1,000 births. These rates were higher for blacks than for whites: 55.8 to 30.0 in 1985 and 47.5 to 25.3 in 1991.

Social Problems. One social problem is illegitimate births. In the United States in 1980 there were 178.1 illegitimate births per 1,000 live births for all races. In 1990, this rate had increased to 280.3. In Rudyville the 1980 rate was 156, and the 1990 rate was 180. A breakdown for the rate in the United States in 1980 by race showed 101.5 for whites, 554.6 for blacks, and 486.5 for all other races. These rates were all higher in 1990: 200.7 for whites; 652.3 for blacks; and 555.3 for all other races (Department of Commerce). A comparable difference showed up in the Rudyville data: In 1980, rates were 90 for whites, 490 for blacks, and 420 for all other races, and in 1990, rates were 150 for whites, 540 for blacks, and 480 for all other races. The Virginia rate for 1990 was 260.4 for all races, 151 for whites, 612.8 for blacks, and 552.8 for all other races (Center for Health Statistics, 1990).

Another social problem is sexually transmitted diseases (STDs). Rates in Rudyville for primary and secondary syphilis were 17 per 100,000 in 1980 and 23.2 per 100,00 in 1990. Rates for all stages of syphilis were 36.2 in 1980 and 53 in 1990. The U.S. rate for primary and secondary syphilis was 12.06 per 100,000 population in 1980 and 18.07 in 1990. The rate for all stages of syphilis was 30.51 in 1980 and 44.94 in 1990.

TABLE 6.17   United States and Rudyville Rates (per 100,000 population) of Selected Communicable Diseases, 1980 and 1989

Disease	1980		1989	
	United States	Rudyville	United States	Rudyville
AIDSᵃ	(2.38)	(3.4)	13.58	16.24
Hepatitis A	12.84	9.4	14.43	11.12
Hepatitis B	8.39	7.4	9.43	8.20
Measels	5.96	9.2	7.33	12.20
Mumps	3.86	3.9	2.34	2.30
Rubella	1.72	1.6	0.16	0.10
Tuberculosis	12.25	18.25	9.46	14.20

a. AIDS data in parentheses are for 1981.

TABLE 6.18   Percentages of Rudyville Population Immunized for Specific Diseases, by Age

Disease	Under 2	2 to 5	5 to 15
Diphtheria	30	65	98
Polio	30	65	98
Smallpox	36	70	98
Tetanus	40	70	98
Measles	30	60	98
Whooping cough	30	65	98

Gonorrhea was also a social problem of concern. In Rudyville the rate was 621.22 per 100,000 in 1980 and 398.21 in 1990. The U.S. rates were 444.99 per 100,000 in 1980 and 297.36 in 1990.

Suicide is another social problem of concern. The rates for 1975 and 1986 in Virginia by age and for 1950 to 1986 by race appear in Tables 6.15 and 6.16. Rates in Rudyville were higher than the state rates at 18 per 100,000 in 1975 and 25 per 100,000 in 1986. These rates showed comparable rises in all age groups and also an increase in each time period for both racial groups with the higher rates in the white population.

Communicable Diseases. Communicable disease rates for selected diseases in the United States and Rudyville for 1980 and 1989 and immunization levels in Rudyville appear in Tables 6.17 and 6.18.

Leading Causes of Death. The leading causes of death by rate for the United States and Rudyville for 1980 and 1990 appear in Table 6.19.

Selected Wellness and Health Promotion Behaviors. The wellness behaviors of the population were assessed by surveys, interviews, and secondary data. The following results were identified: 25% of children aged 6 and over participate

TABLE 6.19 Death Rates per 100,000 Population, by Leading Causes of Death in the United States and Rudyville, 1980 and 1990

	1980		1990	
Cause of Death	United States	Rudyville	United States	Rudyville
1. Diseases of the heart	236.0	250.0	289.5	298.0
2. Malignant neoplasm	183.9	180.0	203.2	198.2
3. Cerebrovascular disease	75.1	78.0	57.9	62.2
4. Accidents	46.7	50.0	37.0	40.0
5. Cardiopulmonary disease	24.7	23.0	34.9	30.2
6. Pneumonia and influenza	24.1	22.0	32.0	30.0
7. Diabetes mellitus	15.4	20.0	19.2	24.2
8. Chronic liver disease	13.5	11.2		
8. Suicide			12.4	16.2
9. Atherosclerosis	13.0	13.0		
9. Chronic liver disease			10.4	10.0
10. Suicide	11.9	13.8		
10. HIV infection			10.1	14.2

regularly in physical exercise for 30 minutes a day; 30% of the population under the age of 20 are regular smokers; police reports show that 80% of the children under the age of 4 are in seat belts and child safety seats; and 20% of the adolescents aged 12 to 19 and 30% of adults over the age of 20 are overweight.

HEALTH SUBSYSTEM

Hospital and Nursing Home Bed Occupancy. There are adequate beds for medical, surgical, maternity, psychiatric, communicable disease, chronic disease cases, and nursing homes in Rudyville as determined by the ratio of beds to population compared with national standards. In addition, there are no waiting lists for admission. However, there are limited rehabilitation beds, and patients needing rehab must travel to surrounding communities.

Ambulance Services. There is adequate and quick ambulance service in Rudyville. The ambulances respond within 15 minutes to most parts of the community, and patients arriving in an ambulance are seen immediately at local emergency units.

Occupational Health Services. Industries in the local area employ occupational health nurses full-time and have physician supervision available. Nurses are prepared at advanced levels and offer a variety of nursing services at all levels of prevention.

School Health Services. School health services were discussed earlier. Because the schools are served by public health nurses from the Rudyville

Health Department who have additional responsibilities, the services to schools are limited. Thus, school services, as discussed earlier, are inadequate.

Health Department Services. As discussed earlier, health department services are being reorganized by a new health director. Many of the services previously offered to low-income families are being transferred or discontinued. Prenatal and infant supervision for those with Medicaid has been transferred to private doctors, and care for those without insurance is limited. In addition, there have been increased efforts to take some preventive screening into the community to reach the population better. This service needs to be expanded. In addition, there has been a shortage of health care for residents without health insurance since the health department closed its medical clinic on January 1, 1996. Because of limited budgets, communicable disease follow-up has been reduced and there is an increase in tuberculosis. There has also been an increase in AIDS, STDs, and suicide. Thus, these services are inadequate. The reader should also review the city budget in relation to health department and other expenditures.

Health Care Staffing. Throughout the city, positions in hospitals for physicians, nurses, social workers, psychologists, aides, and physical therapists are mainly filled. However, to save money, hospitals have reduced the number of budgeted positions for nurses and increased the number of aides. As a result, they have moved away from primary care to an approach in which everyone (people in housekeeping, aides, nurses, dietary personnel) provides some care that was previously performed by nurses. All caregivers wear white uniforms, so it is difficult for clients to determine whether they are nurses or not. Concerns about this pattern of providing care have been expressed by directors of nursing, the state board of nursing, and others.

At the health department, there is a shortage of nurses (discussed previously) and a shortage of environmental health specialists. There have been more rabies cases and more hepatitis outbreaks in restaurants, and no-smoking codes in restaurants are seldom enforced because of a shortage of environmental staff.

COMMUNITY DYNAMICS AS THEY AFFECT THE POPULATION

FIRE PROTECTION

Fire protection in Rudyville is adequate. There is one fire station, located near the oceanfront. This station has four trucks and trained personnel. It may take up to 30 minutes to reach a fire in the most distant part of the city.

POLICE PROTECTION

There are adequate numbers of policemen in Rudyville, and they usually respond quickly to robberies and other emergencies. Less urgent calls, such as barking dogs at night, are answered more slowly. In addition, some laws are rarely enforced, as mentioned earlier. These include laws about activities along the walkway at the oceanfront and on the city streets, such as using skateboards, using in-line skates, and playing ball. For this reason, police services are inadequate. The city has received awards over the last 5 years for being a city with a low rate of crime.

HEALTH SERVICES

These services were rated inadequate. See health department services above.

ENVIRONMENTAL SERVICES

These services are rated inadequate and were discussed briefly above regarding the increased incidence of rabies and hepatitis outbreaks due to a lack of adequate inspections of restaurants and personnel. In addition, waterways are polluted by industries and periodically are closed to fishermen who depend on them for their livelihood. Air pollution has also been a problem, and the city has been put on warning by the federal government. Most of the pollution is from automobiles, but some is from wood- and coal-burning stoves and from the burning of leaves and trash.

TRANSPORTATION SERVICES

These services (buses, taxis, airplanes) are rated adequate, but roads for private automobiles are inadequate and have not kept pace with the increased population numbers. There have been increased numbers of auto accidents, and the frequent stop-and-go traffic during rush hours is frustrating to motorists. Also discussed earlier was a statement by the director of disaster for Rudyville stating that only about 25% of the population would be able to leave the area during a hurricane because of the limited number of roads in relation to the population.

OTHER COMMUNITY SERVICES

Other community services such as social services, community nursing services, ambulance services, hospital services, and educational services were discussed earlier.

EXCHANGES WITH THE NONHUMAN ENVIRONMENT

HOUSING

Rudyville's Housing and Neighborhood Preservation Department has outlined comprehensive strategies to aid in the preservation of housing and to protect health. Census data indicate that the median rent in Rudyville was $484 in 1990. The average utility bill was more than $75 per month. A citywide survey in 1990 by the Rudyville Department of Housing showed that 79% of all housing was standard and 21% was substandard (deficient, deteriorated, or dilapidated). The distribution of housing types in Rudyville is 57% single-family units, 13% townhouses, 1% trailers, 3% duplexes, and 26% multifamily units.

Two organizations provide shelter for the homeless: the Rudyville Christian Homeless Shelter and the Rudyville Samaritan House. These church-sponsored shelters house up to 250 people each year and provide a variety of services to help this population become self-sufficient. However, about 700 people are turned away each year and live in the woods, cars, or other temporary quarters.

Records of housing complaints are not kept by environmental health. Thus, data are not available on numbers and types of complaints.

SANITATION

Air Pollution. Some air contaminants were discussed earlier. In addition to smoke and smog pollution, which were discussed, pollens are an ongoing problem to many in the population every spring and fall. Rudyville is considered to be one of the worst areas of the United States for allergies. Sources of air and water contaminants include industry, vehicles, and homes.

Water Supply. All homes in the northern half and 80% in the southern half of Rudyville are supplied with city water. Others have wells, which along with city water are adequately treated. Because of water shortages and restrictions, many homeowners have dug wells for watering lawns and washing cars. These are regulated by environmental health specialists from the health department, and in 1992 more than 3,400 applications for permits were received.

Sewage and Solid Waste Disposal. The same homes with city water also have sewage disposal. All others have septic tanks. Sewage is adequately treated, and septic tanks are inspected periodically.

Vector Control. Mosquitoes are a problem locally because of the multiple lakes, which are breeding areas. Because of reduced staffing and increased demands, spraying is currently done when requested rather than periodically. This service is inadequate. Rodent control is adequate.

Food Sources. There are more than 1,300 food service permits that require supervision. Because of limited staffing, some restaurants are inspected yearly, whereas others may be inspected more frequently. In addition, multiple oceanfront activities open to the public that serve food require food inspection. As a result of workload and limited personnel, there have been hepatitis and other food-borne outbreaks. This service is rated inadequate.

EXCHANGES BEYOND THE COMMUNITY

Periodically, the community is threatened by outbreaks of influenza and other communicable diseases. At such times, community health nurses organize mass immunization clinics. Thus, this service is adequate. No ongoing threat to the community from other communities, the state, or nation is evident. In addition, resources have been provided by the state and nation on an ongoing basis as well as when needed for epidemics or other disasters.

SURVEYS

Because of the length of this chapter, survey data from Rudyville have been excluded. Survey data would be useful for assessing attitudes and opinions about health concerns and health services and will be discussed in Chapter 7.

Case Study 3

Community Assessment and the Energy Theory

CHRISTINE ELNITSKY

An assessment of a rural county was conducted to obtain information concerning the health care needs of the population and to assist the community in mobilizing resources to achieve maximum wellness (Turner & Chavigny, 1988). The community assessment instrument that was used reflected each of the interdependent subsystems of the community as well as epidemiological measures: *Community Nursing Assessment Guide* (Helvie, 1991). Informant interviews, participant observation, windshield survey, photographic method, and secondary analysis of existing data were combined to provide a holistic picture of the community from the perspective of the people who live and work there (Stoner, Magilvy, & Schultz, 1992).

TOPOGRAPHY AND CLIMATE

Peaceful, quiet creeks meander through rich farmland, extensive pine forests, and scenic marshland in the serene county. According to state documents, the county lies in the northeastern United States on generally flat land with elevations ranging from 20 to 80 feet above sea level. The climate is generally mild, with an average annual temperature of 60 ° and average annual rainfall of 40 inches.

HISTORY

One of several original English shires, the county is predominantly rural, having been farmed since the early 1600s ([Anonymous] Planning Council, 1993). Most of the land in the county is still in agricultural use. The county contains two small incorporated towns.

The first census of the county totaled 50 colonists ([Anonymous County], 1993). A committee of safety was established in the late 1700s. A volunteer fire department was chartered in 1940 ([Anonymous County], 1993). Several major hurricanes and discharge of toxic pesticides took severe tolls on the county's fishing industry ([Anonymous County], 1993).

The county's comprehensive plan set a goal of preserving the rural character and small-town charm, yet the area demographic statistics reveal developmental pressures characteristic of an area changing from rural to suburban in nature ([Anonymous] Planning Council, 1993). Self-reliance, close-knit families, and adherence to tradition are values reflected among long-time residents. The historical roots of the county are apparent in the strong cultural values of independence and self-responsibility.

BOUNDARIES

The county has an area of 300 square miles, of which approximately 50% is farmland ([Anonymous County], 1993) and 25 miles is shoreline ([Anonymous County], 1993). The county is bounded by four other communities and on one side by a river ([Anonymous] Planning Council, 1993).

SUBSYSTEMS

ECONOMIC SUBSYSTEM

Employment distribution data reveal that manufacturing provides 60% of all jobs in the county. According to the State Employment Commission, the unemployment rate in the county (6.7) is higher than that of the state (5.1) and has been higher since 1985 ([Anonymous] Planning Council, 1993). More than one third of the county's working adults commute to jobs outside the county. Principal industries include meat processing, fine paper products, lumber, and manufacturing.

Family income data reveal that the county's poverty percentage rate (14.4%) exceeds that of the state (11.8%). Poverty levels by age group data reveal that those 65 and over have the highest percentage poverty rate (21%), which is also higher than the state rate for this age group (14%). Less than 10% of households receive public assistance income (U.S. Bureau of the Census, 1990).

County budget summaries reveal a concerted effort to improve and expand educational facilities in this growing community. More than 70% of budgeted expenditures for 1993-1994 were for education.

Financial institutions include 11 banks and 1 savings and loan where deposits totaled $180 million in 1992 (Anonymous, personal communication, October 1994). Retail sales have increased in the last 5 years, according to the County Office of Economic Development. Drug sales have increased 160%. Food and general merchandise sales have increased 35% and 34%, respectively.

EDUCATION SUBSYSTEM

Three private and eight public educational facilities exist in the county. Enrollments in public schools revealed show a 4% increase in student population over the last 3 school years.

A small community college has a branch campus in the county that offers associate in arts and sciences programs and continuing education. Five 4-year colleges are within commuting distance of the county. Educational levels of the population were reviewed in 1990 census data, which revealed that fewer adults in the county (48%) are high school graduates than in the state (65%). Median educational level is 11.8 years.

No health personnel training facilities exist in the county. In other words, the county has no medical, nursing, dental, physical therapy, or social work educational institutions.

COMMUNICATIONS SUBSYSTEM

Two daily and two weekly newspapers provide communication in the county. Although the papers do not have health reporters, they cover health issues as broad general information, and as special local health issues occur, they are covered as hard news. Only one radio station originates from the county—one that broadcasts Christian programming. Regional radio stations are available to county residents. No television stations originate in the county. Telephone service commenced in the county in the late 1880s and continues to date ([Anonymous County], 1993). Residents are isolated from the neighboring communities in the region because all telephone calls outside the county are in extended-calling areas requiring additional telephone charges each minute. The county has eight U.S. Post Offices. Communication subsystems do not provide regular preventive health education, and no evidence of a speakers bureau for health topics was identified.

Informal communications systems include bulletin boards in post offices, public health departments, local churches, and the county courthouse. Hand-delivered fliers placed in rural mailboxes are another source of information.

Word of mouth is also a valuable informal communication mechanism.

A branch of the American Red Cross, an exercise and fitness program conducted by the Young Men's Christian Association, and the Commission on Aging provide limited active health programs in the county. County schools have integrated health education into core instruction as a part of science and physical education classes, in accordance with state-mandated health education curricula (Anonymous, personal communication, September 1994). An 18-member school health advisory board is active in health issues related to the school population (Anonymous, personal communication, September 1994).

POLITICAL SUBSYSTEM

A board of supervisors has been the principal governmental agency of the county since the late 1800s ([Anonymous County], 1993). The two incorporated towns have a council-manager form of government. Three members of the current board of supervisors were Democrats and two were Republicans.

Major issues influencing the community's health in the past 5 years include the planning and implementation of connections of various regions of the county to a countywide sewer system. Previously, the majority of residents depended on septic systems. Another issue of importance is a contiguous telephone calling area. State legislation has been introduced to initiate a trial study allowing calls to the region outside the county to be designated as local calls. The inadequate supply of primary care providers has also been an issue of concern for some time. The county was designated a medically underserved area due to the high population-to-provider ratio (> 3,500:1). Although the state is examining the issue, the county remains in need of an estimated 7 to 10 full-time equivalent primary care providers ([Anonymous] Health District, 1991).

RECREATION SUBSYSTEM

The county has a public beach and four boat marinas, a golf course, six tennis courts, two swimming pools, seven ball fields, a museum of county history, a skating rink, three camp- grounds, a wildlife refuge, fishing and hunting clubs, and five parks. Self-guided tours and unsupervised sports with shelters and public restrooms are available at most locations. The county recreation department offers classes in aerobics, dance, martial arts, and tennis for a fee.

RELIGION SUBSYSTEM

There are 75 churches in the county, including one that dates back to the 15th century ([Anonymous County], 1993). Baptists constitute the largest single group of Christians in the county, with 27 churches. In addition, there are 37 Black churches in the county ([Anonymous County], 1993). Time limits did not permit a survey of church members and church sponsorship of health-related activities. The Christian Outreach Program (COP), a coalition of 25 different churches, operates in the county, raising funds for fuel assistance, housing rehabilitation projects, free dental clinics for eligible seniors, and food and holiday gift programs.

TRANSPORTATION SUBSYSTEM

The county has 500 linear miles of roadways (primary, secondary, and dirt) with no interstate or frontage roads. Some roads are only 18 to 20 feet wide, most lack shoulders, and the majority are unlit. There are no painted crosswalks in the heavily populated regions of the county.

Transportation systems to aid the population in reaching health facilities do not exist in the county. The 1990 census revealed that 23% to 32% of county residents are without a vehicle for transportation. Approximately 10% are disabled in terms of mobility and self-care (U.S. Bureau of the Census, 1990).

Local interviews suggested that transportation to health services is a major problem for senior citizens. Area Agency on Aging services are limited due to the availability of only one nurse. The Disability Services Board is addressing the issue of transportation, yet past attempts have not met with success (Anonymous, personal communication, October 1994). Low population density (80 persons/square mile) and long distances between residences and health service locations compound the transportation problem.

WELFARE SUBSYSTEM

State supervised and locally administered social services are provided to county residents in need. Most programs are based on income and resource needs of applicants. Financial assistance includes Aid to Families With Dependent Children, Aid to Dependent Children, general relief, auxiliary grants program, Medicaid, food stamps, and a fuel assistance program. Screening, assessment, information, and referral are provided. For example, referrals are made from Social Services to COP for adults eligible for the dental program administered by the COP (Anonymous, personal communication, October 1994).

Social programs are also provided: family services, child and adult protective services, adult services, employment services, adoption, foster care, and in-home companion care for older adults (Anonymous, personal communication, October 1994).

FAMILIES SUBSYSTEM

The population of the county was 25,053 in 1990, with the majority of the population (53%) located in the northern part of the county. The county's population density (80 persons/square mile) is considerably lower than that of the state (160 persons/square mile) or a neighboring city (1,583 persons/square mile), reflecting its rural character. Changes over the past three decades have resulted in population growth ranging from 6% to 18% per decade in the county. These changes met or exceeded growth in the state. It is important to note that state Employment Commission population projections suggested an expected 22% increase in county population by the year 2000.

There were more than 9,000 households in the county in 1990. Of these, 31% included individual residents living alone. Of those living alone, 61% were females (U.S. Bureau of the Census, 1990). Families accounted for 7,087 (78.5%) of the households, and 3,685 (52%) of these had children under 18 years old. Of the families with children under 18, 20% were headed by females without a husband present. Households with elderly persons accounted for 30% of the total households.

The median age in the county (33.7 years) is higher than that of the state (32.6 years) ([Anonymous State] Employment Commission, 1993). The median age for males is 32.8 years; for females, 34.6 years.

Age Distribution. Age distribution of the population is depicted in Table CS6.1. Of county residents, 28.5% are under 19 years old, 20.9% are 5 to 19 years old, and 11.4% are 65 and older. The proportion of the population that is 65 and over is higher than for either the state (10.7%) or the region (9.0%). Like many nonmetropolitan communities (Krout, 1994), the county has a dependency ratio (66%) almost double that of the state (38%).

Race Distribution. In 1990, the county was 67.8% white and 32.6% nonwhite, compared with the state's race distribution of 77.4% white and 22.5% nonwhite and the nation's race distribution of 80% white and 20% nonwhite (see Table CS6.2). Females accounted for 51% of the total population, 53% of the nonwhite population, and 50% of the white population in 1990 ([Anonymous State] Employment Commission, 1993).

Vital Statistics. Data reveal that the 1992 general mortality rate in the county (8.8/1,000 population) was slightly higher than its 1980 rate (8.7), higher than the district rate (7.1), and higher than the state rate (7.9). Clarification of this statistic would require indirect adjustment of rates by age and by race, which was beyond the scope of this assessment.

Infant mortality rates per 1,000 live births from 1986 to 1990 revealed that the county (12.5) had a higher rate than the state (10.3) but lower than the district (13.4). Data from 1992 revealed that resident infant mortality rates for the county (10.8) have improved, although state (15.6) and district (21) rates have not improved (Table CS6.3).

Social Problems. Although the County Sheriff's Department, a town police department, and the State Highway Patrol all provide services to the county, data on social problems are incomplete due to fragmented information sources and inadequate time for combining all information sources. Interviews revealed that an

TABLE CS6.1   Age Distribution, by Gender, in the County, 1990

Age	Total N	Percentage	Male (N)	Female (N)
Under 5	1,906	7.6	1,020	886
5-9	1,877	7.5	961	916
10-1	1,715	6.8	854	861
15-19	1,658	6.6	886	772
20-24	1,506	6.0	752	754
25-29	2,157	8.6	1,034	1,123
30-34	2,315	9.2	1,156	1,159
35-39	2,109	8.4	1,034	1,075
40-44	1,809	7.2	890	919
45-49	1,607	6.4	822	785
50-54	1,314	5.2	653	661
55-59	1,169	4.7	579	590
60-64	1,103	4.4	540	563
65-69	983	4.0	444	539
70-74	776	3.1	327	449
75-79	518	2.1	195	323
80-84	307	1.2	93	214
85+	224	1.0	60	164
Total	25,053	100	12,300	12,753

SOURCE: U.S. Bureau of the Census (1990).

TABLE CS6.2   Gender and Race Distribution in the County and State, 1990

Race		County N	Percentage	State N	Percentage
White					
	Male	8,493	50.0	2,361,921	49.0
	Female	8,482	50.0	2,429,818	51.0
	All	16,975	67.8	4,791,739	77.4
Nonwhite					
	Male	3,807	47.0	672,053	48.0
	Female	4,271	53.0	732,566	52.0
	All	8,078	32.6	1,395,619	22.5

SOURCE: [Anonymous State] Employment Commission (1993).

estimated 6,500 calls for service are answered each year by the Sheriff's office alone, and trends suggest increases in property crimes over the last 6 years. Current levels were homicides 2 per year, assaults 10 per month, burglaries 11 per month, and larcenies 21 per month. Interviews suggested that the property crime rate is related to an increasing drug problem in the county

TABLE CS6.3 Vital Statistics Rates per 1,000 Population

Category	County		District	State
	1980 N (rate)	1992 N (rate)	1992 N (rate)	1992 N (rate)
Live births	293 (13.2)	371 (14.8)	19,346 (19.1)	96,725 (15.6)
Neonatal deaths	1 (3.4)	2 (5.4)	168 (8.7)	603 (6.2)
Infant deaths	3 (10.2)	2 (5.4)	241 (12.5)	903 (9.3)
Maternal deaths	0	0	1 (0.05)	3 (3.1)
General deaths	189 (8.7)	221 (8.8)	7,372 (7.1)	49,023 (7.9)

SOURCE: [Anonymous State] Department of Health (1993).

TABLE CS6.4 Reported Communicable Disease Cases, by Year

Disease	Number of Cases Reported	
	1981	1991
Aseptic meningitis	—	1
Brucellosis	9	—
Campylobacter infections	—	5
Chicken pox	2	—
Hepatitis		
Type A	1	1
Type B	0	0
Nonspecific A and B	—	1
Unspecified	1	0
Salmonellosis	15	3
Shigellosis	0	2
Tuberculosis	4	2
Typhus Fever	1	0

SOURCE: [Anonymous State] Department of Health (1983, 1993).

(Anonymous, personal communication, October 1994).

Prevention is provided in drug interdiction programs such as DARE, run by the Sheriff's office in the county schools. Community neighborhood watch programs are increasing in popularity, as is the use of home security systems (Anonymous, personal communication, October 1994).

In addition, domestic violence calls are increasing (Anonymous, personal communication, October 1994). A local shelter in a neighboring town anticipated bringing services closer to the county residents through future expansion. The shelter plans to include a transition house in the county.

Health Problems. The communicable disease incidence in the county was recorded for 1981 and 1991 for comparison purposes, and these rates are presented in Table CS6.4. Incidence of brucellosis, chicken pox, tuberculosis, typhus, and nonspecific hepatitis have decreased. Reports on sexually transmitted reveal a rate of 0.17 cases per 1,000 population. Of these, 47% were chlamydia, 38% were gonorrhea, 11% were syphilis, and 3.6% were HIV or AIDS.

TABLE CS6.5   Cause-Specific Crude Death Rates, by Location, 1991 (Rates per 100,000 Population)[a]

Cause of Death	County N (rate)	District N (rate)	State N (rate)
Diseases of the heart	75 (299)	2,850 (278)	15,687 (253)
Malignant neoplasms	55 (220)	1,856 (181)	11,979 (194)
Accidents	13 (52)	289 (28)	2,139 (35)
Cerebrovascular disease	10 (40)	454 (44)	3,297 (53)
Chronic obstructive pulmonary disease	8 (32)	288 (28)	2,004 (32)
Diabetes mellitus	6 (24)	162 (16)	880 (14)
Septicemia	5 (20)	100 (10)	650 (11)
Pneumonia and influenza	4 (16)	214 (21)	1,706 (28)
Chronic liver disease and cirrhosis	4 (16)	90 (9)	585 (8)
Suicide	4 (16)	121 (12)	784 (13)
Atherosclerosis	3 (12)	43 (4)	331 (5)
All other diseases	19 (76)	623 (61)	4,737 (77)

SOURCE: [Anonymous State] Department of Health (1993).
a. Ranked in order of rate in county. Major cardiovascular diseases are broken down by type.

Immunization Levels. Retrospective records review of children entering kindergarten revealed that only 65.7% of county students are adequately immunized by 24 months of age for diphtheria, pertussis, and tetanus; polio; and measles, mumps, and rubella ([Anonymous State] Department of Health, 1994). National objectives call for 90% of 2-year-olds to be adequately immunized (U.S. Department of Health and Human Services [DHHS], 1991).

Data on levels of influenza immunization show that the state's average rate for those 65 years and over in 1993 was 41.4% ([Anonymous State] Division of Communicable Disease Control, 1994). The health district in which the county lies had a reported average immunization rate in the 45% to 59% range.

Leading Causes of Death. The top four leading causes of death in the nation and the state in 1991 were diseases of the heart, malignant neoplasms, cerebrovascular disease, and accidents, ranking first to fourth, respectively ([Anonymous State] Department of Health, 1993). However, vital statistics reveal that the county had a slightly different order of ranking, with diseases of the heart, malignant neoplasms, accidents, and cerebrovascular disease ranking first to fourth, respectively (Table CS6.5).

Proportionate mortality ratios reveal that 7 of 10 deaths in the county in 1991 were due to diseases of the heart (34%), malignant neoplasms (25%), accidents (6%), and cerebrovascular disease (5%). Comparisons of 1981 and 1991 rates reveal an increase in the proportionate mortality ratios for each of the top four causes of death in the county. Both accidents and cerebrovascular disease proportionate mortality ratios doubled in that decade.

The majority of fatal accidents in the county (85%) were motor vehicle accidents. This percentage was almost double that of the state motor vehicle accidental deaths (44.7%) ([Anonymous State] Department of Health, 1993).

A comparison of death rates reveals that county rates were 14% to 65% higher than state or district rates in 6 of the top 10 causes of death. County rates were higher for diseases of the heart (14%), malignant neoplasms (15%), suicide (26%), nephritis (21%), diabetes (41%), accidents (46%), septicemia (51%), and atherosclerosis (65%). These diseases comprise both acute and chronic illnesses.

A comparison of rates also reveals major differences in the rates between white and nonwhite populations within the county. Nonwhite rates of death by cause were higher for all causes except four. White death rates were higher for chronic obstructive pulmonary disease, pneumonia and influenza, chronic liver disease and cirrhosis, and suicide.

HEALTH SUBSYSTEM

Hospital and Ambulatory Services. There are no hospitals or emergency care facilities in the county. Three regional hospitals are within driving distance of the centrally located county courthouse: 26 miles, 23 miles, and 27 miles. Two regional facilities provide outpatient medical centers in the county. Outpatient services include obstetrics and gynecology; cardiology, echocardiography, and vascular testing; orthopedics; urology; ophthalmology; plastic surgery; and psychiatry. Availability of services is limited to daytime business hours and by the fact that specialty physicians are scheduled for a specific day of the week. A 24-hour on-call emergency service is available (through one local physician's private practice), but may require 30 minutes or more to arrive after being called (Anonymous, personal communication, September 1994).

Nursing Home Services. There is one nursing care facility, offering 30 private adult residential care rooms for assisted living and short-term stay services in the county. The 95-bed facility is intermediate care, with no skilled-care beds. Of the 95 beds, 91 are private pay, with 8 people on a Medicaid waiting list for space available in the facility.

Occupational Health Services. Two manufacturing plants offer clinic health programs but no formal occupational health programs. One manufacturing plant has an occupational health program with two full-time staff and one ambulance. The Cooperative Extension Office offers educational services, including pesticide training programs for workers to properly protect themselves from occupational health risks.

School Health Services. The county public schools has five full-time equivalent school nurses on staff for 4,500 students in eight different schools. The ratio of staff to students is 1:900. General services include screening, special service referrals, and medication administration per physician orders. Special services include catheterizations, tube feedings, colos-

tomy care, chest physiotherapy, and oxygen administration (Anonymous, personal communication, September 1994). Emergency first-aid, cardiopulmonary resuscitation, and injury care are provided as needed.

Health Department Services. The resource mothers program uses lay workers, women from the community, to provide support and advocacy for pregnant teens. The women, infants, and children (WIC) program provides vouchers for nutritional food packages for medically and financially at-risk pregnant women and children up to 5 years old. The baby care program provides nutritional counseling, homemaker services, education, and home health care to high-risk pregnant women and infants and children ([Anonymous] Health District, 1993).

In addition, control and follow-up are provided for communicable diseases, sexually transmitted diseases, and tuberculosis. Blood pressure and cholesterol screening and counseling and pregnancy testing are also provided ([Anonymous] Health District, 1993).

The Area Agency on Aging provides homebound clients skilled services, respite services, and nursing visits to those aged 60 years and over who have chronic diseases but do not qualify for skilled home health ([Anonymous] Health District, 1993). Nursing clinics are provided at three community locations.

Child health clinics and children's speciality services, family planning clinics, immunization clinics, and personal care services are provided as well ([Anonymous] Health District, 1993). Environmental health services include sewage disposal permits and water sample testing, restaurant and school cafeteria inspections, rabies control programs, and protection of shellfish growing areas ([Anonymous] Health District, 1993).

Community Health Nursing Agencies. Only one home health agency is located in the county. With a total of six full-time employees, this agency provides services to 60 to 70 clients with duration of services ranging from one visit up to 2 years of visits (Anonymous, personal communication, October 1994).

Residents and community professionals identify the shortage of home health care for seniors as a major problem. "Many of these elderly people fall through the cracks" (Anonymous, personal communication, October 1994). Many residents do not qualify for Medicaid, do not have other third-party insurance, and do not have family members to assist them with living on a daily basis.

COMMUNITY DYNAMICS AS THEY AFFECT FAMILIES

PROTECTION

Five volunteer fire departments provide fire protection, but information on the number and type of calls was not available because of competing demands on fire department personnel time. Volunteer fire personnel in the county make their income by other means, such as farming. At the time of the assessment, personnel were working at harvesting crops (Anonymous, personal communication, October 1994). Police protection was discussed in the section on social problems.

Health services are inadequate according to residents and professionals. Although the range of available services has improved over the last 3 to 4 years, some services remain unavailable to county residents. For instance, there is no emergency care facility in the county.

Environmental services are limited and do not include adequate testing for groundwater contamination, vector control programs, or record-keeping systems that allow comparison and trending. Transportation systems are nonexistent. Social services are inadequate in the area of in-home companion care as evidenced by the 60-person waiting list for these services (Anonymous, personal communication, October 1994). Community nursing services are inadequate due to the low number of agencies providing services within the community.

Ambulance services are inadequate. Of all answered rescue calls in 1993, 70% were answered by the squad in the northern region of the county. Yet resources available to this squad are limited and disproportionate to the level of demand for services when compared with demand and resources for the squad in the southern region of the county.

In addition, rescue squad response times are too long (45 minutes), and sometimes no one is available to respond to a call (Anonymous, personal communication, October 1994). Routing

of 911 calls is slow and restrained due to jurisdictional concerns.

Hospital services are inadequate because there are no hospitals in the county. Residents must travel 23 to 27 miles to reach the nearest hospital, where staff members are not socialized to the county or its residents. As previously stated, transportation barriers also existed.

EXCHANGES WITH THE NONHUMAN ENVIRONMENT

HOUSING CONDITION

Of housing units in the county, 77% are in nonfarm areas (U.S. Bureau of the Census, 1990). Although there is a county building inspections department, there is no housing authority in the county. Thus, classification and tracking of standard and substandard housing is not conducted. In addition, 2% to 3% of housing units in the county have incomplete plumbing facilities (U.S. Bureau of the Census, 1990).

SANITATION

Residents complain of air contaminants whose sources are industry and farming. These include an occasional odor originating from a neighboring paper mill and a more frequent, sporadic odor originating from pig farms in the county.

WATER SUPPLY

The state environmental engineering field office reports that the county has approximately 60 separate groundwater systems. Owners of these sources include the county and private individuals (Anonymous, personal communication, September 2, 1994). Of housing units, 48% have water supplied by the county-owned public system.

No information database of sanitary survey test information exists, only separate, individual records of test results. Groundwater-monitoring reports suggest some pollution, and its most probable source is unlined lagoons located on area pig farms (Anonymous, personal communication, October 1994). Fluoride levels range from 3 to 5 parts per million, a concentration that exceeds the Environmental Protection

Agency guidelines of 2 parts per million. Sodium occasionally exceeds the maximum limits (20 mg/liter), sometimes reaching 100 to 120 mg/liter (Anonymous, personal communication, September 1994).

SEWAGE AND SOLID WASTE DISPOSAL

Sewage systems are present in the two incorporated towns, and extension of the district sewer system is in the process of development for the northern area of the county. Solid waste disposal is in the process of changing from a system of strategically located green Dumpster boxes to a permanent structure system managed by the regional Public Service Authority.

VECTOR CONTROL PROGRAM

Environmental health sanitarians in the county provide only advisory assistance related to control of rodents. The local Public Health Department does not sponsor a vector control program in the county (Anonymous, personal communication, November 14, 1994). The county funds only one control program—for gypsy moths.

FOOD AND MILK

Inspections are conducted by sanitarians at the 64 restaurants with permits in the county. No major outbreaks of food-borne illness have been reported (Anonymous, personal communication, November 14, 1994).

EXCHANGES BEYOND THE COMMUNITY

A perceived health threat is the nuclear power plant in a neighboring county (Anonymous, personal communication, November 1994). State Department of Health, Radiological Health Division environmental assessments show that the county maintains a radon level below the standard guideline value of 4 picocaries/liter recommended by the Environmental Protection Agency (Anonymous, personal communication, September 26, 1994).

Health resources in the region include four area universities for health and social welfare professionals who could serve the county. Students from these universities attend clinical experiences in the county and region. A local community college campus exists in one town of the county. A neighboring county has a free health clinic, intended to provide medical and dental services to indigent clients from the county and surrounding areas.

SUMMARY OF COMMUNITY HEALTH

Despite the general picture of serenity and health, several health-related concerns and potential threats to the community were identified through the analysis of assessment data. Based on the inferences of the analyses, these concerns are presented in the following community diagnoses. Diagnoses are listed according to Helvie's Community Health Nursing Theory (Helvie, 1991).

1. *Community energy deficit related to high accidental mortality* due to (a) unlit, narrow secondary roadways without paved shoulders; (b) an inefficient 911 communication system; (c) the volunteer nature of EMS/rescue squad; (d) long EMS response times or failure to respond; and (e) rapid population growth unaccompanied by commensurate growth in EMS resources, resulting in motor vehicle accident mortality rates higher than state or national rates and motor vehicle accident rates higher than *Healthy People 2000* (U.S. DHHS, 1991) target rates.

2. *Community energy deficit related to high general and specific mortality rates* due to (a) an inadequate supply of health care providers, (b) insufficient availability of health services, (c) a large and growing older and dependent population, (d) the lack of transportation systems, (e) the low educational level of the population, and (f) increased poverty, resulting in general and specific mortality rates that are higher than state and national rates and mortality rates higher than *Healthy People 2000* (U.S. DHHS, 1991) target rates.

3. *Community energy excess related to perceived biological hazards in the environment* due to (a) the lack of mandated testing for pesticides, (b) inefficient record-keeping systems on water tests,

(c) the lack of speakers bureau on health topics and preventive health education in local community, resulting in possible groundwater contamination and high rates in 6 of the top 10 causes of death.

4. *Community energy deficit related to potential increase in the incidence of communicable disease* due to (a) a probable decrease in the level of herd immunity, (b) the low level of immunizations in the population, (c) an inadequate supply of health care providers, (d) the low educational level of population, and (e) the lack of knowledge of available services and resources, resulting in low levels of influenza and pneumonia immunizations among children entering kindergarten and low levels of influenza and pneumonia immunizations among older adults.

REFERENCES

[Anonymous County]. (1993). *Historical notes on [Anonymous] County.* [Anonymous] County: County Board of Supervisors.

[Anonymous County] Planning Council. (1993). *Needs assessment of [Anonymous] County: Vol. 2. Demographic analysis.* [Anonymous City, Anonymous State]: United Way.

[Anonymous] Health District. (1991). *Senate joint resolution: Primary care needs assessment.* [Anonymous City, Anonymous State]: Department of Public Health.

[Anonymous] Health District. (1993). *Your local health department: Caring for you in your home.* [Anonymous City, Anonymous State]: Author.

[Anonymous State] Department of Health. (1983). *1981 State vital statistics annual report.* [Anonymous City]: Center for Health Statistics, Division of Vital Records and Health.

[Anonymous State] Department of Health. (1993). *[Anonymous State] 1991 vital statistics annual report.* [Anonymous City, Anonymous State]: Department of Health, Center for Health Statistics.

[Anonymous State] Department of Health. (1994). *1993 retrospective school enterer survey report 4-3-1.* [Anonymous City]: Author.

[Anonymous State] Division of Communicable Disease Control. (1994). *Memorandum to district directors.* [Anonymous City, Anonymous State]: Department of Health.

[Anonymous State] Employment Commission. (1993). *Population projections 2010.* [Anonymous City]: Author.

Helvie, C. O. (1991). *Community health nursing: Theory and practice.* New York: Springer.

Krout, J. A. (1994). *Providing community-based services to the rural elderly.* Thousand Oaks, CA: Sage.

Stoner, M. H., Magilvy, J. K., & Schultz, P. R. (1992). Community analysis in community health nursing practice: The GENISIS model. *Public Health Nursing, 9,* 223-227.

Turner, J. G., & Chavigny, K. H. (1988). *Community health nursing: An epidemiological perspective through the nursing process.* Philadelphia: J. B. Lippincott.

U.S. Bureau of the Census. (1990). *1990 Census of population and housing: Summary population and housing characteristics.* Washington, DC: U.S. Department of Commerce.

U.S. Department of Health and Human Services. (1991). *Healthy people 2000.* Washington, DC: Government Printing Office.

REFERENCES

Anderson, E. T., & McFarlane, J. (1996). *Community as partner: Theory and practice in nursing.* Philadelphia: J. B. Lippincott.

Barnett, R. (1994). *Using the 1990 U.S. census for research.* Thousand Oaks, CA: Sage.

Berentson, L. (1985). The Orem model applied to community assessment. In Z. Higgs & D. Gustafson (Eds.), *Community as client: Assessment and diagnosis* (pp. 185-194). Philadelphia: F. A. Davis.

Center for Health Statistics. (1990). *Virginia vital statistics: Teenage pregnancies and natural fetal deaths, 1990.* Richmond, VA: Department of Health.

Clark, M. J. (1996). *Nursing in the community.* Stamford, CT: Appleton & Lange.

Clemen-Stone, S., Eigsti, D., & McGuire, S. (1995). *Comprehensive community health nursing* (4th ed.). St. Louis, MO: C. V. Mosby.

Cookfair, J. (Ed.). (1989). *Nursing process and practice in the community.* St. Louis, MO: Mosby Year Book.

Cookfair, J. (Ed.). (1996). *Nursing process and practice in the community* (2nd ed.). St. Louis, MO: Mosby Year Book.

Finnegan, L., & Ervin, N. (1989). An epidemiological approach to community assessment. *Public Health Nursing, 6,* 147-151.

Gordon, M. S., & Kucharski, P. M. (1987). A new look at the community: Functional health pattern assessment. *Journal of Community Health Nursing, 4,* 21-27.

Hanchett, E. (1988). Community assessment according to Roy's adaptation model. In E. Hanchett (Ed.), *Nursing frameworks and community as client* (pp. 61-71). Norwalk, CT: Appleton & Lange.

Hanchett, E. (1989). Nursing models and community as client. *Nursing Science Quarterly, 2,* 67-72.

Helvie, C. (1991). *Community health nursing: Theory and practice.* New York: Springer.

Krieger, N. F., & Harton, M. K. (1992). Community health assessment tool: A pattern approach to data collection and diagnosis. *Journal of Community Health Nursing, 9,* 229-234.

Martin, A. (1988). Community assessment: The cornerstone of effective marketing. *Pediatric Nursing, 14*(1), 50-52.

National Center for Health Statistics. (1992). *Health, United States, 1991.* Hyattsville, MD: Public Health Service.

Neuman, B. (1989). *The Neuman systems model* (2nd ed.). Norwalk, CT: Appleton & Lange.

Orem, D. E. (1980). *Nursing concepts of practice* (2nd ed.). New York: McGraw-Hill.

Polit, D., & Hungler, B. (1993). *Essentials of nursing research: Methods, appraisal, and utilization* (3rd ed.). Philadelphia: J. B. Lippincott.

Roy, C. (1984). *An adaptation model* (2nd ed.). Englewood Cliffs, NJ: Prentice Hall.

Smith, C., & Maurer, F. (1995). *Community health nursing: Theory and practice.* Philadelphia: W. B. Saunders.

Spradley, B. W., & Allender, J. A. (1996). *Community health nursing: Concepts and practice.* Philadelphia: J. B. Lippincott.

Stanhope, M., & Lancaster, J. (1996). *Community health nursing.* St. Louis, MO: Mosby.

Turner, J. (1991). Approaches to the community. In J. Cookfair (Ed.), *Nursing process and practice in the community.* St. Louis, MO: Mosby Year Book.

U.S. Department of Health and Human Services. (1991). *Healthy people 2000: The surgeon general's report on health promotion and disease prevention* (DHHS Publication No. 91-50212). Washington, DC: U.S. Public Health Service.

CHAPTER 7

COMMUNITY ANALYSIS AND COMMUNITY DIAGNOSES

OBJECTIVES

1. Discuss the steps in analyzing community data.
2. Use the steps of community analysis with community data.
3. Evaluate approaches for writing community diagnoses.
4. Use a method to write community diagnoses.

ANALYSIS DEFINED

Although most community health nursing authors discuss analysis of family and community data, few define *analysis.* Anderson and McFarlane (1996) are the exception; according to them, it is "the study and examination of data" (p. 232). This definition is accurate but broad and open to different interpretations about the concepts of study and examination. I would make that definition more specific by defining analysis as the classification, summation, interpretation, and validation of data in order to write nursing diagnoses and establish priorities.

STEPS IN ANALYSIS

During the assessment process discussed and used in two case studies in Chapter 6, a large amount of data was collected. To write nursing diagnoses, these data must be classified, summarized, interpreted, and validated.

CLASSIFICATION

Initially, data are sorted and classified by some system. When a model or theory is used, this classification process is built into the assessment phase and saves time during the analysis. For example, in the Helvie energy theory of community used in Chapter 6, data were classified according to a model of internal characteristics, community dynamics, exchanges with the nonhuman environment, and exchanges beyond the community that was consistent with the theory used. Each of these overall classifications was further broken down into smaller units. For example, internal characteristics of the community included the typography and climate, the history of the community, and the various community subsystems (economic, education, communications, recreation, religion, transportation, welfare, population, and health). These units were further specified for purposes of data collection, and this made classification of data an easy task.

SUMMATION

A second task is to summarize the data by putting them into one of two summary categories on the analysis sheet. These categories are data measurements or statements. Thus, an increase in suicides in Rudyville is a statement, whereas the percentages of unemployment in Rudyville of 2.96%, in Virginia of 3.93%, and in the United States of 4.06% are all measurements.

INTERPRETATION

Interpretation of data often involves comparing a community's data with established standards, state and national statistics, and the community's own statistics for previous years. Collection of comparative data during the assessment phase facilitates this step in analysis. For example, in the community case study in Chapter 6, suicide rates for Rudyville and the state were collected for 1986 and for 1976. These comparison data facilitate interpreting data and making inferences. Otherwise, the nurse must identify the lack of comparative data as a data gap and return to the assessment phase of the process.

In the process of making comparisons, the nurse should first consider the size or magnitude of the problem or concern. For example, an incidence of 130 cases of syphilis per 100,000 population or 0.05 milligrams of lead per liter in the water supply might be sizable problems that warrant attention. A good comparison tool currently is the *Healthy People 2000* (U.S. Department of Health and Human Services, 1991) goals, which establish a standard for the year 2000. For some data, standards are established, such as those for levels of pollutants in air and water, that will determine whether the observations warrant special attention as health issues. For example, what is the acceptable value of lead in the water supply? Does the observed value of 0.05 milligrams of lead per liter exceed safe limits regarding health? Second, the nurse should put the observed magnitude of the problem into perspective by a comparison with past rates to establish trends. Does the incidence of syphilis represent an increase over the last 5 or 10 years? Third, the nurse should compare the observed rate with other communities, the state, or the nation. Is the rate of syphilis in the community higher than that of the state and nation? Is the amount of lead in the water supply higher? Last, the nurse should look at the incidence or condition in relation to structural or demographic variables, such as age, social class, religious group, sex, or geographical area of the community, to specify the inference further.

Such comparisons enable nurses to make inferences—that is, tentative conclusions about the meaning of the data that must be validated for accuracy. For example, an inference might be "a high suicide rate in Rudyville" based on the established goals for the year 2000 and a comparison with state and national rates.

VALIDATION

A part of validation might involve further data collection to resolve gaps or incongruencies in the data. These can be identified as such on the analysis sheets for further action.

Validation of data is necessary to ensure that inferences are correct. Validation data may be collected in a variety of ways. At times, the nurse will need to return to secondary data sources to collect the needed data. At other times, the nurse may wish to solicit input from key community leaders or informants, using either personal interviews or questionnaires. At other times, data for validation may be collected from a sample of recipients of care. For example, if the nurse decides that a service offered by a clinic is inadequate, a sample of the recipients might be surveyed to determine their beliefs about the service. The survey would show that the initial assessment was either correct or incorrect. A sample data validation tool is shown in Table 7.1. This survey would validate or invalidate the nurse's conclusion, from the data collected, that services at the health department are adequate and appropriate.

RUDYVILLE COMMUNITY ANALYSIS

Data collected for Rudyville in Chapter 6 will now be analyzed to demonstrate the concepts of analysis. Following this section, nursing diagnosis, the final step in analysis, will be discussed.

INTERNAL CHARACTERISTICS

TYPOGRAPHY, CLIMATE, AND HISTORY

Table 7.2 shows the summary data and inferences for typography, climate, and history. These data show that Rudyville is a rapidly growing city, has a flat terrain at sea level that creates problems for garbage and trash disposal, has a moderate climate, and has a population influx during the summer. These inferences could easily be validated by a windshield survey and by secondary data.

ECONOMIC SUBSYSTEM

Table 7.3 presents summary data and inferences about the economic subsystem of Rudyville. These data show that a high percentage of the population

TABLE 7.1 A Data Validation Tool for Community Assessment

We wish to evaluate the services of the local health department and would like you to complete the following questionnaire. You do not need to put your name on it. When your data sheet is completed, place it in the box marked "data returns" or mail it to the health department in the attached envelope. Thank you.

Rate the adequacy of the following services on the scale. Put a check under the appropriate rating.

Service	1 (Poor)	2 (Fair)	3 (Good)
Maternity			
Pediatric			
Immunizations			
Adult health			
Communicable diseases			
Chronic diseases (e.g., hypertension, diabetes)			

Would you recommend the service to others?

Service	Yes	No	If Not, Why?
Maternity			
Pediatrics			
Immunizations			
Adult health			
Communicable diseases			
Chronic diseases (e.g., hypertension, diabetes)			

TABLE 7.2 Typography, Climate, and History

Summation/Measurement	Inference
Annual mean temperature, 56.5 °F	Moderate climate
1.8 inches snow annually	Moderate winters
Coastal city subject to hurricanes of increased frequency lately; inadequate roads for evacuation	Disaster potential
Disaster director states that only 25% of the population could be evacuated on present roads in a disaster	
Promoted as a resort with 2.5 million vacationers annually	Population influx in summers
	Seaport
Sea level	Flat terrain
	Garbage and trash disposal problem
Most populous city in Virginia	
Population increased from 125,000 in 1963 to 393,069 in 1990 and is projected to be 500,000 in 2000	Rapid population growth

TABLE 7.3 Economic Subsystem

Statement/Measurement	Inference
Percentage of population over 16 employed: Rudyville 76.8; Virginia: 68.9; U.S. 65.3	High percentage of population working
Percentage employed in armed forces: Rudyville, 13.08; Virginia, 3.48; U.S., 0.89	High military employment
Percentage employed in retail sales: Rudyville, 12.48; Virginia, 10.06; U.S., 10.16	High retail sales employment
Percentage unemployed: Rudyville, 2.96; Virginia, 3.93; U.S., 4.06	Low unemployment rate compared with rates for state and nation
Percentage unemployed: Rudyville, 5.9 in 1992; 2.96 in 1990; 2.4 in 1987	Unemployment increasing
Percentage earning income under $5,000 in 1990: Rudyville, 2; Virginia, 3.1; U.S., 4.	Low percentage of poor families
Percentage earning income over $10,000 in 1990: Rudyville, 96; Virginia, 92; U.S., 90.4	High percentage of more affluent families
Median income in 1990: Rudyville, $39,112; Virginia, $33,328; U.S., $35,225	High median income
Percentage at or below poverty level in 1989 under age 5: Rudyville, 8.5; Virginia, 14.5; U.S., 20.1	Low poverty level for children
Percentage at or below poverty level, Rudyville: 7.7, 1979; 4.6, 1989;	Poverty level decreasing
Percentage at or below poverty level, 1979 and 1989: Virginia: 9.2 and 8.3; U.S., 9.6 and 10	Poverty level decreasing faster than in Virginia and U.S.
Percentage of all families at or below poverty level: Rudyville, 5.9; Virginia, 10.2; U.S., 13.1	Lower percentage of families at or below poverty level than in state and nation
Percentage of female-headed households at or below poverty level: Rudyville, 20.2; Virginia, 26.7; U.S., 31.1	Lower percentage of female-headed households at or below poverty level than in state and nation
Rudyville has 12,000 poor and 13,000 near-poor—88% of whom are without health insurance	Poor and near-poor lack access to health care
1990 report states that 29,000 additional doctor visits are needed annually to provide for the medically indigent	
In 1995, the medical clinic serving 3,000 medically indigent closed	
One free clinic left; has a long waiting list	
Rudyville allocates 0.29% of the city budget to health; two nearby communities comparable in size allocate 3.1% and 2.8%, respectively.	Rudyville allocates more of its budget to schools, police, and public works and less to health, parks and recreation, and libraries than do comparable nearby communities.
Rudyville allocates 1.8% of city budget to parks and recreation; the two nearby communities allocate 2.8% and 3.2%, respectively.	
Rudyville allocates 6.54% of city budget to public works; the two nearby communities allocate 4.2% and 4.0%, respectively.	

TABLE 7.4 Education Subsystem

Statement/Measurement	Inference
More than 50% of city budget is allocated to education	History of mismanagement of school funds
Schools overspent this budget for 2 years; grand jury investigation resulted in some administrators fired and others charged with mismanagement	
74 public and 15 private schools for more than 77,000 students	Adequate number of schools
Additional special and vocational schools	
Four local colleges and 7 additional colleges within 25 miles	
Student-teacher ratio is lower than in schools in surrounding towns	Adequate number of teachers
Health professionals prepared in area colleges for all professions except dentistry	Adequate numbers of locally prepared health personnel, except dentists
58.2% of Rudyville population have at least some college education compared with 47.3% of Virginia population and 48.5% of U.S. population; and only 4% of Rudyville population have under 9 years of education compared with 15.6% of Virginia population and 13.3% of U.S. population	Higher-than-average education level of population

in Rudyville is working and thus that unemployment is low; that the majority are employed in the military, followed by retail sales; that there is a low percentage of poor families; that median income is high; that the population below poverty level is decreasing faster than in Virginia and the United States as a whole; that the poor and near-poor lack access to health care; that a large percentage of the city budget goes to schools, the police, and public works; and that a very low percentage of the budget goes to health, parks and recreation, and libraries. All of these inferences could be validated by secondary data.

EDUCATION SUBSYSTEM

Data on the educational subsystem (Table 7.4) show that there are adequate teachers and schools for the population; that there has been mismanagement in the schools; that there are adequate numbers of health professionals, except dentists; and that the population has a higher-than-average level of education. These inferences could be validated by secondary data and surveys. For example, surveys might be useful to evaluate the adequacy of schools and teachers.

COMMUNICATIONS SUBSYSTEM

Data on the communications subsystem (Table 7.5) show that newspapers have an adequate circulation, that there are adequate mass media communication

TABLE 7.5 Communication Subsystem

Statement/Measurement	Inference
Two major newspapers reach 460,000 adults daily and 550,000 on Sunday	Adequate newspaper circulation; newspapers would be useful for health interventions
Weekly paper reaches 82,655	
One local radio station	Adequate mass communication sources; would be useful for health interventions
Four local television stations	
Two speakers' bureaus; influential community leaders identified	Would be useful for health interventions
Almost no public information on prevention and wellness in mass media; public rates media health coverage as inadequate	Inadequate mass media coverage
Nurses from health department are in schools a half-day to a day per week; they have no time to teach teachers first aid and assessment	Inadequate health education of students and teachers in schools
Some health education classes on hygiene, dental care, nutrition, sick care, and auto and sports safety, but none on other health promotion or prevention and no sex education, first aid classes, or HIV/AIDS and STD education	
Mandatory screening for blood pressure, vision, hearing, and scoliosis	

sources, that health news coverage on wellness and prevention in the mass media is inadequate, and that health education in schools is limited. Surveys would be useful to validate data about health coverage on the TV news and health education in schools.

POLITICAL SUBSYSTEM

Data on the political subsystem (Table 7.6) show that there is an inadequate water supply in Rudyville, that there is a lack of health care for the poor, that there are safety needs for walkers, and that nonsmokers' risk of secondary smoke inhalation has decreased with the passage of nonsmoking laws. Validation data could be collected from secondary data and a windshield assessment.

RECREATION SUBSYSTEM

Summary data and inferences about the recreation subsystem of Rudyville are presented in Table 7.7. These show that some laws are not enforced, creating safety needs for walkers; that there are adequate parks; and that recreation centers are not available to the poor. These inferences could be validated by secondary data and a windshield survey.

TABLE 7.6   Political Subsystem

Statement/Measurement	Inference
Local political division between probusiness/progrowth faction and proresident/slow-growth faction	
Plans for oceanfront shops, malls, amphitheater, sports stadium, additional golf courses	
State-legislature-mandated study showed that many residents lack access to health care; some solutions proposed but not agreed on or implemented	Continuing problem of lack of health care for the poor
No local water supply and residents have been on water restrictions for 4 years	Inadequate water supply
Water is being purchased temporarily from a neighboring city but is limited	
The only option considered by local politicians has been piping water from a distant source, but there are legal complications	
Legislation passed that requires parental notification when minors request treatment of STDs	Law should delay treatment of youths for STDs and raise STD rates
Law passed forbidding smoking in public buildings and restaurants, although enforcement lax	Law may decrease secondary smoke exposure for nonsmokers
Law passed allowing in-line skating on oceanfront walk along with pedestrians	Law should increase pedestrian accidents and injuries

TABLE 7.7   Recreation Subsystem

Statement/Measurement	Inference
Ocean available for swimming	
51 miles of bike trails	
Some bicyclists on roads and walks	Hazards for walkers
In-line skating allowed on pedestrian walkway at oceanfront	
Walkers have been injured	
Lax enforcement of laws	
2 state and 1 regional park	Adequate parks
3 national wildlife refuges	
7 district, 5 community, and 161 neighborhood parks	
6 recreation centers with swimming pool, ball court, and activities: charge a fee, some inaccessible without a car	Recreation centers not available to poor
20 golf courses	
Multiple city tennis courts	

TABLE 7.8 Religious Subsystem

Statement/Measurement	Inference
16 Protestant churches, 10 Catholic churches, and 4 Jewish synagogues	Adequate number of churches for population
Churches involved in politics	
Churches have position of power and are involved in selecting candidates for political offices	Churches are powerful
Church leaders identified	Leaders are resource for surveys, implementation

TABLE 7.9 Transportation Subsystem

Statement/Measurement	Inference
Buses adequate except at rush hour	Public transit adequate except for reaching recreation centers
Buses serve hospital, health and welfare center, and oceanfront; do not serve recreation centers	
90% of population use automobiles	
Increase of 57,350 cars on local roads in past 6 years	Inadequate road system
Increased numbers of auto accidents	
Increased traffic congestion on roads	Increased auto accident

RELIGIOUS SUBSYSTEM

Data on the religious subsystem in Rudyville (Table 7.8) show that there is an adequate number of churches, that churches are powerful, and that religious leaders could be used as a resource for surveys and implementing a community plan. The adequacy of churches could be validated by surveys or personal interviews.

TRANSPORTATION SUBSYSTEM

Transportation subsystem data (Table 7.9) show that public transportation is adequate except for reaching the recreation centers; that roads are inadequate for the increased population; and that auto accidents have increased. The adequacy of mass transportation and roads could be validated by surveys or personal interviews.

SOCIAL SERVICES SUBSYSTEM

Table 7.10 presents summary data and inferences about social services in Rudyville. Inferences show that services are adequate except for housing and

TABLE 7.10 Social Services Subsystem

Statement/Measurement	Inference
Reports identify a shortage of housing and medical care for the poor	Inadequate housing and medical care for poor
Reports estimate 1,000 people without shelter and most of these without health care	
One local social services center, open weekdays, sees clients on first-come, first-served basis	
Short waiting list for services	Adequate accessibility of social services
Center provides all services, including food stamps, Aid to Families With Dependent Children, general relief, fuel assistance, counseling and employment services	
Center located on bus line	

medical care for the poor. These data could be validated by secondary data and interviews or by surveys with clients and with providers in the homeless shelters.

POPULATION SUBSYSTEM

Data on the population subsystem (Table 7.11) show that the population of Rudyville is growing rapidly; that Rudyville is a high-density area; that there are large increases in the population under the age of 5, between the ages of 35 and 49, and over the age of 65; that the largest population is in the 20- to 34-year-old age group and that the median age is lower than the state and nation; that there is a moderate dependency ratio; that population diversity has been increasing; that there are more Hispanics and Asians than in Virginia as a whole; and that the white population is decreasing. The data also show a high birth rate; a high infant mortality rate, which is two times greater in the black population; an increasing neonatal death rate, which is lower than that for the state and which is two times greater for blacks; a high percentage of low-birth-weight babies; a higher black than white abortion rate; an increasing illegitimacy rate, which is lower than that for the state and three times greater in the black population but which shows a decreasing gap between white and black; a high syphilis rate, which is increasing; and a high gonorrhea rate, which is decreasing. Data also show a high suicide rate, which is increasing and is higher in the white population and in those between the ages of 55 and 74, followed by the ages of 25 to 54; a high AIDS rate, which is increasing; a low hepatitis A rate, which is increasing; a hepatitis B rate that is low and decreasing; a high measles rate, which is increasing; a low and decreasing mumps and rubella rate; a high but decreasing tuberculosis rate; a low immunization level in those under the age of 1 and a moderate rate for those aged 1 to 5 and over the age of 15; an increasing and high death rate for diseases of the heart, chronic obstructive pulmonary disease (COPD), diabetes mellitus, suicide, and HIV/AIDS; a low but increasing death rate for malignant neoplasms, pneumonia, and influenza; a high but

TABLE 7.11   Population Subsystem

Statement/Measurement	Inference
Percentage of population increase from 1986 to 1991: Rudyville, 18%; Virginia, 8%; U.S., 4%	Rapid growth of population
Rudyville, 50% to 100% increase in population every 10 years	
Population density in 1990: Rudyville, 1,565 people/square mile; Virginia, 156/square mile; Lise (rural county) 79/square mile; Metro area around Rudyville, 1,410 people/square mile	High population density for area
	Large population increases for groups aged under 5, 35 to 49, and over 65
	Percentage changes in population for all age groups were higher than those for state
	Largest population is in 20- to 34-year-old age group
34% of population under age 19 or over age 65	Moderate dependency ratio
Racial distribution in Table 6.13	Population racial diversity has increased from 1980 to 1990; white population has decreased
	Proportions of population who are Hispanic, Asian, or white are greater in Rudyville than in Virginia as a whole
Median age, 1990: Rudyville, 28.9; Virginia, 32.6; Lise County, 33.6; Devon, 33.8	Median age lower than in state and surrounding communities
Birth rate in 1990 for Rudyville was 18.5/1,000 compared with Virginia's rate of 15.6/1,000	Higher birth rate
Infant mortality in Rudyville, 13.4 in 1988 and 12.8 in 1991 compared with Virginia's rates of 10.1 in 1988 and 10 in 1991	Rudyville infant mortality rate higher than state and *Healthy People 2000* goals
All infant mortality rates above *Healthy People 2000* goal of 7/1,000	
Infant mortality rates by race for 1991 in Virginia were 8.3 for whites and 20.9 for blacks	Black infant mortality more than twice the rate of whites and more than national goal
Rudyville rates were similar	
Black rate above *Healthy People 2000* goal of 11/1,000	
Neonatal rates, 1983 and 1990: Rudyville, 3.4 and 5.4/1,000 live births compare with Virginia, 6.8 and 6.2	Neonatal mortality rate increasing but below state rates
Neonatal rates by race 1980 and 1990: Virginia (1980) W = 8.4 and B = 15.2; (1990) W = 7.5 and B = 15.2	Neonatal rates in blacks more than twice the rate for whites
Similar rates in Rudyville	
Percentage of total births that were low birth weight in 1991: 7.2%, a figure higher than state and *Healthy People 2000* goals	High percentage of low-birth-weight babies
Social Problems	
Legal abortions per 1,000 births, 1985 and 1991 in Rudyville: 35.4 and 34.4; black rate almost double white rate	Higher black than white abortion rates
Illegitimate births per 1,000 live births, 1980 and 1990: Rudyville, 156 and 180 compared with U.S. rates of 178.1 and 280.3	Increasing illegitimate birth rate but lower than that for the U.S.
Illegitimate rate by race, 1980 and 1990	

Statement/Measurement	Inference
U.S. in 1980: white, 101.5/1,000 live births; black, 554.6; other, 486.5	
U.S. in 1990: white, 200.7; black, 652.3; other, 555.3	Black rate more than 3 times white rate, but the gap is decreasing
See discussion in chapter 6 on Rudyville and Virginia	
Venereal disease, primary and secondary per 100,000 for 1980 and 1990: U.S., 12.06 and 18.07; Rudyville, 17 and 23.2	Syphilis rate high in Rudyville
Syphilis, all stages, 1980 and 1990 per 100,000: U.S., 30.51 and 44.94; Rudyville, 36.2 and 53.0	Syphilis rates high in Rudyville and increasing
Gonorrhea rates per 100,000, 1980 and 1990: U.S., 444.99 and 297.36; Rudyville, 621.22 and 398.21	Gonorrhea rates high in Rudyville but decreasing
Suicide: for Virginia, 1975—15.3/1,000; 1986—14/1,000	High suicide rate
Rudyville, 1975—18/100,000; 1986—25/100,000	Suicide rate increasing and higher in white population
Higher rates in all ages and the white population, similar to state	
Rate of 28/100,000 for Rudyville in 1990 is above the goal of 8.2 by *Healthy People 2000*	Suicide rate highest between ages 55 and 74 and then between ages 25 and 54
Health Problems	
Communicable diseases—see Table 6.17	AIDS rate high and increasing
	Hepatitis A rates low but increasing
	Hepatitis B rates low and decreasing
	Measles rate high and increasing
	Mumps and rubella rates low and decreasing
	Tuberculosis rate high but decreasing
Immunization level for acute communicable diseases	
Immunization level below *Healthy People 2000* goal of 90% immunized by age 2	Immunization levels are low for under age 2
See Table 6.1 for immunization status	Immunization levels are at a moderate level for ages 1 through 5 and over age 15
Leading causes of death	
See Table 6.19 for data	The following diseases have high death rates and are increasing: diseases of the heart, COPD, diabetes mellitus, suicide, and HIV infections
	The following diseases have low death rates but are increasing: malignant neoplasms, pneumonia, and influenza
	Death rates are high but decreasing for accidents and CV disease
	Death rates are low and decreasing for chronic liver disease

TABLE 7.12 Health Subsystem

Statement/Measurement	Inference
Adequate numbers of beds—Rudyville, in med/surg, psychiatric, communicable and chronic disease based on ratio of beds to population	Adquate beds for most conditions Shortage of rehab beds
No waiting lists for hospitals	
Limited numbers of rehab beds	
Adequate nursing home beds	
Adequate and quick (within 15 minutes) ambulance service	Adequate ambulance services
Full-time occupational health nurses in industry prepared at graduate level and physician available	Occupational health services are adequate
Nurses from health department in schools for one-half to 1 day a week; limited focus on teaching wellness, prevention, and health promotion	School nursing services are inadequate
Health department services include care for children and pregnant women; some preventive services in community need to be expanded	Inadequate preventive services Inadequate prenatal and child care
Shortage of health care for the medically indigent; deficits reflected in rising rates of TB, AIDS, VD, and suicides; limited budget from city.	Inadequate services for some communicable diseases Inadequate budget to meet health needs
Hospital staffing: most health professional positions filled. Reduced positions for nurses, which were filled by aides to save money.	Nursing care patterns may affect quality of patient care
Everyone (nurses, aides, housekeeping) provides nursing care and all wear white	
Concerns about this by directors of nursing and state board of nursing.	
Health department and environmental health staffing, shortage due to budget limits	Inadequate environmental health services
Increased numbers of rabies cases and hepatitis outbreaks	Increase in rabies and hepatitis outbreaks
Nonenforcement of no-moking laws	Smoking laws unenforced

decreasing death rate for accidents and cardiovascular disease; and a low and decreasing death rate for chronic liver diseases. These data are primarily secondary data and if validation is needed, it could be obtained from other secondary data.

TABLE 7.13 Selected Health Promotion and Wellness Behaviors

Statement/Measurement	Inference
25% of those age 6 and over participate in physical exercise 30 minutes daily. This is below the *Healthy People 2000* goal of 30%.	Inadequate numbers of children and adults exercising
30% of the population under age 20 are regular smokers. This is over the *Healthy People 2000* goal of 15%.	High numbers of smokers in population
80% of children under age 4 are in seat belts and child safety seats. This is below *Healthy People 2000* goal of 95%.	Safety hazards due to nonuse of seat belts
20% of adolescents age 12 to 19 and 30% of adults over 20 are overweight. This is above the *Healthy People 2000* goal of 15% for adolescents and 20% for adults.	Excessive overweight in adolescents and adults

HEALTH SUBSYSTEM

Summary data and inferences about the health subsystem of Rudyville are presented in Table 7.12. Inferences show adequate beds in hospitals for all conditions except rehabilitation; adequate ambulance services; adequate industrial health services, inadequate school health services, and a limited focus on wellness and prevention; inadequate prenatal and child services; inadequate care for the poor; inadequate services for some communicable diseases; an inadequate budget to meet health needs; nursing care patterns in hospitals that may affect the quality of care; inadequate environmental services; increased cases of rabies and hepatitis outbreaks; and lack of enforcement of no-smoking laws. Some data could be validated by secondary sources, and personal interviews and surveys might also be needed.

SELECTED HEALTH PROMOTION AND WELLNESS BEHAVIORS

Inferences from Table 7.13 on wellness and health promotion behaviors in Rudyville are inadequate numbers of children and adults exercising; high numbers of smokers; safety hazards due to nonuse of seat belts for children; and excessive numbers of overweight adolescents and adults. Surveys or personal interviews of a random sample of the community would be useful to validate the inferences.

COMMUNITY SERVICES

Inferences on community services for Rudyville (Table 7.14) are adequate fire protection; inadequate police services despite the low crime rate; inadequate environmental health services, resulting in some preventable diseases and pollution; and an inadequate transportation system, causing stress, increased

TABLE 7.14 Community Services

Statement/Measurement	Inference
Fire—One fire station, services adequate	Fire protection adequate
Police—Adequate numbers of police who respond quickly to emergency but not to nonemergent situations	Police services inadequate
Some laws not enforced. City given awards past 5 years for low crime rates.	Low city crime rate
Environmental health services—increased incidence of rabies, hepatitis outbreaks, minimal inspections of restaurants and personnel. Waterways polluted from industries periodically, and rivers closed to fishermen. Air pollution problematic with pollutants from cars, and coal and wood burning. City was placed on warning from federal government. Failure to enforce smoking ban.	Environmental health services inadequate, resulting in preventable disease and pollution
Transportation—Roads inadequate for population increases. Increased numbers of autos and accidents. Increased frustration due to stop-and-go traffic. Inadequate roads to evacuate the population in a disaster.	Roads inadequate for population Stress due to inadequate roads Potential disaster due to inadequate roads Increased auto accidents
Other community services	Adequate

accidents, and a potential for disaster. These conclusions could be validated with secondary and survey data.

EXCHANGES WITH THE NONHUMAN ENVIRONMENT

Inferences about exchanges with the nonhuman environment in Table 7.15 are that housing in Rudyville is inadequate; sanitation is inadequate; water and sewage treatment are adequate; and food inspection and vector control are inadequate. Survey data would help to validate these inferences.

EXCHANGES BEYOND THE COMMUNITY

Information about exchanges beyond the community (Table 7.16) indicates that the internal response of external threats to the population in Rudyville is adequate and that external services respond and are adequate when needed.

NURSING DIAGNOSIS

The final step in analysis after validating inferences is to write a nursing diagnosis. A nursing diagnosis provides direction for planning.

TABLE 7.15 Exchanges With Nonhuman Environment

Statement/Measurement	Inference
Housing	
Median rent of $484 in 1990.	
City survey in 1990 revealed housing is 79% standard; 21% substandard	Inadequate housing for some
Two organizations provide shelter for homeless: 250 people are provided shelter each year and 700 are turned away.	
Sanitation	
Air—smoke and smog; pollen an ongoing allergy problem; city considered one of worst allergy areas in country; air and water pollution from homes, industry, and vehicles.	Inadequate sanitation
Water supply—All northern area of city has city water and 80% of southern area has; 20% of southern area has wells that are adequately treated. Additional wells for lawns and cleaning.	Adequate water treatment
Sewage and solid waste—All northern homes and 80% of southern homes have city sewage. Others have septic tanks that are treated.	Adequate sewage treatment
Vector control—Mosquitoes problematic; spraying when requested.	Inadequate vector control
Food services—Over 1,300 food service permits needing inspection; limited personnel to inspect. Diseases resulted.	Inadequate food inspection

TABLE 7.16 Exchanges Beyond the Community

Internal response to external threat—Services implemented efficiently and are effective when problems are introduced into and threaten the community, such as a flu epidemic.	Internal response adequate to external threat
External services—External services have responded to external threats and have provided resources. In addition, state and federal government provide ongoing funding for programs such as the lead poisoning prevention program and immunizations.	External services respond when needed and are adequate

DEFINITION

Yura and Walsh (1988) define nursing diagnosis as

the judgment or conclusion reached by the nurse based on assessment data that indicate the potential for or actual human need fulfillment alteration viewed as an excess, disturbed pattern of expression, or a deficit, lack, or limitation for the client as person, family or community. (p. 129)

This definition fits very well with these authors' emphasis on human need theory. The North American Nursing Diagnosis Association (NANDA) redefined nursing diagnosis in 1990 as "a clinical judgment about an individual, family, or community response to actual or potential health problems/life processes" (McFarland, 1993, p. 10).

NURSING DIAGNOSIS CLASSIFICATIONS

Several classification systems for nursing diagnosis have been developed. One is the NANDA system, developed in 1973 and refined frequently since. The initial classification system was directed toward the needs of individual sick patients. This system was criticized for its lack of usefulness with families and communities and its lack of emphasis on health promotion and wellness. It has been broadened in an attempt to make it more useful to community health nurses. Wellness diagnoses have been added but are still inadequate for positive states of health. Ways to address the aggregate or community have included developing a new classification taxonomy similar to the Omaha system, (see below), adding new diagnoses to the NANDA classification, or modifying the existing NANDA system to make the diagnosis applicable to aggregates (Ridenour, 1992). Neufeld and Harrison (1990) say that any approach to aggregate diagnosis should include the aggregate affected, the identified response or health state, the contributing factors, and data to substantiate the diagnosis. As recently as 1994, only one potential aggregate diagnosis had been submitted to NANDA for development. That was "effective community coping" (NANDA, 1994).

A second classification system is the human needs theory nursing diagnosis developed by Yura and Walsh (1988). Although this is easy for most nurses to use because of their background with human needs, it has the same fault as the NANDA system. These include its emphasis on individuals and on sick behaviors, which makes it difficult to use with groups and communities and to address wellness behaviors.

A third classification system is the Omaha system, which uses four categories for identifying individual and family needs: environmental, psychosocial, physiological, and health behavior. This system includes some wellness behaviors and is more useful to community nurses than other systems. However, it also fails to address communities and aggregates.

Helvie (1993) did a survey to determine whether community health nurses use nursing classification systems for making nursing diagnosis with groups and communities. A survey tool was sent to all schools of nursing and all health departments in Maryland, Virginia, and North Carolina ($N = 200$ respondents). Respondents were asked if they used the NANDA, human needs theory, Omaha systems for making diagnosis with groups and communities and, if so, which ones were used. They were also given six aggregate or community situations and asked to write diagnoses for them. Demographic data on the nurse respondents, such as age, type of educational background, and years of practice, were collected. There was a 44% return rate. Results showed that nurses do not usually use the systems, but when they do, they most often use the Omaha system. Nursing diagnoses written for the six situations showed that nurses can write aggregate- or community-focused diagnoses.

DIAGNOSIS USING NURSING THEORY

Although nursing diagnosis classification systems for nursing theories have not been developed, with the exception of the human needs nursing theory (Yura & Walsh, 1988), nursing theories often dictate a format for writing nursing diagnosis. Some of the nursing theories discussed in Chapter 6 for community assessment will be evaluated below for nursing diagnosis.

Anderson and McFarlane (1996) use the Neuman theory of community and develop nursing diagnosis based on a system of joining inferences together. In this system, they use inferences to describe the problem, to list the etiological factors, and to identify the signs and symptoms characteristic of the problem. Thus, a nursing diagnosis using this framework would be "A high infant mortality related to inadequate resources (inaccessible services) as manifest by women delivering without prenatal care or self delivering."

Krieger and Harton (1992) developed an assessment tool called the Community Health Assessment Tool (CHAT), based on Gordon and Kucharski's (1987) 11 functional patterns. Community diagnoses were developed consistent with this model for practice. Using the problem identified above, high infant mortality, the diagnosis for this model would be "Dysfunction in sexuality-reproductive pattern: Higher mortality for Black infants compared to White infants related to under-utilization of community services by the Black population" (p. 233).

Most authors who use the Orem (1980) or Roy (1984) models usually use NANDA diagnosis. Thus, a nursing diagnosis for high infant mortality using Orem's model might be "Self-care deficit in health maintenance related to inadequate information and inadequate resources resulting in high infant mortality that is even higher in the black population." The nursing diagnosis using Roy's model would be the same except that "self-care deficit" would be replaced by "altered health maintenance."

The Helvie energy theory used throughout this book focuses on the concept of energy. Thus, nursing diagnosis would incorporate energy in any diagnosis. The nursing diagnosis for high infant mortality would be as follows:

Community energy deficit related to high infant deaths due to (a) inadequate facilities and manpower to provide prenatal services; (b) inadequate budget for health; (c) lack of time to teach about pregnancy, childbirth, child care, and prevention and health promotion of pregnant women and children (e.g., effects of prenatal smoking, medications, infections, need for exercise and proper nutrition), resulting in

1. A higher percentage of infant deaths than at the state and federal levels
2. A higher infant death rate than the *Healthy People 2000* goal
3. A high percentage of deliveries without prenatal care
4. Twice the infant death rate among blacks
5. A 6- to 8-week waiting period for pregnant women who wish to attend a clinic
6. Lack of awareness of health promotion and preventive activities during pregnancy among 75% of all mothers delivering, as determined by survey data.

FORMAT FOR COMMUNITY NURSING DIAGNOSIS

Although the above approaches to nursing diagnoses are similar, some may be easier for the community nurse to use than others. Thus, the community nurse should use the framework that is comfortable as long as it summarizes the assessment data and can be used for planning services.

There is no one format for nursing diagnosis. However, a diagnosis should include, at least, the problem or condition and the causal factors related to the problem. The problem must be identified, and without the related factors, it would be difficult to plan for solving the problem. For example, the mention of a high infant mortality rate in the example above identifies the problem but does not identify the causal factors that will direct planning. The causal factors of inaccessible services and resources provides direction for planning. Thus, in any assessment, the nurse should also try to determine the basis for the statistics or behaviors assessed. Also a diagnosis frequently includes a statement related to the size or duration of the problem, as in the statement above that 75% of all mothers delivering lack awareness of health promotion and preventive activities during pregnancy.

The format used with the Helvie energy theory is as follows: "There is a community energy balance or deficit (identifies how well the community is doing regarding the particular problem) related to (the problem or behavior and community or aggregate affected), due to (community factors that cause the energy balance or deficit), resulting in (the effect of the balanced or deficit energies on the population)." If any of these pieces are missing, the nurse may need to identify a data gap and assess further to obtain additional data.

Some diagnoses identified in a community assessment may not be amenable to nursing interventions and thus are not nursing diagnoses. Such diagnoses should be shared with the appropriate colleagues for solution when identified.

The energy of the client can be balanced, excessive, or deficient depending on the findings of the assessment. For example, an individual may have excess energy or a deficit in relation to nutrition. However, most diagnoses for the community will describe a balance or a deficit because the focus is on how well the community (all the efforts of the private and public sectors) has prepared for or responded to the community's actual or potential problems. Thus, in the nursing diagnoses of Rudyville below, community energy is deficient with respect to preparation for hurricanes because the community is not adequately prepared for a possible disaster from a hurricane. With respect to the summer population influx, the community's energy is balanced because the community is prepared for and adequately deals with that. Although the community nurse usually does not plan interventions for nursing diagnoses that deal with balanced energies, they are identified so that the positive aspects of community health can be supported. In addition, surveillance must continue so that any change in these areas will be noted.

Some deficits may be identified in a community assessment may not be amenable to nursing interventions and should be shared with and resolved by other disciplines. For example, in the case of Rudyville's inadequate preparation for hurricanes, the nurse might plan to resolve the knowledge deficit of the population and might establish a coalition of community people to encourage better roads for evacuation. However, the deficit in roads would also need to be explained to public works or city officials, who would assume the responsibility for planning.

NURSING DIAGNOSES FOR RUDYVILLE

Selected nursing diagnoses for Rudyville using the Helvie theory are presented next.

TYPOGRAPHY, CLIMATE, AND HISTORY

There is a community energy deficit related to the disaster potential of hurricane destruction to the community population, due to (a) increased frequency of hurricanes on the coast, (b) inadequate roads for evacuation, and (c) a knowledge deficit of the public, resulting in predictions that only 25% (100,000 of 400,000) of the population could be evacuated on present roads in a disaster and findings that only a small percentage of the population knows what to do and where to go in a disaster, as obtained from a survey of a random sample of the population.

There is a community energy balance related to increased population influx in summers, due to the community's proven ability to meet shelter, food, safety, and other population needs.

ECONOMIC SUBSYSTEM

There is a community energy balance related to employment of the adult population, due to the community's ability to provide adequate employment resulting in (a) a high percentage of the population working, (b) a low percentage of poor families, (c) a low percentage of the population below poverty level, (d) a high median income, (e) a high percentage of more affluent families, and (f) low unemployment.

There is a community energy deficit related to inadequate and inappropriate health care for the poor and near-poor, due to (a) a lack of facilities for free health treatment, (b) inadequate knowledge of wellness and prevention, and (c) long waiting lists for the one free clinic, resulting in a large proportion of the 3,000 poor or near-poor without health care, 90% (2,700 people) of this population going to the emergency room for nonemergent problems, and 90% of the poor population being unable to discuss prevention and wellness behaviors.

EDUCATION SUBSYSTEM

There is a community energy balance related to access of the school-age population to public education, due to (a) adequate numbers of schools at all levels and (b) adequate student-to-teacher ratios, resulting in a better-than-average-educated population and adequate numbers of most health professionals prepared locally.

COMMUNICATIONS SUBSYSTEM

There is a community energy balance related to access to daily information on local and world events, due to the community's provision of adequate newspapers and mass media sources, resulting in (a) two major newspapers with a circulation of between 460,000 and 500,000 readers, (b) a weekly paper with a circulation of 82,655, (c) 18 AM and 26 FM radio stations, (d) one local radio station and one university radio station, (e) three television stations and one religious station, and (f) 90% of the adult population who know current events, according to a random sample survey.

There is a community energy deficit related to the lack of information on prevention and wellness for the community population, due to the community's failure to provide adequate health information on wellness and prevention on mass media sources, resulting in (a) no information on prevention and wellness presented on mass media channels, (b) only 10% of the population surveyed being knowledgeable about wellness, and (c) only a small proportion of the population surveyed practicing wellness behaviors.

There is a community energy deficit related to the lack of health information in schools for the school-age population, due to (a) nursing time in schools being limited to 4 hours a week, (b) limited budget for health and health personnel, (c) no other personnel to teach this content, and (d) no information in the school curriculum on health promotion, wellness, sex education, first aid, and sexually transmitted diseases (STD), resulting in (1) only 10% of a random sample of the school population having knowledge in these areas, (2) only 20% of the students sampled participating in ongoing exercise, (3) only 25% of the sample eating nutritious foods, (4) an increase of 3 to 20 cases per 100,000 population for STDs over a 7-year period, and (5) higher rates for STDs in the Rudyville school population than in the state and nation.

POLITICAL SUBSYSTEM

There is a community energy deficit related to a potential severe water shortage for all citizens, due to the community's failure to provide for an adequate water supply, resulting in water restrictions for 4 years, high cost of water to citizens, and pressure applied by the adjacent community that is temporarily supplying water to reduce water consumption.

There is a community energy balance related to exposure to secondary smoke, due to the community's passage of laws forbidding smoking in public buildings and restaurants, resulting in no-smoking sections in all restaurants and no smoking in any public building.

There is a community energy deficit related to safety needs of walkers, due to the community's passage of laws allowing in-line skating on pedestrian walkways, resulting in 20 pedestrian injuries in 1 year.

RECREATION SUBSYSTEM

There is a community energy balance related to recreation and exercise available in parks, due to the community's provision of adequate parks for the population, resulting in parks being accessible and available to all people.

There is a community energy deficit related to safety needs of walkers, due to failure of the police to enforce local laws about prohibiting bicycles, skateboards, and balls in pedestrian areas, resulting in an average of 25 injuries each year for the last 3 years, which represents an increase from no injuries of this kind 5 years ago.

There is a community energy deficit related to indoor recreational activities for the poor, due to lack of free recreation center membership and lack of accessibility to recreation centers by public transportation, resulting in 3,000 people being ineligible for and not participating in recreation center activities.

RELIGIOUS SUBSYSTEM

There is a community energy balance regarding accessibility of religious activities, due to adequate numbers of churches of all faiths located on public transportation routes.

TRANSPORTATION SUBSYSTEM

There is a community energy deficit related to intracity travel and highway safety, due to (a) inadequate roads for the current population, (b) no funds allocated to increase roadways, (c) infrequent testing of drivers, and (d) limited enforcement of speeding laws, resulting in (1) double the amount of time to access work or shopping by automobile; (2) increased stress on the public on highways, according to a survey; (3) increased automobile accidents; and (4) increased car insurance rates.

SOCIAL SERVICES SUBSYSTEM

There is a community energy balance related to social services' meeting most physical needs of the poor, due to the community's provision of adequate social services, resulting in the availability of food stamps, AFDC, general relief, and other programs to all who need them.

There is a community energy deficit related to the lack of housing and health care for the poor, due to (a) inadequate funding for housing and health care, (b) one free clinic for 3,000 poor, (c) one 6-family unit complex for 3,000 poor, and (d) a long waiting list for assistance with housing or health care, resulting in 3,000 people with little or no health care, 25% of the population (100,000 people) living in substandard housing, and 800 people without housing.

POPULATION SUBSYSTEM

There is a community energy deficit related to high infant mortality, due to (a) inadequate facilities and personnel to provide prenatal services; (b) inadequate budget for health care; and (c) lack of time to teach about pregnancy, childbirth, child care, and disease prevention and health promotion for pregnant women and children (e.g., effects of prenatal smoking, medications, infections, need for exercise and proper nutrition), resulting in a (1) higher percentage of infant deaths than for the state and nation, (2) a higher infant death rate than the *Healthy People 2000* goal, (3) a high percentage of deliveries without prenatal care, (4) twice the infant death rate among blacks, (5) a 6- to 8-week waiting period for pregnant women who wish to attend a clinic, and (6) survey results showing that 75% of all mothers delivering are unaware of health promotion and preventive activities during pregnancy.

There is a community energy deficit related to births of low-birth-weight infants, due to (a) an inadequate budget for health care, (b) inadequate facilities and personnel for prenatal care, and (c) lack of information on prenatal care and needs, resulting in a low-birth-weight rate higher than the state and nation and a low-birth-weight rate higher than the *Healthy People 2000* goals.

There is a community energy deficit related to STD rates, due to (a) inadequate funding for health care, (b) a shortage of nurses for treatment and contact follow-up, (c) a lack of knowledge of the public about prevention and treatment of STDs, and (d) a lack of recreational opportunities for some segments of the population, resulting in increased rates of syphilis, gonorrhea, and AIDS in 1990 over 1980; higher rates of STDs than for the state and the *Healthy People 2000* goal; and survey results showing 70% of the population being unaware of prevention and treatment measures.

There is a community energy deficit related to suicide rates in all age groups of the white population, due to (a) inadequate funding of mental health services, (b) inadequate number of mental health facilities, (c) a long waiting list for care, (d) no mental health facilities for the poor, and (e) a lack of community education on how to cope and deal with stress, resulting in (1) only 25% of population being able to identify coping mechanisms and ways to deal with stress, (2) a higher suicide rate than for the state, (3) a higher suicide rate than for the *Healthy People 2000* goals, and (4) a higher suicide rate in 1986 than in 1975.

There is an energy deficit related to the rate of measles in children and the immunization rate for all people, due to inadequate funding for health care personnel and inadequate information on immunizations and prevention provided to the public, resulting in (a) an increase in the measles rate from 9.2 in 1980 to 12.2 in 1990; (b) a rate above the U.S. rate of 7.33 and the *Healthy People 2000* goal; (c) only 30% of the mothers with children under 5 being able to state the importance of immunizations, resources for obtaining them, and diseases prevented by them; (d) immunization level in the community of about 35% for infants under the age of 1, 65% for those under the age of 2, and 60% for those over the age of 15; and (e) immunization levels below the state and the *Healthy People 2000* goals.

There is a community energy deficit related to death rates for cardiovascular disease, COPD, diabetes mellitus, suicide, and HIV/AIDS, due to inadequate health funding for health care personnel to provide treatment and a lack of public education on treatment and prevention of these preventable diseases, resulting in (a) increased rates from 1980 to 1990 for cardiovascular disease (250 to 298), COPD (23 to 30.2), diabetes (20 to 24.2), suicide (13.8 to 16.2) and HIV infections; (b) higher rates in Rudyville than for the United States for cardiovascular disease, accidents, diabetes, suicide, and AIDS; and (c) only 45% of the population knowing prevention and treatment aspects of the listed diseases.

HEALTH SUBSYSTEM

There is a community energy balance related to the availability of hospital beds for most conditions and for ambulance service, due to the community's provision for adequate numbers, resulting in no waiting lists and rapid response to calls and transport to hospital by ambulances.

There is an energy deficit related to the availability of rehabilitation treatment, due to the community's failure to provide rehabilitation beds, resulting in (a) no local rehab beds or services (b) long waiting lists for care outside the community, and (c) travel required to attend rehab facilities.

There is a community energy deficit related to school nursing services, due to an inadequate budget for school nurses, resulting in (a) limited nursing time in schools, (b) no teaching of health promotion and disease prevention, (c) only 25% of the students being knowledgeable about health promotion and wellness, and (d) only 20% of the students practicing wellness behaviors consistently.

There is a community energy deficit related to environmental health services, due to the community's failure to provide adequate personnel for protection against rabies, hepatitis A outbreaks, air and water pollution, and enforcement of nonsmoking and other health-related laws, resulting in (a) an increase from no rabies cases in animals 5 years ago to 10 annually now, (b) a rabies rate higher than that of the state, (c) an increase from no hepatitis outbreaks in restaurants 5 years ago to three annually now, (d) a higher rate of hepatitis outbreaks than that for the state, (e) a pollution level (air and water) above that for the state, (f) the community's being placed on warning by the federal government for pollution levels, and (g) frequent smoking violations in restaurants, as reported on a survey.

HEALTH PROMOTION AND WELLNESS BEHAVIORS

There is a community energy deficit related to exercising in the over-age-6 group, due to the failure of the community to provide education on the need for, benefits of, and ways to exercise, resulting in (a) only 25% of the population over the age of 6 exercising daily for 30 minutes or more, (b) an exercise level in Rudyville below the *Healthy People 2000* goal of 30% and below the state level of 40%, and (c) 85% of the population over the age of 6 being uninformed about the need for, benefits of, and ways to exercise.

There is a community energy deficit related to cigarette and cigar smoking in population under the age of 20, due to (a) the community's failure to provide adequate information on the harmful effects of and ways to stop smoking, (b) limited knowledge of and inadequate facilities for smoking cessation programs, and (c) no information on ways to increase self-esteem and avoid peer pressure, resulting in (1) high numbers of smokers in the population, (2) the percentage of smokers under the age of 20 (30%) being higher than the *Healthy People 2000* goals of 15% and the state percentage of 20%, and (3) 90% of the population under the age of 20 being unaware of the harmful effects of smoking, ways to stop, facilities to assist with smoking cessation, and ways to increase self-esteem, according to a community survey.

There is a community energy deficit related to the failure of parents to use safety seats and seat belts with children, due to (a) the community's failure to provide adequate information about the use and importance of seat belts as a prevention of injury, (b) inadequate resources for purchasing safety seats for low-income families, and (c) a lack of enforcement of seat belt and safety seat laws, resulting in (1) only 80% of children under the age of 4 using seat belts, a figure below the *Healthy People 2000* goals of 95% and the state level of 87%, and (2) 70% of parents with children under the age of 4 being unaware of the importance of seat belts to prevent injury and of resources available to assist with purchase of safety seats.

There is a community energy deficit related to a high percentage of over-weight adolescents and adults, due to the community's failure to provide education about nutrition, dealing with stress and peer pressure, and ways to feel good about oneself, resulting in (a) 20% of the adolescents aged 12 to 19 being overweight and 30% of adults over the age of 20 being overweight, percentages above the *Healthy People 2000* goals of 15% for adolescents and 20% for adults, and (b) inability of 40% of a random sample to discuss proper nutrition, how to deal with stress and peer pressure, and how to develop self-esteem.

COMMUNITY SERVICES

There is a community energy balance related to fire protection, due to the community's adequate provision for this service, resulting in (a) quick response by the fire department to fire calls and (b) no loss of life in fires for many years.

EXCHANGES WITH THE NONHUMAN ENVIRONMENT

There is a community energy balance related to water and sewage treatment, due to the community's adequately meeting this population need, resulting in no waterborne or sewage-related diseases identified over the past 5 years.

There is an energy deficit related to infrequent food and food preparation inspection due to the community's failure to provide adequate numbers of personnel to inspect food establishments on a routine basis, resulting in increased numbers of food-borne illnesses, such as hepatitis.

EXCHANGES BEYOND THE COMMUNITY

There is a community energy balance related to internal response to external threats due to community mechanisms to deal with external threats.

There is a community energy balance related to the response of external services for internal threat due to adequate mechanisms to deal with community needs, resulting in assistance provided when needed by the state and federal government.

REFERENCES

Anderson, E., & McFarlane, J. M. (1996). *Community as partner: Theory and practice in nursing.* Philadelphia: J. B. Lippincott.

Gordon, M. S., & Kucharski, P. M. (1987). A new look at the community: Functional health pattern assessment. *Journal of Community Health Nursing, 4,* 21-27.

Helvie, C. (1993, June). *Use of nursing diagnosis with groups and communities.* Paper presented at the Sigma Theta Tau International Conference, Madrid, Spain.

Krieger, N., & Harton, M. (1992). Community health assessment tool: A pattern approach to data collection and diagnosis. *Journal of Community Health Nursing, 9,* 229-234.

McFarland, G. K. (1993). Nursing diagnosis: The critical link in the nursing process. In G. K. McFarland & E. A. McFarland (Eds.), *Nursing diagnosis and intervention: Planning for patient care* (2nd ed., pp. 10-20). St. Louis, MO: Mosby Year Book.

Neufeld, A., & Harrison, M. J. (1990). The development of nursing diagnoses for aggregates and groups. *Public Health Nursing, 7,* 251-255.

North American Nursing Diagnosis Association. (1994). *Nursing diagnosis: Definitions and classifications.* Philadelphia: Author.

Orem, D. E. (1980). *Nursing concepts of practice* (2nd ed.). New York: McGraw-Hill.

Ridenour, N. (1992, April). *Examples of possible approaches to aggregate diagnoses.* Paper presented at the 10th Conference on Classification of Nursing Diagnoses of the North American Nursing Diagnostic Association, San Diego.

Roy, C. (1984). *An adaptation model* (2nd ed.). Englewood Cliffs, NJ: Prentice Hall.

U.S. Department of Health and Human Services. (1991). *Healthy people 2000: The surgeon general's report on health promotion and disease prevention* (DHHS Publication No. 91-50212). Washington, DC: U.S. Public Health Service.

Yura, H., & Walsh, M. (1988). *The nursing process: Assessing, planning, implementing, evaluating* (5th ed.). Norwalk, CT: Appleton & Lange.

PART IV

COMMUNITY PLANNING AND INTERVENTIONS

CHAPTER 8

PLANNING COMMUNITY INTERVENTIONS

OBJECTIVES

1. Identify the steps in the planning process.
2. Discuss the energy theory in planning.
3. Discuss methods for setting priorities for nursing diagnoses.
4. Discuss community goals, objectives, and planned interventions.
5. Define and differentiate three models of community development.
6. Discuss the major concepts of community development and relate them to planning.
7. Discuss multilevel intervention approaches to community change.
8. Apply planning concepts to Rudyville.

Planning is the step in the nursing process between the nursing diagnosis and nursing interventions. Its purpose is to meet the established needs of the community population effectively by using a logical decision-making process for developing a detailed plan. It has been defined as "the determination of a plan of action to assist clients toward the goal of optimum wellness" (Yura & Walsh, 1988, p. 138). Archer, Kelly, and Bisch (1984) define it as "a collaborative, orderly, cyclic process to attain a mutually agreed-on desired future goal" (p. 14).

STEPS IN PLANNING

Planning consists of several steps: (a) prioritizing the community diagnoses, (b) establishing goals for expected outcomes of interventions, (c) determining objectives to meet the established goals, and (d) determining nursing interventions to meet the objectives.

Some authors describe a health planning process similar to the above process that includes (a) *preplanning and assessment,* which is similar to assessment, analysis, and priority setting; (b) *policy development,* which includes establishing goals, objectives, action plans, and timetables to meet goals, and identifying resources to accomplish the actions and deal with potential obstacles; and (c) implementation and evaluation.

PLANNING AND THE ENERGY THEORY

The purpose of the planning process from an energy theory frame of reference is to assist the community to establish or reestablish a balance of energy (community adaptation toward health) in specific areas. These areas are identified in community inferences in the case study and are later developed into nursing diagnoses as energy deficits. The community problem identified in the "related to" part of the nursing diagnosis identifies the actual or potential problem that is not being adequately cared for by the community. For example, "Community deficit related to high infant mortality" identifies the inadequacy of the community in caring for the problem of infant mortality. A goal related to this diagnosis would be "Establish a balance of energy in the community by decreasing infant mortality." The "due to" part of the diagnosis identifies the specific areas where the community (all parts, public and private) has failed to provide for the identified population adequately, thus causing the deficit. For example, in the "high-risk infant mortality diagnosis" these include (a) inadequate facilities and numbers of personnel to provide prenatal care; (b) inadequate budget for health care; and (c) lack of time to teach about pregnancy, childbirth, child care, and preventive care and health promotion for pregnant women and children.

The way to reestablish a community balance is by developing objectives in relation to the effects of the imbalance on the population or aggregate. These effects are identified in the "resulting in" part of the definition. For example, in the high infant mortality example, the "resulting in" part of the diagnosis includes (a) a higher percentage of infant deaths than the state or nation, (b) a higher infant death rate than the *Healthy People 2000* objectives, (c) a high percentage of deliveries without prenatal care, (d) twice the death rate among blacks, (e) a 6- to 8-week waiting period for prenatal care, and (f) lack of awareness of health promotion and preventive activities during pregnancy among 75% of all mothers delivering, according to survey results.

Objectives should be written in relation to these effects. Thus, one of the objectives related to the knowledge deficit about health promotion might be as follows: "Ninety percent of all mothers delivering in Rudyville will state five health promotion activities within 1 month of delivering." This information could be collected by survey during hospital confinement. For mothers to have this information, interventions should be planned. There are numerous ways to intervene, and the nurse usually selects the best of the alternatives identified. For example, newspaper articles could be written, television or radio programs could be presented, or group discussions could take place in prenatal clinics. It might also be necessary to collect additional community data to identify which of these methods would reach the largest number of pregnant women.

In addition to planning actions identified in the objectives (presented below), one must plan how the actions will be implemented, who will implement each action, who will obtain the needed resources for implementation, when the actions will be implemented, where they will take place, how much time will be involved, how implementations will be evaluated, and who will provide feedback to the community on the accomplishments.

Goals and plans for some additional nursing diagnoses developed for Rudyville will be presented at the end of this chapter. This should assist the reader in using this theory.

PRIORITIZING COMMUNITY DIAGNOSES

It is never possible to work with all identified community diagnoses because of limited resources (personnel, money, time). Thus, it is important to establish a method of prioritizing community diagnoses to determine the order in which they should be addressed.

Several such methods have been proposed. The American Public Health Association (1991) suggests five factors to consider when setting priorities: (a) the extent of community concern, (b) resource availability to deal with the problem (money, personnel, time, equipment, supplies), (c) how solvable the problem is, (d) the need for special education, and (e) whether additional resources and policies are needed.

PRIORITY-SETTING MODELS

HUMAN NEEDS MODEL

Yura and Walsh (1988) suggest a classification system of high, medium, or low priority. Maslow's (1954) hierarchy of needs has also been used as a model for priority setting. Maslow stated that needs exist on a hierarchy and as one set of needs is met, the next set demands attention. The most basic human needs, which are considered to be needs that must be satisfied and that motivate behavior for all people, are physiological needs, such as food, oxygen, physical activity, rest, elimination, water, and sexual satisfaction. The next set of needs consists of safety and security needs, which include needs for sameness, familiarity, and trustworthiness in people, places, events, and things. The next level consists of love and belonging needs, which include needs for affection, warmth, kindness, and consideration in relationships. The fourth level consists of indicators of self-esteem, which include respect, status, prestige, and a good reputation. The last level consists of the need for self-actualization.

If one used this hierarchy to establish priorities, physiological needs would take precedence over safety needs, safety needs would supersede the need for love, and so forth. In a broader sense, physical threats such as actually or potentially life-threatening situations would take precedence over mental and social health problems. Yura and Walsh (1988) have developed nursing diagnoses related to human needs that, theoretically, could be placed within this framework of priority setting.

HANLON'S COMMUNITY PRIORITY SETTING MODEL

Hanlon (Pickett & Hanlon, 1990) proposes another method of priority setting that focuses specifically on community health needs. The model uses the following factors for priority setting of community diagnoses:

1. The magnitude of the problem identified: Problems that affect large numbers of people ordinarily supersede those that affect only a few.

2. The severity of the disease: Diseases that are severe in terms of mortality and morbidity should supersede those that are not; thus, although more people might be identified with the common cold than with tuberculosis, the severity of tuberculosis would give it priority.

3. Existence of sufficient scientific knowledge and techniques for treating and preventing the disease process if it is to be given priority

4. The availability of resources such as money and personnel: The job should be completed with the least amount of time, energy, and money that is consistent with an agreed-on quality of work. If resources are not available to carry out a program, it should not be included, and the priority might be to locate resources to carry out the program later.

5. Readiness of the population for the proposed program: For example, if the plan is to immunize all children under the age of 5 for measles and this is unacceptable to the community, it should not be a priority. Instead, the priority might be to work with the community to determine and remove the blocks to this plan if it is important.

Pickett and Hanlon's formula can be used with these and other factors to set priorities. Although it is directed toward setting community priorities based on medical diagnosis, it is equally appropriate for prioritizing community nursing diagnosis.

Some examples of priorities in Rudyville appear at the end of this chapter with their rationales. Priorities are set using the Pickett and Hanlon method.

ESTABLISHING COMMUNITY GOALS AND OBJECTIVES

Following priority setting, goals should be established for the nursing diagnoses. Goals are broad guidelines and, according to McKenzie and Jurs (1993), do not indicate the way to achieve the desired outcome. At the community level, most goals for primary prevention can be stated in terms of reducing the incidence or prevalence of disease or injury or increasing the numbers or percentage of the population group at the particular time and place who practice a positive health behavior. For example, the nurse might identify a low immunization level in a certain census tract related to a lack of knowledge of the importance of and resources for immunizations on the part of the population. In this instance, the goal might be, "Increase the immunization level of all people (or children under the age of 5 or minority children under the age of 5 or whatever constitutes the identified population at risk) in Census Tract X."

When one is using the energy theory, the emphasis is always on balancing the community energies in the particular area of concern. Thus, in the above example, the goal would be to balance community energies regarding the immunization level of children under the age of 5 in Census Tract *X*.

DETERMINING HOW TO MEET THE GOALS

The "how to" accomplish the goal is described in the objectives. Objectives describe the precise behaviors or changes required to reach each goal. For community nursing diagnoses, objectives would be directed toward the community population or aggregate.

An objective has four basic components: (a) the client, (b) the activities to meet the goal, (c) a time frame for the activities' accomplishment, and (d) a standard. A standard is appropriate only with community activities and usually represents a proportion of the population who will accomplish the activity. For example, considering the potential disaster threat facing Rudyville (see Chapter 7) due to possible hurricanes, inadequate roads, and an uninformed public (only 25% of the population could be evacuated from the city in time to avoid the disaster), a standard of 90% of the population evacuated might be set for the community. Selected goals and objectives will be identified for Rudyville at the end of this chapter.

PROGRAM EVALUATION AND REVIEW TECHNIQUE

Often, when planning takes place over a long time, it is helpful to break objectives into subobjectives and place them on a time axis along with the planned activities related to each. The longest path in terms of time through a network from the beginning to the final objective is the *critical path*. A program evaluation and review technique (PERT) chart allows the planner to evaluate progress at each stage (subobjective) to determine if appropriate progress is being made. For example, a final objective might be, "90% of children under the age of 5 in Rudyville will be immunized by January 31, 1999." If resources such as facilities, equipment, and personnel are unavailable for the activity, obtaining them will make up one set of subobjectives that might include purchasing land and contracting for a building and equipment installation. Time periods would be established for each subobjective: For example, obtaining facilities might take a year. A second set of subobjectives might involve advertising for, interviewing, and hiring personnel. A third set might involve activities to make the public aware of the program. Others could also be identified. Whichever activity took the longest to complete prior to the initiation of the program would be the critical path.

ALTERNATIVE ACTIONS TO MEET GOALS

Another step in planning is a consideration of alternative actions to reach the goal. Following the selection of the best alternative, the nurse arrives at planned interventions. Most of the data for considering alternative possibilities for meeting objectives will be found in the community assessment. Some questions the nurse might consider in relation to the objective of immunizing 90% of the children under the age of 5 might be these: Are adequate facilities available for immunization programs? Are they conveniently located? Are they used? Do parents know about the services? Do they view the services as valuable? Is the population able to pay for the service? Could they obtain immunizations from private physicians, or should the health department provide them? Do staff nurses see value in immunizations?

Answers to these questions should open up consideration of still other alternatives. If, for example, facilities are adequate but are not being used because the community is uninformed about the need for and resources available for immunizations, education could be provided by (a) TV or radio programs by nurses, (b) programs in schools, (c) meetings of key people with neighborhood groups such as civic leagues in each area of the city, and (d) phone calls or door-to-door visits by volunteers. From these and other alternatives, the nurse selects the best one and plans for implementation.

COMMUNITY INTERVENTION PLANS

Community interventions differ from individual or family interventions because the focus is on aggregates or the total community. Some aggregate- or community-focused interventions discussed in later chapters include using the mass media subsystem to reach the population with health education; using the political process to bring about community change; establishing partnerships on behalf of community activities; special mass immunization, screening, or other aggregate- or community-focused activities; coalition building; and empowerment of community aggregates using community organization principles.

COMMUNITY INVOLVEMENT

An important aspect of community work is the involvement of the community. Some authors suggest involving the community from the assessment step onward, whereas others involve the community after data collection but during planning, intervention, and evaluation. This concept is emphasized below as part of community organization and will be discussed in Chapter 10.

COMMUNITY ORGANIZATION

DEFINITIONS

Community organization is an important concept to consider when planning for the health of communities. It has been defined as "The process whereby community change agents empower individuals and aggregates to solve community problems and achieve community goals" (Swanson & Albrecht, 1993, p. 131). It was defined by Bracht (1990) as a planned process to activate a community to use its own social structure and any available resources (internal-external) to accomplish community goals, decided primarily by community representatives . . . interventions are organized . . . from within the community to attain and then sustain community improvements. (p. 67)

Both definitions are basically the same in that one identifies community empowerment and the other "activating a community"; one says the community "solves community problems and accomplishes goals," and the other identifies communities' attaining and sustaining community improvements. As the reader will discover shortly, these definitions relate to only one model of community development, that of locality development.

MODELS OF COMMUNITY ORGANIZATION

There are three models for effecting community change: (a) locality development, (b) social planning, and (c) social action.

LOCALITY DEVELOPMENT MODEL

This model has also been called the community development model. Community development was defined by the United Nations (1981) as "a process designed to improve conditions of economic and social progress for the whole community with its active participation and the fullest possible reliance on the community's initiative" (p. 8). This model is based on the assumption that a wide spectrum of local people should be involved in goal setting and actions to maximize community change. Themes emphasized in the model include democratic procedures, voluntary cooperation, self-help, development of indigenous leadership, and education.

SOCIAL PLANNING

The second model of effecting community change, social planning, emphasizes a technical approach to solving social problems. In this model, change is believed to require expert planners, who, using technical abilities and skills, including the ability to manipulate large bureaucratic organizations, can bring about complex changes. The planner usually establishes, arranges, and delivers goods and services to people who need them. Building community capacity (locality development) and fostering radical social change (social action) are not integral to this approach.

SOCIAL ACTION MODEL

This model assumes that a disadvantaged segment of the population needs to be organized, at times in alliance with others, to make adequate demands on the larger society for increased resources or treatment more in accord with social justice or democracy. Practitioners push for changes in major institutions or community practices and for a redistribution of power, resources, community decision-making privileges, or policy changes in formal organizations. Examples of groups who have used this approach include civil rights groups such as the National Association for the Advancement of Colored People (NAACP), Congress of Racial Equity (CORE), and Southern Christian Leadership Conference (SCLC); some white antiracist organizations; student groups associated with the new left, such as Students for a Democratic Society (SDS); and recent groups, such as nonsmokers rights groups and groups fighting for the rights of gay men and lesbians, tenants, or the homeless.

The three models are not discrete but may overlap in practice. For example, a social planner (Model 2) who has met resistance in implementing a program for obese adolescents may decide that wide discussion between and participation of community members is necessary to obtain success with the program (Models 1 and 2). Rothman (1970) recognized this overlap: "Having isolated and set off each of these models, . . . it would be well to point out we are speaking of analytical extremes and that in actual practice these orientations are overlapping rather than discrete" (p. 23). Nevertheless, organizations tend to be guided by one of the three models.

DIFFERENCES BETWEEN THE MODELS

Bracht (1990) identifies a few variables in the three models. He says the locality development model is a process model that emphasizes self-help and the development of community capabilities and cooperation; the social planning model is a task model that emphasizes solving community problems; and the social action model combines process and task to emphasize a redistribution of power, resources, and relationships and changes in basic institutions.

Rothman and Trotman (1987) similarly argue that the locality development model is process focused with an emphasis on cooperation and system capabilities, increasing participation and local leadership, whereas the social development model is task oriented (a category comprising both social planning and social action models here), with an emphasis on completing a concrete task and solving problems such as providing services, establishing new services, or getting legislation passed.

Another difference involves assumptions about community structure and problem conditions. In the locality development model (Model 1), the planner sees the community overshadowed by the larger community and the problem as a lack of relationships and democratic problem-solving abilities, whereas in the social planning model (Model 2) the planner sees the community as having major social problems, such as physical or mental health or housing problems or some other problem of interest to the planner, and in the social action model (Model 3), the planner views the community as a system of privileges and power with a disadvantaged population and the problem as social injustice, deprivation, and inequity or exploitation at the hands of oppressors such as the "power structure," "big government," or "society."

A third difference between the models is in the change strategies used. In Model 1, the strategy is to have a broad section of people get together to determine and then solve the community's problems. The approach is, "Let's meet and talk this over." In Model 2, the planner gathers facts about a problem and decides what to do about it. The approach is, "Let's gather the facts and solve the problem." The strategy in Model 3 is to identify the issues so people know who the enemy is and then to organize mass action to pressure the enemy. The enemy may be an organization, such as the housing and urban renewal authority; a person, such as the city manager; or an aggregate, such as slum landlords. The approach is, "Let's crystallize the issue, organize mass action, and bring pressure on the selected targets."

There are also characteristic change tactics with the three models. The change tactic for Model 1 is consensus through discussion and communication. In Model 2 the change tactic is consensus or conflict, and Model 3 uses change tactics of conflict or contest, such as confrontation and direct action or negotiation.

The role of the practitioner also varies in the three models. In Model 1, the practitioner is an enabler-catalyst who encourages problem solving, expressions of concerns, organizational skills, and interpersonal relationships. In Model 2, the practitioner's role is more technical or that of an expert in which he or she gathers data, implements programs, and interacts with bureaucracies. In Model 3, the practitioner is in an activist or advocacy role and organizes groups and manipulates organizations and movements to influence the political process.

The practitioner's orientation toward the power structure also varies. In Model 1, the members of the power structure collaborate in a common venture, whereas in Model 2, the power structure is often the sponsor or employer of the practitioner, and in Model 3, the power structure is viewed as an external target of action or an oppressor to be coerced or overturned.

The boundary definition of the community client also differs. In Model 1, the client system is the total community, such as a city or neighborhood. In Model 2, the boundary is the total community or segment of a community, such as the mentally ill, aged, or Jewish community, and in Model 3, the boundary is a community segment that is deprived.

The conception of the client population or constituency also varies. In Model 1, the clients are the citizens of a community, whereas in Model 2, they are the consumers of services, and in Model 3, they are the victims of the system.

Typically, in the past, health planners used Model 2. But because this method has been found to be ineffective or partially effective in dealing with current community problems, there has been more emphasis on the use of Model 1. This has led to the timeliness of concepts such as empowerment, community competence, and partnerships. Although these concepts will be enlarged on in the next section of the book, they will be discussed briefly here because they relate to community organization.

MAJOR CONCEPTS IN COMMUNITY ORGANIZATION

Several concepts are important in current community organization practice when focusing on Model 1—locality development. This model has been found to be the most effective way to bring about community change.

EMPOWERMENT

Rappaport (1984) defines *empowerment* as "a process by which individuals, communities and organizations gain mastery over their lives" (p. 1). Empowerment allows communities to transform their lives and environment.

The concept of empowerment operates on two levels at the same time in community organization practice. At one level, individuals involved in community organization efforts experience increased social support, which increases their sense of control. This sense of control, in turn, may have positive health effects. For example, Leighton and Stone (1974) found that community involvement was a significant psychosocial factor in improving people's perceived confidence, coping capacity, and satisfaction in life. Studies by Cohen and Syme (1985) and Thomas, Goodwin, and Goodwin (1985) showed that social participation may affect the defense system of the body and decrease its susceptibility to illness. Thus, participation in community organization may influence physical health.

The second level operating during community empowerment affects the community and has been operationalized partially as community competence. Empowerment of communities has had a positive effect on health and social indicators and may be reflected in lower community rates of alcoholism, divorce, and other social problems. In addition, Minkler (1985), Israel (1985), and Thomas, Israel, and Steuart (1985) say the empowered community working effectively for change may effect changes in some of the problems that contributed to its ill health in the first place.

COMMUNITY COMPETENCE

Community competence is an expected outcome of community development and is closely related to the concept of empowerment. It can be defined as the community's ability to engage in effective problem solving (Iscore, 1980). Cottrell (1983) states that it is operative in the community when

> the various members of the community are able to collaborate effectively on identifying the problems and needs of the community; can achieve a working consensus on goals and priorities; can agree on ways and means to implement the agreed upon goals; [and] can collaborate effectively in the required actions. (p. 403)

Cottrell (1976) also proposed eight conditions that were essential for community competence: (a) commitment, (b) self-other awareness and clarity of situation definitions, (c) articulateness, (d) communication, (e) conflict containment and accommodation, (f) participation, (g) management of relations with the larger society, and (h) machinery to facilitate participant interaction and decision making. These are a combination of individual characteristics and community processes that facilitate participation in community activities.

The development of leadership is an important aspect of community competence. The community needs people who can assist others to think through the steps of identifying problems, setting goals, implementing plans, and so forth. Leaders should also be able to facilitate the process of group discussion and the attainment of consensus among community members.

PARTICIPATION AND RELEVANCE

Two additional concepts of importance in community organization are participation and relevance. *Participation* relates to the need for community members to be active rather than passive in the learning process and is a concept rooted in the social psychology theories of learning. These theories are reinforced by cognitive theory principles, which stress the importance of feedback and understanding rather than memorization. Dewey (1946) and Lindeman (1926) looked at participation in adult education as the process of enlarging the understanding of people by getting them actively involved and helping them make and implement decisions for themselves. These ideas are closely related to community development.

Bracht (1990) identifies three ways to increase community participation in community health projects: (a) establishing work groups or task forces to work with specific components of the project, (b) involving target group members in selection of intervention strategies, and (c) providing staff to carry out details and to offer technical assistance and consultation as needed to community members. Case studies later in Part IV will show how community participation has been obtained in community projects.

According to Green (1986), community organization is based on the "principle of participation" and large-scale behavioral changes require that people heavily affected by a problem be involved in defining it, planning and initiating steps to resolve it, and establishing structures to ensure that the desired change is maintained (Green, 1986; Vandevelde, 1983). Community participation is so important in community work that much of Chapter 11 is devoted to it.

The concept of *relevance* is also important. To be considered, the proposed change must be relevant; that is, people must experience a need for change if change or learning is to occur. Lewin (1958) discussed the need for unfreezing of old attitudes and beliefs as a prerequisite for trying new ones, and Hochbaum (1960) focused on the need for a "psychological state of readiness to learn" (p. 15) before a change will take place. Nyswander (1966) articulated the concept of relevance by introducing the concept of starting where people are. The practitioner who starts with the community's felt needs and concerns is more likely to experience success with change than the practitioner who tries to impose an agency agenda from outside.

SELECTION OF COMMUNITY ISSUES

Another important concept in community development is *issue selection.* This involves separating problems that are troubling but of minor importance from those that the community feels strongly about (Bracht, 1990). Important criteria for good issues include winnability, simplicity, and specificity. Winning issues builds confidence and competence. Issues should also be simple and specific so that community members can explain them in a few sentences. Issues should unite people, involve them in achieving resolution of the issue, and build community organization (Bracht, 1990).

Methods used to help groups obtain information about issues to select include nominal group process (Delbecq, Van de Ven, & Gustafson, 1975), door-to-door surveys, and Freire's (1973) problem-posing dialogue method. Freire's method is so useful, it is discussed here in detail.

Freire developed a methodology in which groups discuss common problems, and through a problem-posing dialogue, look for the root causes behind the problems that they initially identified. They are then helped to explore the relationships between various aspects of their reality and to develop action plans based on critical reflections, to help transform that reality (Freire, 1973). In one application of this method discussed by Minkler and Cox (1980), women in rural Honduras discussed with the Catholic priests some common problems, such as worms in children. From their discussion of causes behind the problem, they identified factors such as poverty and lack of education. They then developed an action plan that included the building of a village school by the women. In New Mexico, Wallerstein and Bernstein (1988) used this method with high-risk teenagers (low-income minorities and Anglos with drinking and driving problems and higher suicide rates than the national average) in a substance abuse program. The goal was to empower these teenagers by having them visit emergency rooms and jails and then discuss the experience in a safe environment. These teenagers were encouraged to analyze discussions with hospital patients and each other to identify the root causes of problems in their communities and their possible role in solving the problems they identified. Some interventions included presentations of this material to others at risk.

COMMUNITY ORGANIZATION IN PRACTICE

Although not a pure community organization project in which the practitioners assisted the community to identify its problems and then solve them, the project to be discussed here used strategies of community involvement to improve its chances of success. It exemplifies what is probably the approach more often used in health projects—that is, a combination of Model 1 (locality development) and Model 2 (social planning) discussed earlier. According to Carlaw, Mittelmark, Bracht, and Luepker (1984), the program had to balance the need for a scientific project that ensured investigator control and measurable results with an emphasis on local ownership and responsibility as required for a successful community-based program. Thus, this project was initiated from outside the community by researchers who knew what they wanted to address and did not "start where the people were." With the exception of problem identification, however, efforts were made to involve the community: for example, in setting objectives and choosing issues for mobilization.

The Minnesota Heart Health Project (Mittelmark et al., 1986) was a large-scale, population-based project aimed at the primary prevention of cardiovascular disease. Goals of the project were to achieve a reduction in risk factors and in morbidity and mortality from cardiovascular diseases by improving the behavior of the community population. The study took place in three communities with a total population of about 250,000 people and compared three reference communities having a comparably sized population (Carlaw et al., 1984). The population focused preventive interventions included (a) smoking cessation, (b) detection and control of hypertension, and (c) dietary and exercise pattern changes (Mittelmark et al., 1986).

Community members worked jointly with the research team in making decisions and implementing programs to ensure that community partnership was an integral part of the project. The "hypothesis was that educational interventions planned with, through, and for communities would lead to changes in individual and family behaviors conducive to heart health" (Carlaw et al., 1984, p. 245). Early efforts to initiate a community partnership included community analysis and "mapping," data gathering from community leaders, and the formation of community advisory boards in each study community. Later, small group structures (board membership, functional task forces, and committees) were used to allow citizens to identify actions to be taken and groups to be targeted. In addition to providing for community participation, this approach also allowed for the continued diffusion of the interest and awareness in cardiovascular disease prevention in the community (Mittelmark et al., 1986).

In addition to community organization concepts and principles, mass media and face-to-face education were used. One of the three communities was added to the project each year and provided with a 5-year intensive education program. The first phase of the program involved community awareness of the heart health concept, and the second phase involved opportunities to practice behaviors that would improve cardiovascular health (Carlaw et al., 1984).

Community competence was increased by the development of an effective network of community groups and support systems that progressively assumed more planning and funding roles and demonstrated increased problem-solving skills (Blackburn, 1983). The program contributed to individual and community empowerment in several ways and moved from a social planning to a locality development model. Carlaw et al. (1984) say, "Sustained volunteer interest and assertiveness of community leadership for heart health" (p. 248) and the community's assumption of roles that were increasingly "initiating" were indicators of the project's success in empowering the community.

The overall evaluation goal of the project was to "measure the changes in disease, risk factor distributions, and behaviors and to relate these changes to components of the educational program" (Blackburn, 1983, p. 415). Although the extent to which these goals have been met has not yet been reported, there has been some success in terms of community organization. According to Bracht (1990), community leadership has remained relatively stable, and more than 50% of the founding executive committee members from each community remain on the committee; 42% of the heart health programs within communities are currently run by local community sponsors, and another one third are in transition. Thus, community retention rates for volunteers, community ownership, and continuity all indicate success in the application of community organization concepts and principles.

COMMUNITY ORGANIZATION STEPS

Bracht (1990) identifies five steps in the community organization process that are similar to the nursing process and that involve citizens at each step. The first step is *analysis,* which involves an accurate evaluation of community data and early involvement of community members and organizations to ensure collaboration and broad community involvement. Key elements of this step include

(a) defining the community; (b) collecting data; assessing the capacity of the community to change, including the driving forces and support for change; (c) assessing community barriers to change or the restraining forces; (d) assessing readiness for change; and (e) synthesizing the data and setting priorities. It should be noted that Bracht does not have separate steps for assessment, analysis, and planning.

The second step is the *design and initiation*. It involves beginning implementation and formal activities to mobilize the citizens. Key elements include (a) establishing a core community planning group and a coordinator or local organizer; (b) choosing an organizational structure; (c) identifying, selecting, and recruiting for boards or committees, depending on structure; (d) defining the mission of the organization; (e) clarifying the roles and responsibilities or members of the board, staff, and others; and (f) training and recognizing members as needed.

The third step is *implementation* and is the action step. The key elements are (a) broad participation of citizens, (b) developing a sequential work plan, (c) using comprehensive strategies that integrate multiple actions, and (d) making sure that the program, materials, and messages are consistent with community values.

The fourth step is *program maintenance-consolidation*. Key elements include (a) integrating interventions into networks of the community, (b) establishing a favorable organizational culture, (c) starting an ongoing recruitment plan, and (d) disseminating the results of the project.

The fifth step is *dissemination-reassessment*. Key elements include (a) updating the community analysis, (b) evaluating the effectiveness of the programs, (c) determining future direction of the program and making modifications, and (d) summarizing and disseminating the results.

MODELS AND CONCEPTS OF COMMUNITY CHANGE

A major purpose of planning is to bring about change in a community's health. For example, in the community diagnosis of high infant mortality discussed earlier in this chapter, the goal was to reestablish an energy balance in the community by reducing the infant mortality rate. Ways to bring about this change were identified in objectives.

The following are models and concepts for community change that have been provided in the literature.

MULTILEVEL INTERVENTION MODEL

Simons-Morton, Simons-Morton, Parcel, and Bunker (1988) present a multilevel intervention model that focuses on personal and environmental changes. They say that both personal factors and the environment (direct environmental influences and environmental influences on personal factors) are important determinants of health and that interventions should be directed toward both.

Personal and environmental factors influencing health operate at the individual, organizational, and governmental levels. Individual health is affected by personal behavior. Organizational health—the well-being of its members, clients, or patients—is affected by the policies and practices of the organization. Governments affect the health of their constituents by public action and legislation. Thus, interventions in community health should consist of "(1) influencing individuals to reduce personal risk factors for disease and (2) influencing organizations and governments to reduce environmental risk factors for disease" (Simons-Morton et al., 1988, p. 27).

Multilevel Approaches Toward Community Health (MATCH) similarly addresses the three levels of intervention and is used following community assessment, analysis, and priority setting. It is an organizing framework providing structure to interventions and accommodating a variety of theoretical perspectives and intervention approaches.

The model comprises four phases with two or three components in each phase. During Phase 1, health goals are selected. These may relate to a specific population defined by place (clinic, school) or by health condition (cancer, heart disease). The target population consists of those who have health problems (individuals, a group of individuals, or members of a community) and is identified by community assessment or some other method. Health goals can be selected from 1 of the 15 national priorities and may involve reductions of morbidity and mortality or increases in wellness.

Phase 2 is intervention planning to achieve goals through personal and environmental changes. The objectives will differ depending on the level of intervention. Objectives at the individual level include reducing disease risk factors in individuals, whereas objectives at the organizational level involve changing or establishing organizational policies, programs, practices, and resources. Objectives at the governmental level involve changing establishing local, state, or federal governmental policies, programs, and legislation. Achievement of objectives requires influencing the knowledge, skills, attitudes, beliefs, and behaviors of the intervention target. Intervention targets are people with authority, power, and influence who can create change at the targeted level.

Phase 3, the intervention phase, involves developing and testing the needed materials for the intervention, hiring needed personnel, and scheduling sites for meetings, classes, or other interventions. Selected interventions identified in a model to influence the three levels include (a) individual—screening, medical care, health education, counseling, and persuasive communication; (b) organizations—organizational changes, consulting, training, and networking; and (c) governmental—political process, social action, social change, and community development.

Phase 4 of the model is evaluation of the process, impact, and outcome of the intervention to determine how the intervention approaches were applied and whether or not the health goals and intervention objectives were achieved (see Chapter 14).

One example used was a hypothetical intervention to decrease the prevalence of untreated hypertension in a community. At the individual level, practitioners can help individuals to learn about the importance of hypertension in health, to obtain testing and treatment, and to comply with prescribed treatment;

at the organizational level they can help organizations to establish screening programs, initiate education programs about hypertension, and provide financial incentives for hypertensive screening and treatment (e.g., lower health or insurance costs); and at the governmental level, they can encourage legislators to fund hypertension screening, education, and research.

Another example presented considered a multilevel intervention to reduce coronary heart disease in a community. At the individual level, the focus was on encouraging a diet low in fat and salt, a regular schedule of aerobic exercises, and not smoking; at the organizational level, the focus was on providing low-fat and low-salt foods for purchase in cafeterias or machines, establishing exercise facilities, and implementing smoking restriction policies; and at the community or governmental level, the focus was on funding research on dietary practices to lower coronary heart disease, providing food commodities that met the dietary recommendations of lowering coronary heart disease, instituting community education programs, and passing laws and ordinances restricting smoking in public places.

HEALTHY CITIES: MODEL OF COMMUNITY CHANGE

The Healthy Cities model discussed by Flynn (1992) is a multilevel model for community change. This model proposes that community change be evaluated at the following levels: (a) individual—how much individuals were influenced by the project; (b) subsystem level—what changes took place within community organizations and groups; (c) interrelationship among subsystems level—how important "social connectedness" in the community was; and (d) total community level—whether there have been changes in norms and values, such as policy changes. Some aspects of the subsystem (structure and activities of the committees described) and interrelationship among subsystems (description of projects developed) levels were evaluated.

The framework for analysis of social change used was Etzioni's (1976) four levels of social change: (a) knowledge of the community, (b) effective goals and organization, (c) committed power bases to support change, and (d) community participation and consensus.

Community leaders on committees in six cities were given data (vital statistics) on their cities and asked to identify problems and strengths in each community as well as gaps in knowledge and ways to obtain the needed data. Staff assistance was available to assist with survey development and other related tasks. Top priorities ranged from environmental health to teenage pregnancy to community safety. The committees for the six cities varied from 2.73 to 3.13 on a Healthy Cities Committee Effectiveness Inventory that evaluated five components of group dynamics: "maintenance of morale, sharing, leadership, maturity or self readiness, and task or work accomplishment" (Flynn, 1992, p. 18). Each item was rated from 1 to 4, with 1 being low effectiveness and 4 being high effectiveness. The committees were also at various stages of establishing organizational procedures ranging from none for one city to rules established, beginnings of bylaws, and plans to incorporate and gain tax-exempt status in another.

The third level is a power base to support change, and again, committees operated at various stages of effectiveness in gaining support for their action plans. These ranged from a city that ranked low as far as having a broad-based committee but had two proposals submitted and one funded and had strong support of the mayor and local health officer on the committee to a city that was high as far as having a broad-based committee and had submitted and received funding for one proposal and also had strong support on the committee from the mayor and local health officer.

The fourth step is community participation and consensus, which is measured by the numbers of steering committees and short- and long-range action programs. Cities varied from having two to six steering committees. Short-term actions included 2-minute radio messages addressing topics such as immunizations, leaf burning, humor and healing, fever, and smoking. Long-term strategies included a school teen parenting program combining education and health and a program for recycling of solid waste.

This program is less than 3 years old, so it is too early to carry out a complete analysis of social change. This report, which focused on two levels of social change, subsystem and interrelationships among subsystems, found variations in two levels of social change: (a) goal setting and organization and (b) power bases to support change. All cities addressed two of the four levels of social change, and some addressed all four levels. Although the committees all identified priorities, there was variation in the ability of committees to organize themselves. Some have formalized structure, whereas others have delayed this task. In addition, there was variation in committee functioning and in obtaining broad-based community participation on the committees.

BRACHT'S SOCIAL CHANGE MODEL

Bracht's (1990) social change model of community is based on systems theory, which is also the theoretical focus of this book. It assumes that social structures are long-lasting, functional, interdependent, and relatively stable systems based on a degree of consensus about goals, norms, and values. The community system is described as being made up of subsystems such as the political and economic subsystems discussed in Chapter 2. Bracht adds to these the community's voluntary civic groups that are interested in health matters as well as political action and grassroots groups specific to the community.

Change in one segment of a system leads to an adjustment or response in another part of the system. Thus, change can be introduced at any level of the community. However, change beginning in one subsystem may take a long time to affect the whole community, and in the process, various factors may divert or stop the change process.

From the perspective of community organization, change of the total community is the usual target because that maximizes dissemination of change throughout the subsystems. New rules of behavior required by the change must become a part of the total system. Concepts about how and why change is likely to occur follow.

CONCEPTS OF COMMUNITY CHANGE

According to Moore (1963), social change is "the significant alteration of social structures (that is, patterns of social action and integration), including consequences and manifestations of such structures embodied in norms (rules of conduct), values, and cultural products and symbols" (p. 34). Social change has been explained by two different types of theories, functionalist and conflict. *Functionalist* theories focus on patterns and processes that maintain the stability of the system and see social change as a slow, gradual process. There is cooperation and consensus within the system regarding societal goals, norms, and values, and norms hold the system together. Social change is a result of the breakdown of part of the system that is no longer able to contribute to system maintenance or the overwhelming of the system by external or environmental changes. New rules of conduct that help maintain the changed system then occur along with the social norms changes. Moore uses the example of cigarette smoking: Scientific change (accumulation of evidence on the dangers of secondhand smoke) is leading to smoking restrictions in public places, and thus, smokers must learn new rules for smoking.

Conflict theories of social change see imbalance and ongoing adjustment as part of any system. The community is made up of interest groups, and change occurs when a particular interest group becomes dominant. Social norms are still believed to help maintain the stability of the system, but this is a coercive rather than a consensual process. Dominant groups, especially the economic and political sectors, determine social norms and resist attempts to change those norms. Moore again used tobacco as an example: Tobacco companies have a strong economic and political base through lobbying and have been able to maintain advertising privileges and price support from the government. They have also influenced social norms by defining smoking as a matter of individual choice or as an individual problem. Changing this social norm would require an opposing group such as a nonsmokers' rights group to exert more influence than the tobacco industry over that part of the system.

COMMUNITY CHANGE PROCESS

Process theories for community change include the individual, organizational, community, and environmental levels. Theories related to each of these levels are presented in Bracht (1990).

BRACHT'S MODEL

Bracht's model uses all material presented previously. His system is stable (functionalist theory), and most of the subsystems (including families) agree on the goals, norms, and values of society. There are also interest groups who act to maintain the status quo and groups who engage in collective action to bring about change (conflict theory). There is interaction with the external community because laws, policies, or critical events external to the community may influence community norms and values. These external forces may also be the impetus for group action to change community behavior and may be planned within or outside the community. External organizations may use social planning or locality development models to bring about change and may work in partnerships with internal and external resources.

Organizations work together for change at the subsystem level, and social network and organizational theories explain how these relationships are initiated and sustained. The process of diffusion of the changes to other groups is explained by diffusion theory (see Chapter 9), community development (discussed earlier in this chapter), and organizational development. Some organizations may provide more leadership than others, and key subsystems that should be involved include economics and politics.

Individuals interacting with subsystems are exposed to changing norms and practices that may be reinforced by role models who have made the changes. Social learning theory explains how this change in individuals occurs. Eventually, changes in subsystems and organizations and their relationships will influence widespread individual changes.

MEASURING COMMUNITY CHANGE

Bracht's model identifies areas of measurement to evaluate community change. At the individual level, the researcher would be interested in obtaining the following data from survey: individuals' awareness of project, their understanding of problems, their participation in the project, and their changes in behavior as a result of the project.

Community change at the subsystem level would focus on organizational and group changes and might include policy changes that relate to the problem, support for and participation in the project, and other activities related to the problem of concern. Community changes in interrelationships between subsystems should also be evaluated and would indicate changes in the amount of involvement of organizations and groups with each other, or their "social connectedness." These changes could be evaluated by the development of coalitions, participation of subsystems in community boards and task forces, and communitywide involvement of subsystems.

The last area of evaluation involves communitywide changes in norms and values. Areas of assessment include community policies related to the area of concern, enforcement procedures of the community, and shifts in norms perceived by the public.

RUDYVILLE'S PRIORITIES, GOALS, AND OBJECTIVES

By Pickett and Hanlon's model (1990), the diagnosis "community energy deficit related to disaster potential" would definitely be a high priority to address because a disaster would affect a large number of people and could be severe, because there is knowledge available to prevent damage to people (evacuation), and because the readiness for the population for better roads has been established. However, this could be an expensive intervention and would require taking resources from somewhere else in the budget. The goal might be expressed as "to balance community energies by decreasing the potential effect of the disaster on the population." Obviously, at this stage in technology, a change in a hurricane's path cannot be accomplished to prevent property and people destruction. Thus, the emphasis would be on preventing injury to the population.

Objectives using the "resulting in" part of the nursing diagnosis might include the following: (a) 90% of the population will be safely evacuated after the next hurricane warning; (b) 90% of the population will know when and where to go and what to do following the next hurricane warning. Alternative interventions for the first of these objectives might include coalition building to bring pressure on local and state politicians to shift budget allocations to provide adequate roads and evacuation plans; using the political process for this purpose; and notifying the highways and disaster departments and letting them move forward with a plan. Notification of the public could also be done by a variety of approaches similar to those discussed in the example used earlier involving immunizations.

Some other high priorities to address in Rudyville would be the lack of health care for the poor, the lack of health information in schools and on mass media, the lack of housing for the poor, low infant birth weights, and high STD rates.

Moderate-priority areas to address would include the unavailability of rehab beds and the exercise needs of those over the age of 6.

Those areas identified as showing an energy balance would be low priority at this point but would need to be evaluated periodically for change.

REFERENCES

American Public Health Association. (1991). *Healthy communities 2000—Model standards: Guidelines for community attainment of the year 2000 national health objectives.* Washington, DC: Author.

Archer, S. E., Kelly, C. D., & Bisch, S. A. (1984). *Implementing change in communities: A collaborative process.* St. Louis, MO: Mosby.

Blackburn, H. (1983). Research and demonstration projects in community cardiovascular disease prevention. *Journal of Public Health Policy, 4,* 398-421.

Bracht, N. (1990). *Health promotion at the community level.* Newbury Park, CA: Sage.

Carlaw, R. W., Mittelmark, M., Bracht, N., & Luepker, R. (1984). Organization of a community cardiovascular health program: Experiences from the Minnesota Heart Health Program. *Health Education Quarterly, 11,* 243-252.

Cohen, S., & Syme, S. L. (Eds.). (1985). *Social support and health.* Orlando, FL: Academic Press.

Cottrell, L. S. (1976). The competent community. In Kaplan, B., Wilson, R., & Leighton, A. (Eds.), *Further explorations in social psychiatry.* New York: Basic Books.

Cottrell, L. S. (1983). The competent community. In R. W. Warren & L. Lyon (Eds.), *New perspectives on the American community.* Homewood, IL: Dorsey.

Delbecq, A., Van de Ven, A. H., & Gustafson, D. H. (1975). *Group techniques for program planning: A guide to nominal group and Delphi processes.* Glenview, IL: Scott, Foresman.

Dewey, J. (1946). *The public and its problems: An essay in political inquiry.* Chicago: Gateway.

Etzioni, A. (1976). *Social problems.* Englewood Cliffs, NJ: Prentice Hall.

Flynn, B. (1992). Healthy cities: A model of community change. *Family and Community Health, 15*(1), 13-23.

Freire, P. (1973). *Education for critical consciousness.* New York: Seabury.

Green, L. W. (1986). The theory of participation: A qualitative analysis of its expression in national and international health politics. *Advances in Health Education and Promotion, 1,* 211-236.

Hochbaum, G. (1960). Modern theories of communication. *Children, 7,* 13-18.

Iscore, I. (1980). Community psychology and the competent community. *American Psychologist, 29,* 607-613.

Israel, B. (1985). Social network and social support: Implications for natural helpers and community level interventions. *Health Education Quarterly, 12,* 66-80.

Leighton, D. C., & Stone, I. T. (1974). Community development as a therapeutic force: A case study with measurement. In P. M. Roman & H. M. Trice (Eds.), *Sociological perspectives on community mental health.* Philadelphia: F. A. Davis.

Lewin, K. (1958). Group decision and social change. In E. Maccoby, T. Newcomb, & E. Hartley (Eds.), *Readings in social psychology* (3rd ed.). New York: Holt, Rinehart & Winston.

Lindeman, E. (1926). *The meaning of adult education.* New York: New Republic.

Maslow, A. H. (1954). *Motivation and personality.* New York: Harper & Row.

McKenzie, J., & Jurs, J. (1993). *Planning, implementing, and evaluating health promotion programs: A primer.* Philadelphia: W. B. Saunders.

Minkler, M. (1985). Building supportive ties and sense of community among the inner-city elderly: The Tenderloin Senior Outreach Project. *Health Education Quarterly, 12,* 303-331.

Minkler, M., & Cox, K. (1980). Creating critical consciousness in health: Application of Freire's philosophy and methods to the health care setting. *International Journal of Health Services, 10,* 311-322.

Mittelmark, M., Luepker, R., Jacobs, D., Bracht, N., Carlaw, R., Crow, R., Finnegan, J., Grimm, R., Jeffrey, R., Kline, F., Mullis, R., Murray, D., Pechacek, T., Perry, C., Pirie, P., & Blackburn, H. (1986). Community-wide prevention of cardiovascular disease: Education strategies of the Minnesota Heart Health Program. *Preventive Medicine, 15,* 1-17.

Moore, W. E. (1963). *Social change.* Englewood Cliffs, NJ: Prentice Hall.

Nyswander, D. (1966). The open society: Its implications for health educators. *Health Education Monographs, 1,* 3-15.

Pickett, G., & Hanlon, J. (1990). *Public health administration and practice* (9th ed.). St. Louis, MO: Time Mirror/Mosby.

Rappaport, J. (1984). Studies in empowerment: Introduction to the issue. *Prevention in Human Services, 3,* 1-7.

Rothman, J. (1970). Three models of community organization practice. In F. M. Cox & J. E. Trotman (Eds.), *Strategies of community organization* (pp. 20-36). Itasca, IL: F. E. Peacock.

Rothman, J., & Trotman, J. E. (1987). Models of community organization and macro practice: Their mixing and phasing. In F. M. Cox & J. E. Trotman (Eds.), *Strategies of community organization* (4th ed.). Itasca, IL: F. E. Peacock.

Simons-Morton, D., Simons-Morton, B., Parcel, G., & Bunker, J. (1988). Influencing personal and environmental conditions for community health: A multilevel intervention model. *Family and Community Health, 11*(2), 25-35.

Swanson, J., & Albrecht, G. (1993). *Community health nursing: Promoting the health of aggregates.* Philadelphia: W. B. Saunders.

Thomas, P., Goodwin, J. M., & Goodwin, J. S. (1985). Effects of social support and stress-related changes in cholesterol levels, uric acid levels, and immune function in an elderly sample. *American Journal of Psychiatry, 142,* 735-737.

Thomas, R., Israel, B., & Steuart, G. W. (1985). Cooperative problem solving: The neighborhood self-help project. In H. P. Cleary, J. M. Kitchen, & P. G. Ensor (Eds.), *Advancing health through education.* Mountain View, CA: Mayfield.

United Nations, International Children's Emergency Fund/World Health Organization Joint Committee on Health Policy. (1981). Community involvement. In *National decision making for primary health care.* Geneva, Switzerland: Author.

Vandevelde, M. (1983). The semantics of participation. In R. M. Kramer & H. Speck (Eds.), *Readings in community organization practice* (3rd ed., pp. 95-105). Englewood Cliffs, NJ: Prentice Hall.

Wallerstein, N., & Bernstein, E. (1988). Empowerment educator: Freire's ideas adapted to health education. *Health Education Quarterly, 15,* 379-394.

Yura, H., & Walsh, M. (1988). *The nursing process* (5th ed.). Norwalk, CT: Appleton & Lange.

CHAPTER 9

PLANNING FOR DIFFUSION AND MAINTENANCE OF COMMUNITY CHANGE

OBJECTIVES

1. Define diffusion and institutionalization.

2. Discuss factors influencing the innovation process.

3. Evaluate the innovation-development process.

4. Discuss categories of innovation adopters.

5. Evaluate approaches to change with innovation adopters.

6. Discuss organizational diffusion.

7. Discuss the institutionalization of a program.

Planning the best way to reach the most people when initiating community changes is important and is the subject of diffusion theory. In addition, after interventions directed toward changing health behaviors of aggregates or the community are completed on a trial basis or after funding has ended, it is important to maintain the changes introduced. Planning for maintaining those changes is addressed by institutionalization. The concepts of diffusion theory and institutionalization are covered in this chapter.

ENERGY THEORY, DIFFUSION, AND INSTITUTIONALIZATION

Diffusion theory involves planning the best way to reach the most people with community interventions to influence health. From an energy frame of reference, these plans assist the community to establish or reestablish a balance of energy (community adaptation toward health) in a specific area that has been identified from a community assessment. Following the assessment, inferences are made and developed into nursing diagnoses. Diffusion theory, then, assists in identifying the best ways to implement plans to establish or reestablish a balance of energy for the identified problem. Institutionalization involves the best way to maintain changes initiated to improve community health. From an energy point of view, institutionalization involves ways to maintain an energy balance in a community in a specific area after it is achieved.

DEFINITIONS

Diffusion is defined as "the process by which an innovation is communicated through certain channels over time among members of a social system" (Rogers, 1983, p. 333). An innovation is "an idea, practice, service or other object that is perceived as new by an individual or other unit of adoption" (p. 11).

Innovations may be accepted by individuals and organizations. Use of seat belts is an example of an innovation adopted by individuals, and a large increase in this behavior when the intervention is new indicates diffusion of the seat belt behavior. At the organizational level, an increase in fitness programs in a significant number of businesses and organizations would indicate diffusion of fitness as a change in behavior of organizations. Diffusion is most effective if organizations, individuals, and communities are targeted concurrently (see discussion of multilevel interventions in Chapter 8). Thus, diffusion should involve organizations, mass media channels, the political process, and other means of changing health behavior and the environment.

SPEED AND EXTENT OF THE INNOVATION PROCESS

Rogers (1983) identifies several attributes of an innovation that influence its diffusion: its relative advantage, compatibility, complexity, trialability, and observability. The *relative advantage* of the innovation is its superiority (actual or perceived) over existing practice or ideas. If the innovation is considered to be superior to current practices, it is more likely to be adopted. Dimensions of superiority include unique benefits, usefulness, economic factors, convenience, satisfaction, prestige factors, and time involved.

Compatibility is the effects (actual or perceived) of the innovation on existing values and norms and its cultural, psychological, and sociological aspects. Adoption and diffusion of an innovation are greater if the innovation is more compatible with the existing social system (economic, sociocultural, and philosophical value system). Many of the proposed community changes for health presented in Benjamin Paul's (1955) book, discussed in Chapter 5, failed because practitioners did not consider their compatibility with the existing social system.

The *complexity* of an innovation is also a factor in its adoption and diffusion. A complex innovation is more difficult to communicate and to understand and use and is therefore less likely to be adopted than one that is less complex and less difficult to understand and use.

Trialability is the degree to which an innovation can be tried or implemented on a limited basis. New ideas or innovations that can be tried or experimented with on a limited or trial basis are more likely to be adopted and diffused than those that cannot.

Observability is the visibility of the innovation's results to others. Innovations that generate visible results and, consequently, stimulate positive communication about the innovation promote greater adoption and diffusion than those that are not observable.

Other attributes identified by Kolbe and Iverson (1981) include reversibility, risk, cost-effectiveness, and modification. *Reversibility* is the ease of discontinuing an innovation with few or minor lasting consequences. Those innovations that can be terminated by individuals or organizations without discomfort will be more easily adopted and diffused than those that lack such reversibility features.

Modification refers to the ability to update and adapt an innovation to changing times. An innovation that can be easily updated is more likely to be adopted than one that lacks this feature.

Risk is the degree of uncertainty introduced by an innovation. Innovations involving higher risks are less likely to be adopted and diffused in a population.

Cost-effectiveness relates to the benefits of an innovation over the cost. A desirable innovation is one in which the perceived benefits (tangible and intangible) outweigh the costs.

It is generally accepted that for the best chances of adoption and diffusion, these attributes should be included in any planned community change. However, Orlandi, Landers, Weston, and Haley (1990) argue that this belief is based on the assumption that the attributes of the innovation and the characteristics of the adopter determine the success of adoption and diffusion of an innovation, whereas this is only a part of the process. They say that looking at the characteristics of the innovation and the decisions of the adopter as an intact package does not consider the concept of innovation refinement as an influence in adoption. Second, they say that the above model of attributes does not incorporate the role and efforts of the resource system (source of knowledge and expertise from which the innovation originated) or user system in influencing diffusion. Third, they say that the model does not recognize that the adoption decision is only one step in a process that extends from the adoption decision to program maintenance—a process in which failure is possible at any step.

POTENTIAL POINTS OF SYSTEM FAILURE IN DIFFUSION

Points of possible failure are, in order, innovation failure, communication failure, adoption failure, implementation failure, and maintenance failure. All of these potential failures must be prevented to ensure a lasting and meaningful impact from the innovation (Orlandi et al., 1990).

Innovation failure is a failure of the innovation to bring about an intended effect and may lead to system failure. This might occur when an innovation is poorly designed, inadequately evaluated, or dishonestly represented, even though it may be highly regarded.

Communication failure is a result of ineffective communication about an innovation, even though it may be efficacious and have good potential for achievement. This failure usually results from a lack of awareness of the innovation or lack of awareness of its availability by the user subsystem.

Adoption failure may result from a variety of factors, such as a differing value and belief system or the user's lack of necessary resources. Thus, despite the development of an efficacious innovation that is properly communicated, failure may occur because of poor adoption.

Implementation failure occurs when the innovation is improperly implemented or not implemented at all. This may occur when an aspect of the program, such as instructor training, that is instrumental to the program's efficacy is omitted or condensed. This most frequently occurs when the innovation is adopted by an organization and implemented among its members.

Maintenance failure results when a successful program loses its momentum and rapidly dissipates. Program maintenance for most community changes is important (see "Institutionalization" below).

INNOVATION DEVELOPMENT PROCESS

The innovation development process comprises all the decisions, activities, and effects that occur from the beginning stage of an idea's generation and development through its production, diffusion, adoption, and consequences (Rogers, 1983). Rogers (1983) describes six stages of this process: (a) recognizing the problem or need; (b) using basic or applied research; (c) developing the idea in a form expected to be acceptable to the adopter; (d) producing, marketing, and distributing the innovation through commercial efforts; (e) diffusing and adopting; and (f) the consequences. According to Kolbe and Iverson (1981) and Patton (1978), however, there is little evidence that more successful diffusions result from using this process than from not using it. Some factors that may cause inconsistencies in diffusion are (a) limited involvement of the user systems in developing the innovation, (b) gaps in translating knowledge from controlled studies to the real world of practice, and (c) the failure of research to consider long-term intervention effects and program maintenance.

INTEGRATION OF INNOVATION DEVELOPMENT AND DIFFUSION

Many barriers discussed above have the potential to undermine the objectives of innovation development or the innovation diffusion process. Orlandi et al. (1990) say many of these barriers are not addressed in projects and that there is frequently a gap between the goals and outcomes of planned innovations, resulting in uncompleted projects. This gap may be between the point at which innovation development ends and diffusion begins. They argue that some of the factors that account for the success of innovation development and diffusion and the factors that account for the success of diffusion show some similarities and that there are strategies to address these factors together. These would bridge the gap that exists when the two processes are considered separately. The linkage approach to innovation development and diffusion planning that attempts to bridge this gap was first described by Havelock (1971) and later expanded by Kolbe and Iverson (1981) and Orlandi (1986, 1987). This approach integrates three separate but interactive systems—the resource system, the linkage system, and the user system—into a single systems model.

The *resource system* includes researchers, innovation developers, trainers, consultants, services, products, and materials. The diffusion process comprises the activities implemented specifically to result in the spread of the innovation in a selected group, the user system. The linkage system includes members of the resource system, members of the user system, change agents who facilitate the collaboration between the previous two systems, and strategic-planning activities. The exchange of information within the linkage system uses concepts from community organization (see Chapter 8) and theories of social change (see Chapters 8 and 14) and is closely related to social marketing as described by Bloom and Norvelli (1981) and Norvelli (1990). Social marketing research techniques include a variety of methods to collect relevant quantitative and qualitative data to optimize the effectiveness of the innovation development and diffusion planning processes by addressing group preferences, perceived needs, expectations, limitations, and other user issues so that innovations are sensitive to sociocultural factors. Two key concepts in this process are segmentation of a population into subgroups and tailoring of an innovation to the identified characteristics of the targeted population segment.

Three ideas, then, are important in innovation development and diffusion. First, the resource system should be aware of the multiple steps of developing and diffusing an innovation and the steps at which the process can fail. Second, Rogers's (1983) six-step innovation development process model (discussed earlier) is applied and attention is given to the objectives at each step. Third, the identified gaps and limitations of these models are considered and minimized by the use of a linkage approach and social marketing to increase user participation in planning.

Interventions may be carried out by user system or resource system members. The implementation process and the innovation are developed jointly by the user and resource systems to increase the efficacy of the innovation and diffusion.

CATEGORIES OF AND APPROACHES TO INNOVATION ADOPTERS

CATEGORIES OF INNOVATION ADOPTERS

The adoption of innovations follows a consistent pattern throughout a population (Green, Gottlieb, & Parcel, 1987). This pattern can be described in terms of a sequence of adoption categories by different population groups. Rogers (1983) identifies five mutually exclusive adopter categories: innovators, early adopters, early majority adopters, late majority adopters, and laggarts. The ideal types of each of these follow.

Innovators will take risks, are anxious to try new things, and have a major role in introducing new ideas to the community, although they may not be respected by community members. They can also deal with a high degree of uncertainty and occasional setbacks such as the loss of financial or other resources.

Early adopters command the greatest degree of opinion leadership because they are respected members of the community or social system and thus serve as role models. They can also speed the diffusion process and decrease the uncertainty of others by adopting the innovation and communicating with others about it. Early adopters are viewed by others as discreet users of new ideas.

Early majority adopters are seldom leaders in a social system. They deliberate for a long time before reaching a decision about the innovation and are just a step ahead of the average member of the social system. However, they are an important link in the diffusion process.

Late majority adopters are a step behind the average member of the social system in adopting innovations. They respond to increased pressure from others, to the new norms of the group, and to economic necessities. Members of this group are skeptical and require a clear understanding of the usefulness of an innovation before they feel safe in using it.

Laggarts are the last members of a social system to adopt an innovation. This group is traditionally minded and suspicious of innovations. They are bound to the past, view the world in terms of what has been done in the past, and are somewhat isolated from the social system.

FACILITATING INNOVATION ADOPTION

Green et al. (1987) discuss how innovation interventions can be directed toward specific adopter categories. Early adopters would require a cognitive approach, whereas the majority adopters would need a motivational approach. Late adopters would require efforts to remove barriers to the adoption of an innovation. These barriers might be environmental, economic, or behavioral.

Parcel, Perry, and Taylor (1989) draw on social learning theories to identify strategies for facilitating innovation changes, including modeling, incentives, guided mastery, self-application of the acquired skills, and social contracting.

MODELING

According to Bandura (1986), modeling is the major way that people learn about an innovation. In this process, individuals observe others using the innovation, they learn about it, and they begin to develop expectations and values for their own use of the innovation. In addition, modeling may increase or decrease inhibitions associated with a previously learned behavior. Several factors will affect the quality and success of learning through modeling: (a) the characteristics of the model and (b) the clearness of the outcomes of the innovation. When models are similar to the potential user, learning is more effective. Models who demonstrate the behavior or who demonstrate overcoming an obstacle or who easily perform a difficult behavior are most effective. Also, clear outcomes for the modeled behavior are more effective than ambiguous outcomes.

INCENTIVES

Because knowledge and skills gained through modeling may not be sufficient to cause a person to use the new behavior, incentives may be a necessary addition. There are three types of incentives: direct, vicarious, and self-produced (Kolbe & Iverson, 1981). An external outcome happening to an individual directly when a behavior is performed is a direct incentive. The distribution of rewards and punishments to others as a result of their behavior that a person observes is a vicarious incentive. An incentive that a person determines for himself or herself for performing a particular behavior according to internally set standards is a self-produced incentive.

GUIDED MASTERY

Guided mastery is a strategy in which behavioral skills are taught and an individual's self-efficacy is increased (Bandura, 1986). This strategy allows the person to practice the behavior in a simulated situation in which the fear of making mistakes is minimized. The behavior may be modeled during the practice session and the user may receive feedback.

SELF-APPLICATION OF ACQUIRED SKILLS

This strategy involves practicing the behavior in a natural environment without a model and with responsibility for self-monitoring. During the initial practice, an environment conducive to success should be chosen. Repeated successful performances will increase efficacy.

SOCIAL CONTRACTING

This strategy may provide the structure for self-monitoring and for self-application of the behavioral skills. A contract is a written agreement between two or more people and demonstrates a commitment. The following information is usually included: (a) the parties involved, (b) behaviors each will perform, (c) goals to be achieved, (d) how goals will be measured, (e) incentives for successful performance, and (f) signatures of the involved parties. Additional information about contracting and examples of contracts are presented in Helvie (1991).

DIFFUSION IN ORGANIZATIONS

Because of the current emphasis on multilevel interventions (see Chapter 8) as the most effective way to assist communities to improve health behavior, concepts and theories of diffusion in organizations are important also. Different factors are operating in organizational change and individual change related to health behavior. "Although organizational change results from individual decisions, these decisions are made in the context of the individual's organizational role" (Basch, 1984, p. 59).

Some insights about organizational diffusion can be obtained from a study of planned diffusion within 12 schools in 10 states by Huberman and Miles (1984). They found that diffusion was most successful if two factors were present: "mandated, stable use" and "skillful, committed use" (p. 48). "Mandated, stable use" refers to pressures to implement the program by administration, a lack of serious resistance, and harmony between teachers and administrators. Thus, the successful program may require a management-to-employee approach in which the implementer of the program works with management initially to obtain a commitment for the program.

"Skillful, committed use" refers to the use of the innovation by the user system and requires assistance on the part of the implementer to increase the user's mastery and commitment of the program. Thus, diffusion and maintenance are enhanced when training is provided, and training and proficiency increase commitment.

MODEL FOR ORGANIZATIONAL DIFFUSION

Rogers and Shoemaker (1973) and later Rogers (1983) identified five stages in the diffusion process: knowledge, persuasion, decision, implementation, and confirmation. Parcel et al. (1989, 1990) used these stages to develop a process framework for organizational diffusion. Their process has four steps: dissemination, adoption, implementation, and maintenance. During dissemination, knowledge and persuasion are used; during the adoption step, a decision is made; and during implementation and maintenance of the innovation, there is confirmation. These stages are discussed next.

DISSEMINATION

During the dissemination stage, information is provided about the innovation, and potential users are motivated to adopt the program. Modeling, as discussed earlier, may serve as a major force in learning about an innovation (Bandura, 1977). Modeling can be informational and motivational. For example, when a successful program on smoking prevention in a school is viewed by teachers and administrators in another school, they obtain information about the program and are motivated by its potential use for positive results.

Modeling serves as a determinant of diffusion in two major ways: through media channels and through interpersonal channels. In what Bandura calls the "dual-link model," modeling occurs through both channels. People learn about the innovation from mass media, and then influential people inform others about it through personal communication. For example, a program introduced into a school district might start with media such as videotapes and printed materials. Then interpersonal means such as demonstrations, meetings, and classroom observations could be used to continue the dissemination.

ADOPTION

Interventions during this stage are for obtaining a commitment from an organization's administration and key decision makers to adopt and use the program. Although knowledge and motivation are necessary for adoption, they are not sufficient. According to Bandura (1986), environmental inducements may create favorable conditions that induce and support the decision of the organization to adopt the program. Two strategies may be used: (a) demonstrating how the program benefits the user and fits within the current activities and goals of the organization and (b) creating vicarious incentives that provide benefits to individuals and the organization.

For example, if schools are mandated to carry out a certain school program such as smoking prevention, the intervention strategy to be used by the resource system would be to demonstrate how the new program would meet the mandate and how it could fit easily within the current teaching curriculum. In addition, incentives would be used such as financial incentives (free training of teachers and low-cost supplies and materials) and social incentives (recognizing the school as a leader on mass media and providing certification for teacher training). Efforts should be made to reach early adopters and give them visibility as models of the program.

IMPLEMENTATION

Two necessary aspects of any innovative program being introduced are completeness and fidelity (Parcel et al., 1990). *Completeness* refers to the delivery of the complete program to participants. Incompleteness can lead to failure of a program. *Fidelity* refers to the program's reflection of the intent and methods designed. For example, modifying a program to use teacher lectures for smoking prevention after peer teaching had been found effective and had been planned could jeopardize the program's adoption by changing the method.

During this stage, staff members and others implementing a program should be trained in the skills and provided with the resources needed to conduct the program so that all components are included and fidelity is maintained. Staff training and technical support are therefore important at this stage. During staff training, modeling should be used, and practice with feedback should be provided. Technical support to answer questions is important. In an evaluation of a school health program, Connell, Turner, and Mason (1985) found a relationship between the training of staff and the extent to which a program was implemented and students learned.

MAINTENANCE

During this stage, the emphasis is on moving the program to an institutionalized status in the adopting organization. This is accomplished when the program is used beyond the initial trial period. Often, resources decrease following the trial period, and attention in the user organization shifts to other concerns. The resource system should be aware of these customary changes and provide incentives to staff to continue the activities and to administrators for supporting the activities. Incentives that may be used are performance feedback, recognition reinforcement, and putting a monitoring and feedback system in place. These are discussed further by Parcel et al. (1990).

SELECTED DIFFUSION STUDIES

Shea, Basch, Lantigua, and Wechster (1992) discuss a healthy heart program implemented in a disadvantaged urban setting and identify six potential barriers to diffusion of this community-based disease prevention program: (a) scale and complexity, (b) model adaptation to a community without a geopolitical boundary, (c) cultural diversity, (d) competing problems, (e) the evaluation role, and (f) sustainability of the program. Strategies for addressing some of these problems are discussed, and the authors conclude that the diffusion model can be useful.

Puska et al. (1986) discuss a project that used lay opinion leaders to promote diffusion in the community. More than 800 lay opinion leaders were trained for working with a population to institute changes to reduce risk factors for heart disease. After 4 years, the self-reported effects and long-term feasibility of the project were reported from a survey. The authors concluded that lay opinion leaders significantly influenced the program.

Oppewal (1992) describes the multiple-site case implementation of a Bone Up on Arthritis Program at the organizational level. Three research questions were answered involving the diffusion process of the program, how it was adapted to the specific organizations and community, and the attributes identified as important during the initial implementation of the innovation. In addition, implications for practice were identified. A case study on this program by Dr. Oppewal is provided at the end of this chapter.

PROGRAM INSTITUTIONALIZATION

Another name for program maintenance, discussed briefly above, is *program institutionalization.* It is the final step of the innovation diffusion process and ensures that a program continues after funding or the trial period has been discontinued. Often, successful institutionalization continues the program in the adopting organizations but also attracts others (late adopters) to the program. According to Goodman and Steckler (1989), this is the most neglected stage of innovation research, and consequently, it has a weak theoretical basis. This step will be discussed in greater depth below.

DEFINITIONS

By Goodman and Steckler's (1989) definition, institutionalization is "the attainment of longevity" (p. 63). Successful programs become an integral part of the host organizations during this step, and there is mutual adaptation between the program and the institution as a result of their interactional changes with each other (Berman, 1978). According to Kanter (1983), "It is when the structures surrounding a change also change to support it that we say that a change is 'institutionalized'—that it is now part of legitimate and ongoing practice, infused with value and supported by other aspects of the system" (p. 299).

MODELS OF INSTITUTIONALIZATION

EXPLANATORY MODEL OF INSTITUTIONALIZATION

Goodman and Steckler (1989) propose a model to explain how institutionalization occurs that includes six factors: (a) standard operating routines, (b) a cluster of critical precursor conditions, (c) mutual adaptation of the actors' aspirations, (d) the action of a program champion, (e) mutual adaptation of the program and organizational norms, and (f) a fit between the program and the organization's mission and operation.

STANDARD OPERATING ROUTINES

Standard operating routines refers to typical ongoing interactions within the organization, such as receiving reports being part of the program at regularly scheduled meetings of administrators, organizational boards, and supervisors and regular interactions between members of these groups and staff of the program, as well as client groups using the program.

CRITICAL PRECURSOR CONDITIONS

The cluster of critical precursor conditions includes problem awareness, a concern for the problem, receptivity to change, availability of solutions to the problem, adequate program resources, and program benefits observed. When the first five conditions are present, recognition of program benefits usually follows. One example provided by the authors is that of a school that successfully built coalitions for tobacco prevention programs because personnel developed an awareness of the harmful effects of smoking, fostered concern that students might use tobacco, accessed a validated national curriculum on tobacco use prevention (availability), and provided teacher in-service education by a national expert (adequacy). By consolidating the program on tobacco prevention education with other classroom responsibilities of teachers, administrators could see the program as an asset rather than a burden (benefit). This led to active support for the program.

Programs that meet the personal, professional, or organizational aspirations of individuals may also influence their perception of benefit over cost and lead to advocacy for the program. To illustrate this, the authors describe how the physician director of school health services eventually came to support the inclusion of the curriculum on tobacco use prevention in schools because she wanted the health care delivery and education in the school district to be comprehensive (aspiration). Her initial nonsupport was a result of her perception that the tobacco use prevention program was too narrow and used too many resources (cost outweighed benefits). Following increased visibility and acceptance of the program, district administrative personnel were more interested in including other health areas in the curriculum, and the director realized that the smoking program could be a stepping-stone to other programs, a development that would meet her goal for more comprehensive programs. As a result, she became an advocate of the program (benefit outweighed cost). Thus, if all critical precursor conditions are present, the benefits are perceived and lead to program advocacy.

MUTUAL ADAPTATION OF ACTOR'S ASPIRATIONS

Coalitions or "natural marriages" between constituents of programs result from program advocacy. A necessary component of these "natural marriages" is to satisfy the aspirations of each actor or partner in the marriage. This requires a mutual accommodation of the various aspirations of the program constituents, or *mutual adaptation of aspirations.* An example offered by the authors involved a senior citizen exercise program that was moderately institutionalized in a department of health, education, and recreation within a university. The administrator and department head held different aspirations. The administrator wanted to increase grants, publications, and revenue from the program, whereas the department head wanted to add a community health component to the program. Both saw the benefit but had different aspirations. As a result, they accommodated to each other. The administrator accommodated to the department head's aspirations by providing start-up funds for the program, and the department head agreed to market the program aggressively to generate revenue and research. Continued meeting of aspirations is important and "natural marriages" or coalitions may dissolve if this does not occur or if aspirations change.

ACTION OF A PROGRAM CHAMPION

According to Goodman and Steckler (1989), institutionalization and the forming of coalitions requires a broker or program champion who can blend the various aspirations. Key characteristics of these program champions are (a) an important organizational link or location, (b) the ability to determine the various aspirations of constituents by using sophisticated analytical and intuitive skills, and (c) outstanding interpersonal and negotiation skills used in coalition building. This person is most effective if he or she is at a middle to upper level in the host organization, with access to program planners and to important organizational decision makers such as board members and agency directors.

MUTUAL ADAPTATION OF THE PROGRAM AND ORGANIZATION'S NORMS

Mutual adaptation of norms occurs as a consequence of the forming of the coalition. Whereas the adaptation of aspirations occurs among key people, the adaptation of norms occurs between the program and the organization and increases the program's fit within the organization. Structures, functions, beliefs, and behaviors are all part of the accommodations made between the program and organization.

The authors offered the following illustration from the case of the senior exercise program at the local university discussed earlier. The administrator of the university and the department head joined forces and established a coalition within the university. As they advocated for the program, an adaptation of norms was manifested by changes in several structures, functions, beliefs, and behaviors: Off-campus housing for the program was established (structure), experienced staff were hired (function), and other programs within the university such as nursing recognized the program of health promotion as a distinct enterprise (belief and behavior). These initial efforts at institutionalization led to further institutionalization, such as permanent housing on campus, staff line positions in the budget, and a permanent committee to coordinate health promotion activities.

FIT TO THE ORGANIZATION'S MISSION

Institutionalization requires a fit between a program and the organization's mission and core operations. Low fit leads to shallow institutionalization, whereas high fit leads to a deeper institutionalization. In complex and segmented organizations, the program's fit may be to one division rather than to the whole organization.

MARKETING MODEL OF INSTITUTIONALIZATION

Lefebvre (1990) developed a marketing model of institutionalization that has four steps: (a) deciding on the target for institutionalization, (b) producing a marketing plan, (c) deciding action strategies, and (d) refining the plan by analyzing the strengths and weaknesses of the program.

DECIDING ON THE TARGET

Efforts to institutionalize or maintain a program may be directed toward individuals, organizations, networks, or coordinating agencies. Members of the general community may be targeted, especially key community members such as political or business leaders who may assume leadership in continuing the program maintenance as a result of the personal commitment developed while volunteering during the trial or funded period. This group may help others learn the desired behaviors by serving as role models for knowledge and motivation. But although individuals are important for continuing programs, they are not sufficient to continue the program alone.

Schools, companies, civic and voluntary organizations, governmental agencies, churches, fitness centers, restaurants, and grocery stores are important organizations to target for institutionalization efforts. Although their personnel may initially require training, they may later be able to carry on the program themselves.

Networks of social support are important in continuing individual and organizational commitment and ultimately institutionalizing a program. Thus, it is important to provide regular opportunities for individuals and organizations involved with the program to interact and discuss issues of mutual concern, to develop coordinated plans, and to reinforce each other.

One can also create new structures such as community boards, private foundations, or a single agency to coordinate institutionalization efforts and assume responsibility for maintaining the program. This model is considered the most effective way to continue programs but is also the most costly in terms of resources.

As is the case of community interventions, a multilevel approach is probably the most effective, and individuals, organizations, networks, and coordinating agencies should all be targeted.

PRODUCING A MARKETING PLAN

Institutionalization involves marketing because its goal is to convince people and organizations to make long-term commitments to the program. Marketing consists of assessing the consumer's needs and implementing services and products that meet those needs in a way that also meets organizational objectives. The plan for marketing should consider objectives, audience for messages, channels for messages, message content, products, services, and resources.

Objectives. The marketing plan for institutionalization requires setting a variety of objectives concerning practices, relationships, values, and outreach. Objectives related to practice of the components of a program might include teachers' incorporation of education on nutrition into the school curriculum, restaurants' continuing to offer healthy foods, and individuals' continuing to practice behaviors related to good nutrition. Objectives related to relationships might stipulate desired forms and frequent communication between volunteers, in church or worksite committees, or in other networks to support the program. Objectives related to values would stipulate the desired values for adoption by individuals, groups, or organizations that would guide future decisions, such as an individual's choice to patronize shops that offer lean meat or an organization's choice to offer a daily exercise routine to its employees. Finally, outreach objectives would be those concerning the establishment of new connections with interested and organizations, such as those who performed or offered health programs.

Audience. In general, the audiences chosen for messages are those already discussed in the section "Deciding on the Target" above. However, specific marketing efforts will require selection of specific audiences within the larger, general audience, such as a particular company, school, clinic, or neighborhood association.

Channels. Channels are the methods for reaching the audiences with messages, programs, or services. The most influential method, as discussed earlier, is personal contact—for example, outreach by peers to some segment of the general public, outreach by board and committee members to other important community people and resource managers, or outreach by volunteers who stimulate grassroots community organizing. Another channel is the mass media, which may highlight individual and organizational efforts toward institutionalization, reinforce participation in the program, and report program activities. Finally, there are organizational channels. Large organizations can be helpful in diffusing and institutionalizing the program or service through bulletin boards, newsletters, and other forms of in-house communication.

Messages. Messages should promote the following:

1. Self-efficacy—a sense that one can change one's risk behavior; help others do the same; effectively help to change the behavior of groups, organizations, and the community by one's own efforts; and maintain the program
2. Collective efficacy—a group's sense that its members can help themselves and others, create healthier organizational or community environments, and sustain a program
3. Organizational self-sufficiency—an organization's sense that it can carry out programs relatively independently that are cost-effective
4. High outcome expectations—an organization's determining its success from an evaluation that motivates further involvement
5. Stakeholders, a group that should have the broadest base possible—people who believe in the program and who have been actively involved in its implementation

Products. Self-help kits, scores, group programs, curricula, and other such products are the most tangible and visible aspects of the program. Four product features are important for promoting the product's adoption and use: (a) usefulness to the needs of individuals and organizations; (b) low cost or affordability to consumer groups; (c) adaptability, such that products can be used immediately by individuals or organizations but have audiovisual, printed, or curricular components that can be added or subtracted to meet the needs of different populations; (d) packaging that is attractive and that offers clear instructions, readable information, and the right amount of information.

Services. Services offered during institutionalization may differ from those offered during diffusion. Program staff move from service delivery to consultation and training in an effort to facilitate the assumption of responsibilities by the user. Whereas previously, they carried out the functions themselves, they now offer *referral* to continuing organizations. Finally, they offer *direction,* which involves the timing of transfer of services or products to other organizations. Two factors determine when transfer will take place: quality and positioning. For example, when a product or service is effective, as determined by evaluation, is in a usable form, and is reasonably priced and appropriately packaged, it is of high enough quality to be ready for institutionalization. When it is viewed as necessary, it is well positioned. At this point, the program can be transferred.

Resources. During movement from diffusion to institutionalization, there may be a shortage of resources. Some resources for institutionalization that can be generated from the community are people, messages, services, products, and money. Some possible people resources are volunteers, faculty and students in universities, hospital staff, news reporters, and civic organizations. Some message resources are worksite newsletters, church bulletins, school curriculums, local newspapers, and television interests. Services may be available from existing programs in local nonprofit and voluntary organizations. Similar products that have the same goals may be used to preserve the services or program to be institutionalized. Financial resources may be obtained from United Way, corporate foundations, local private foundations, and public and private organizations, among others, and from external sources (state and national organizations) such as the American Cancer Association, the American Lung Association, the American Heart Association, depending on the program and services to be institutionalized.

DECIDING ACTION STRATEGIES

At this point, one develops specific strategies to fulfill the objectives of the marketing plan. Action strategies for institutionalization of a program are (a) identifying the audience, such as key leaders, worksites, and schools; (b) segmenting this audience by adopter status (innovators, early adopters, etc.), (c) determining the needs of each group; (d) directing institutionalization messages, products, and services to each group; (e) developing a broad base by diffusion techniques; and (f) obtaining long-term financial support.

REFINING THE PLAN

This step involves reviewing each program product and service to determine its fit with organizational institutionalization strategies. This can be done by portfolio analysis, described by Kotler and Andreasen (1987) as involving three steps: (a) partitioning similar products and services of an organization; (b) assessing the market condition, current performance, and market share for each group; and (c) forecasting the future of the product or service.

The case study that accompanies this chapter applies the concepts of diffusion theory.

Case Study 4

Implementing *Bone Up on Arthritis* Within the Great Lakes Chapter

SONDA RIEDESEL OPPEWAL

This case study describes how members of a voluntary health organization implemented a community-based innovation, the Bone Up on Arthritis (BUOA) program, for the first time. Nurses developed the innovation, led the dissemination efforts at the national level of the Arthritis Foundation (AF), and led the implementation efforts at the local organizational level. A nurse, working as Program Director for an AF chapter, was responsible for diffusing the program to community members. This description of how the Great Lakes AF chapter implemented the BUOA program highlights some of the challenges the diffusion process presents to health care organizations and specifically to organizational and community members involved with this process.

AUTHOR'S NOTE: The research reported here was funded by an Arthritis Foundation Health Professions Traineeship.

BACKGROUND TO THE CASE STUDY

An opportunity existed to examine directly how a voluntary health organization implemented an innovation for the first time. These organizations are established community agencies with an interest in health promotion (Goodwin, 1986; Hamlin, 1965) and represent ideal vehicles for disseminating innovative health programs to the clients they serve. The AF is a voluntary health organization whose national office supplies and recommends different educational programs to local chapters for dissemination to community members (Boutaugh & McDuffie, 1984). Employed staff members and volunteers work at the AF National Office in Atlanta, Georgia, and in 73 local chapters and branches across the country. The organization's primary mission is to promote arthritis research and health care (AF, 1986).

AF leaders at the national office were eager to disseminate a community-based arthritis self-care education program titled BUOA soon after nurse researchers evaluated it in 1987. Developed by nurse researchers in 1984 and updated in 1988, this program enabled participants to listen to six audiotapes about arthritis self-care management in their homes. Instructional booklets accompanied each audiotape, and trained community coordinators (CCs), lay or professional volunteers, provided assistance when requested by participants. The program's curriculum content was based on a needs assessment of persons with arthritis. Given the past success of the BUOA program in improving arthritis knowledge, self-care behaviors, learned helplessness, and pain control (Goeppinger, Arthur, Baglioni, Brunk, & Brunner, 1989), leaders at the AF National Office decided to offer this program to local chapters to disseminate to community members with arthritis.

A case study follows to show how a nurse used diffusion theory concepts in practice. Pseudonyms replace the names of persons interviewed as well as the name of the AF chapter. Interviews were conducted with the following organizational and community members:

- Chapter executive director (Tim)
- Chapter volunteer (Tina)
- Chapter program director (Joan)
- Chapter volunteer coordinator (Kate)

- Branch directors (Tara, Lee)
- BUOA volunteer coordinator (Nancy)
- BUOA community contact volunteers (Sybil, Pat, Helen, Elaine, Gwen)
- BUOA participants (Penny, Violet, Vanessa, Rachel, Nora)

THE ARTHRITIS FOUNDATION, GREAT LAKES CHAPTER

The Great Lakes Chapter office is located in the metro Ridgecrest area in a large business building on a major highway. One suite houses the chapter office, and the office for the Metro Ridgecrest Branch is in a suite across the hall. Chapter and branch staff members and volunteers interact frequently, sharing resources as needed in tastefully decorated and well-equipped offices. Two rooms in the chapter suite are designated for volunteer use.

The chapter office provides services to the entire state of Great Lakes, 83 counties in all, with people from diverse ethnic backgrounds. Almost half of the state's population lives in the three counties making up the metro Ridgecrest area. The city of Ridgecrest has an estimated population of 1,200,000. The chapter supervises six branch offices and two volunteer-directed units. Each branch office has a full- or part-time branch director, and most have secretarial assistance. Chapter and branch employees number 26; there are approximately 600 volunteers throughout the state.

Joan is a registered nurse who has worked as the chapter program director for the past 5 years. She is convinced that the organization's main strength is "the people who work" for the chapter, both volunteers and staff. Even though the organization is highly centralized and formalized, a family-like atmosphere exists. In addition to the strong support from volunteers and staff, Joan especially appreciates working with Kate, a volunteer who is the chapter volunteer coordinator for programs. Kate works 20 to 30 hours every week recruiting and coordinating volunteers, which gives Joan more time to write or revise branch guidelines for program implementation and to supervise the current 20 to 22 programs in operation across the chapter. Joan finds written guidelines crucial for successful program implementation; she describes herself as the type of person who "likes things in black and white." As program director, Joan has a certain degree of autonomy supervising the arthritis programs offered throughout the chapter. She attributes her autonomy, in part, to her efforts to keep the chapter executive director informed of her progress by giving him a copy of every memo she sends out.

Despite working in an organization that is goal directed and that maintains a family-like atmosphere, one challenge that Joan faces is working with people who have different ideas and personalities. Sometimes, it is difficult to maintain the level of control that Joan thinks is necessary when she supervises programs.

> One of the detrimental things about working with branches is they often want to go off and do their own thing, and they see [the] chapter coming in as interference rather than assistance, at times, for certain things. And for me in programs, my biggest challenge is to work with a branch in a way that everybody concerned with the branch sees what I do as an asset to them, not as something that the chapter sitting off down here somewhere else says we have to do this.

PRESSED FOR TIME: APPLYING FOR BUOA

In early February, after reading the memo from the national office about the BUOA program, Joan immediately recognized a problem. The deadline date for applying was only a few weeks away. There was little time for BUOA to undergo the chapter's normal review procedure, a requirement before implementing new programs. The protocol, outlined in a written document titled "Guidelines for Review of a New or Existing Program," calls for several Patient and Service Education Committee members to rate the program in three areas: value, feasibility, and effectiveness/benefits.

Joan immediately called staff members at the national office to request a copy of the BUOA material and any program guidelines. The final booklets were not yet ready, nor were program guidelines, but a draft of a BUOA booklet was better than nothing. With the committee expecting a full review of the program before even considering it, Joan described her predicament: "If I walk into that committee and give what National originally sent to the chapters and say,

'Would you decide whether or not we can do this?' the committee will laugh at me." The additional material from the national office arrived promptly, and Joan handed it over to two committee members who agreed to review the program before the next Patient and Education Service Committee meeting in March. One volunteer became ill, so only one person, the chair of the committee, completed the review.

Tina liked the BUOA booklet and recognized that the content was basically the same as the arthritis self-help course (ASHC) but at a lower reading level. Her primary concern, however, was whether the program would be useful to that target audience—people with low reading levels. There was only one way to find out. She decided to test the program on a group of sixth graders and adults with low literacy skills, thinking, "If it works with those two groups and they like it and they respond to it, then there's probably a very good chance that the target audience for BUOA will take to it."

With the help of a few contacts, Tina lined up the two groups and asked them to read the BUOA booklet and then discuss how difficult or easy it was to read and understand. Members from both groups said they had no difficulty with the material. The booklet sparked thoughtful questions from the sixth graders, and the adults liked the tone of the program, which was not perceived as condescending.

After completing the review on March 7, Tina presented a favorable report to Patient Service and Education Committee members, who agreed with her recommendation to apply as a BUOA pilot site. Important information missing from the description of BUOA from the national office was an estimated budget. The program seemed expensive to Joan because of postage and telephone costs. Without knowing how the chapter would cover the costs for BUOA, Tim, the executive director, agreed to find the funding needed if the chapter was selected as a pilot site. They could apply for grants to help fund BUOA in the future. After little discussion, chapter board members approved the recommendation to apply as a BUOA pilot site.

PROGRAM PREPARATION BEGINS

After hearing at the end of April that the chapter was accepted as a pilot site, Joan recalled feeling a "little confused." She had not received any program material from the national office. "I really felt I needed a lot more clarification of Where do we go now? And I felt that everything was having to move too fast." Because national office members had not sent a written job description for the volunteer coordinator, she could not begin recruiting. She needed more information. The BUOA orientation meeting scheduled for June 6 left little time for recruitment efforts.

In mid-May, the job description arrived. Kate reviewed the information and then turned to her files of potential volunteers. She selected six people she thought would enjoy working with BUOA, telephoned several people for their response, and then gave three biographical forms in the order she recommended to Joan. Nancy was Kate's first choice. Although Nancy had never volunteered for the AF because of time constraints while in graduate school, she had undergone training for the Helpline program, a telephone counseling and support service. After thinking about Kate's request to become the volunteer coordinator and reading the BUOA information, Nancy discussed the idea with her school adviser, who approved the project for her thesis requirement. The idea was more enticing to Nancy. Joan interviewed Nancy and asked her to take the position. Nancy agreed, feeling somewhat "flabbergasted" that the chapter even considered her for such a major role when she had not yet volunteered for the AF. Nancy also remembered how difficult it would have been to give Kate any phony excuses. In her words, "Kate's hard to turn down."

As recruitment efforts for a volunteer coordinator were under way, Joan realized that she needed to decide where the pilot program would take place. To give each of the six branches an opportunity to participate, Joan mailed a description of the BUOA program and application to the six branch directors, asking if they would like to participate as a pilot site for BUOA. They would be responsible for recruiting two to four CCs and 20 BUOA participants by July 31, as well as compiling a list of community resources.

Joan was careful to communicate clearly with branch members, distinguishing between their responsibilities for BUOA and the chapter's responsibilities. Because chapter members wanted to maintain control over the lesson delivery, to see how participants were doing and to allow participants adequate time for absorbing individual lessons, they decided to mail the lessons one at a time. By experiencing what it was like to do this for 50 participants, chapter staff members would be in a better position to help the branches eventually take over this responsibility.

Two branch directors applied—Tara, from the Metro Ridgecrest branch, and Lee, from the Fairview branch. The decision to participate in BUOA was easy for both directors. Tara explained, "We submitted our application based on our need to have a program that would meet a minority population and an underserved area and an economically deprived area." The ASHC had not been successful in Ridgecrest; few people attended. Tara speculated that some people lacked transportation, that some were homebound or bedridden, or that the ASHC content was too difficult to read. Metro Ridgecrest branch members responded with enthusiasm to the proposal to participate with BUOA because "this was a program that would meet needs." By taking the course to the home setting, Tara thought some barriers were removed for persons who were perhaps less motivated to learn through self-help education. Branch members anticipated that the number of BUOA participants would exceed, by far, the number of ASHC participants after the program was established. Although the Ridgecrest and Fairview branches would target different populations—inner city and rural—Lee applied for BUOA for the same reason as Tara. She thought it would meet the needs of the people living in the rural farming villages in her area.

The week following an orientation meeting provided by Dr. Goeppinger and AF National Office staff members, Joan, Nancy, and Kate spent a day adapting the national office's guidelines for implementing BUOA from the chapter office but using the two branches as pilot test sites. They separated the steps for which the chapter would remain responsible and developed a working set of guidelines for the two branches. After the pilot program's evaluation, they would later revise the guidelines for general use by any of the six branches interested in offering BUOA. The group also developed a packet of information for the branch directors that included suggestions for recruiting volunteers and participants.

Joan and Nancy agreed to meet on a weekly basis to discuss BUOA plans, divide the work, and meet with Kate if they were discussing volunteer recruitment. Kate would focus on volunteer recruitment for the Ridgecrest area because she had information on volunteers in that area. She had scant information on potential volunteers in the Fairview area, and Lee thought she could recruit one volunteer without difficulty. Joan, Nancy, Kate, and Tara decided that after Kate identified potential volunteers in the Ridgecrest area, they would mail packets of information and then follow up in a week with a telephone call to each prospective volunteer. If the person was interested, then Nancy would conduct an interview face-to-face or by telephone. Joan recognized it was not always easy finding chapter or branch volunteers who adhered to program requirements and had the required time commitment; volunteers in one AF program could not be "taken away" for a new program.

Understanding who was doing what for the BUOA program was important to Joan. She described her role as "knowing what's going on all the time," and a major responsibility was developing explicit, clear program guidelines. To fulfill this second goal, Joan, with assistance from Kate and Nancy, outlined 21 objectives that chapter members "needed to do to fulfill our obligations and have a good, successful pilot." This document, the "Arthritis Foundation Program Review and Evaluation Tool," illustrated the timetable for the objectives and specified possible strategies or tactics for each objective along with a priority rating and a start and target finish date. Joan outlined action steps according to date and person responsible, and the form included columns to summarize how each step was evaluated, the time needed for completion, and financial cost.

Before BUOA reached any participants, Joan summarized her plans for the program: "What I'm aiming for is when we get done with the national pilot and we get ready to go and hit 83 counties, that we have some sort of a systematic way to follow through on an ongoing basis." Volunteers would be crucial so that the program could be ongoing, starting whenever a new person was ready for the lessons. After the branches began delivering the lessons within their regions, chapter members would assist them if needed, and provide the program to people living in areas not covered by branches. Joan envisioned BUOA taking as much volunteer time and budget as the AF literature distribution, which occurs daily: "I'd like within two years to see that we have at least 1,000 requests a year for this program. And then I'd have a volunteer in here working every day on some aspect of the program."

VOLUNTEER RECRUITMENT IN RIDGECREST: SCRAPING FOR FIVE

Nancy and Kate developed an application form for potential community contact volunteers (CCVs) to complete if they were interested in attending the training on July 25 and 26. In addition, a description of BUOA, the CCV job description, and a letter from Tara were mailed to 37 persons whom Kate identified as possibly interested in volunteering. Tara or Kate telephoned each of the potential CCVs a week later to explore their interest.

To some degree, the response of the potential CCVs was not surprising. Not one person agreed to volunteer. The job description stated that home visits might be needed for delivering a tape recorder or demonstrating an exercise. No one was willing to make a home visit in the Ridgecrest area—it was not considered a safe place. Joan thought this reluctance to visit homes even in their own neighborhoods was justified. "Right now it's pretty much considered that in this area . . . there is a crack house on every block, one in ten people is carrying a gun, and probably every other person is carrying a weapon. That's what the city of Ridgecrest is."

By the third week of July, not one CCV had been recruited. Time was running out, even though the national office changed the CC training to mid-August because of a delay with materials. After several discussions, the chapter staff members agreed to eliminate the home visit expectation from the CCV job description (as it was originally conceived by the innovator developers). The CCVs could make their contacts with participants over the telephone. If a home visit was needed for some reason, chapter staff members rather than volunteers would be responsible.

Another problem that some of the potential CCVs voiced after reviewing the job description was the expected time commitment. The job description stated, "Four to ten (4-10) hours per week to make home/phone contacts with Home Study participants. And, two to four hours per week to report on project status to Volunteer Coordinator and to record contacts." Nancy realized this time expectation was too high; potential volunteers viewed it as "outrageous." One person likened it to a full-time job, and another anticipated having a very sore ear from talking on the telephone for that many hours. Nancy revised the job description by prefacing the time commitment as a "maximum" expectation. Chapter staff tried to allay concerns expressed by potential CCVs that the program would be time-consuming.

After chapter members sent the revised recruitment packets to another set of selected persons, four persons in the metro Ridgecrest area agreed to volunteer for BUOA. Each had turned down the request initially but reconsidered after the job description was changed.

RECRUITING PARTICIPANTS: COVERING ALL THE ANGLES

Efforts to recruit BUOA participants started in June with volunteer recruitment because Joan wanted the CCVs to begin working with participants as soon as possible after the training, when their enthusiasm for the program would be high. The first recruitment strategy was submitting press releases to area newspapers. One press release, submitted to an office in Bath County, where Ridgecrest is located, was immediately picked up by a newspaper office in neighboring Franklin County. An error appeared in the story, however, asking participants from outside Bath county to join the program. Within a week, about 40 people from Franklin County called to sign up for BUOA. Chapter staff decided to include this group with the pilot even though they were not from the urban area. One of the CCVs who volunteered in the chapter office each week for the Helpline program agreed to work with the Franklin County participants if she could use the office telephone for the long-distance calls.

Other strategies for recruiting participants included a 10-minute radio interview with Joan about the BUOA program and short public service announcements on radio. Nancy called all of the newspaper offices to follow up on the status of the press releases. In urban areas, where newspapers are inundated with press releases, not all are published: "Here you send it and you hope it shows up in the paper, and if it doesn't you contact the person and do a little begging."

After developing a flier about BUOA, Tara, Kate, and Nancy mailed it to different senior centers and neighborhood churches. The fliers were also available at AF displays for interested persons to read. Kate had used similar recruitment methods in the past for the ASHC and found that publicizing AF programs in church bulletins or newsletters was quite effective. She had even "tested" whether pastors were more likely to post or publish the program announcements if the AF letter was addressed "Dear Pastor" or with his or her specific name. She found that the salutation did not make a difference, because the announcement was usually printed if space was available.

When some BUOA press releases remained unpublished and after she had contacted newspaper offices to inquire about their status, Kate resorted to "Plan B." She reviewed the last 6 months of information and referral forms from persons who inquired about the ASHC but did not attend, as well as any other requests from persons who suggested they might be interested in self-help information. She also scanned records of persons in the Ridgecrest area who called the national office's toll-free telephone number with a question about arthritis. All of these target individuals, about 150 people, received a "Who, What, Where, When" flier about BUOA and a participant application form in the mail. Kate also tried to initiate cable television announcements and a spot on a local television station's "We Care" program to describe BUOA. Volunteers working with the chapter's Helpline program were also asked to inform appropriate "call-ins" about the opportunity to participate in BUOA.

THE COMMUNITY CONTACT VOLUNTEER TRAINING

Four CCVs—Helen, Elaine, Gwen, and Sybil—from metro Ridgecrest, Pat from Fairview, and Joan, Nancy, and Kate attended the volunteer training August 10 and 11. All five CCVs had arthritis. Whereas Pat was new as an AF volunteer, the others had volunteered in the past for the ASHC, a mutual support group, or the Helpline program. Pat was the only CCV with a health-related background. One of the Ridgecrest CCVs lived downtown, and the other three lived within the tricounty metro Ridgecrest area.

Despite little time to review the BUOA materials before the training, most comments about the training were positive. Sybil thought the training was work but fun. Elaine agreed: "We got a chance to go through what the other persons with arthritis would be going through and getting a feel for it on our own, so we'd know more or less what they're doing and how it's probably feeling to them." Helen, a mutual support group leader and trained ASHC leader, found the training well organized and observed the trainers using the same adult learning principles they reviewed with the CCVs. Pat appreciated the exercise demonstrations and thought the "hour after hour of role playing" was helpful. For Gwen, however, "Everything was repeated, repeated, repeated." Nancy agreed that if volunteers had previous AF training in a similar program, it "may not be necessary to go through the materials line by line."

During the training, Joan, Kate, and Nancy presented their plans for delivering the BUOA materials to participants and then asked if the CCVs approved. They agreed to mail the lessons one at a time from the chapter office via United Parcel Service. A stamped, addressed envelope would be included for the participant to return the completed audiocassette to the chapter office. Once the tape reached the chapter office, the next booklet and tape would be mailed. This method allowed time for the information to "settle in," preventing participants from going through the lessons too quickly. It also gave the chapter greater control to assess how participants liked the program and to determine how long the participants needed to complete the lessons. Although postage costs were higher with this method, Tim agreed with Joan that "this way we have more control over the program."

After discussing how participants would receive the lessons, the issue of making home visits reemerged at the CCV training. The trainers from the national office, Lisa and Janice, mentioned that a home visit might be in order if a participant required a tape recorder or an exercise demonstration. Joan differed. A better solution in her opinion was to encourage participants who requested an exercise demonstration to ask their local physician or physical therapist and take their BUOA booklet to their appointment. If a tape recorder were needed, it could be mailed rather than delivered in person. Joan thought these suggestions were "better than a

home visit because, when this program's over, we aren't still going to be running out to the home. So if we have referred them to their current support health care team for answers, aren't we modeling something better for them than their dependence on us?" She realized that some home visits might be necessary or even desirable: "You're dealing with individuals, [so] you could have just about anything come up. And you might determine that 'Gee, I'd like to make a home visit.' "

IMPLEMENTATION BEGINS: GAINING MOMENTUM

A week after the training, Joan sent a list of 22 potential participants to the University of Michigan (the research site). A month later, 60 names had been mailed to U of M and 2 people were ready for the BUOA lessons. Nancy remembered the impatience and excitement she and other chapter members shared:

It seemed like forever before the first person went through the enrollment process. We were all excited here in the office. You should have seen us, we were all bouncing around in here and shouting. Then we got down to business in terms of getting the lessons out to them.

Nancy spent one day devising the BUOA delivery system with Joan's assistance. Even though the system was somewhat cumbersome and "kind of labor intensive" because of the many papers that were processed initially, it worked. To the file of each participant, they taped a form on which to log the dates the BUOA lessons were sent and returned and to document any contacts the chapter staff made with participants or with the CCV. Mailing the first BUOA lesson and audiocassette was most time-consuming. When a BUOA audiocassette was returned, two envelopes were labeled, one for the participant and one for the chapter office, and the second tape and booklet were mailed after noting the date on the chapter contact record. A display of the delivery system was posted on the bulletin board over Nancy's desk so other volunteers could help with the process.

By October 10, Joan reported that 21 participants were enrolled in the program; more than 70 persons had applied. Four participants had dropped out during the enrollment process, probably because they found the consent forms intimidating. One participant's wife refused to sign the consent form, a physician advised one person against participating, another person dropped out because he was having surgery, and another was not feeling bad and was no longer interested.

By early November, there were 76 potential participants. Nancy halted participant recruitment efforts in order not to exceed 50 participants, but some factors were not under her control. On November 8, staff members at the *Ridgecrest Free Press* published the BUOA announcement, even though the cutoff date for the press release was October 15. Unsure of how to deal with too many participants, Nancy and Joan decided to keep the names and addresses of any interested persons responding to the newspaper article and later mail them a letter with information about when BUOA would be restarted after the pilot study ended.

In addition to mailing out the BUOA lessons, Nancy called the five CCVs occasionally to check on their progress or sent them a letter. For example, she mailed the CCVs a copy of the "Mr. Sun" newsletter that she received each month from University of Michigan researchers. She also included a more personal note to the CCVs.

In addition to words of encouragement, Nancy included in her monthly letters a list of participants and the lessons they were on so the CCVs could see how their participants were progressing through the program. At first she organized the list of participants by county but later according to their CCV, which resulted in a "flood of tapes coming in." Nancy attributed the participants' progression with the lessons, in part, to the number of contacts the CCVs made with them. For example, Nancy suspected that one CCV was not contacting her participants because they were not progressing to Lesson 2. After discussing this problem briefly with Joan, Nancy met with the volunteer to remind her of how important her telephone contacts were—she was the only person in contact with the participants; the chapter staff were not. According to Nancy, the talk worked and the CCV "started making her calls." Recognizing that it is easy to procrastinate, Nancy viewed the monthly letters as a way of encouraging the CCVs to telephone their participants. By letting the volunteers know how the program was progressing, she instilled in them a "stronger sense of ownership."

BUOA FROM THE VOLUNTEER'S PERSPECTIVE: CATCH AS CATCH CAN

On November 1, the AF chapter hosted a meeting for the CCVs with the purpose of sharing experiences, problems, or concerns with Nancy, the BUOA volunteer coordinator. Three of the five CCVs attended: Elaine, Gwen, and Sybil. Helen and Pat were interviewed by telephone later that month.

Although the CCVs recognized they were helping themselves by helping others as BUOA volunteers, their enthusiasm for the program varied. Each experienced some uncertainty about her role as a CCV and some frustration. For example, Sybil asked at the meeting how long she should talk with her participants and how frequently she should call. She found that one participant who seemed very depressed was very difficult to "get off the phone." Nancy suggested telling the participant about some of the community resources outlined on the BUOA resource sheet. When Nancy reassured the CCVs that their telephone conversations did not have to be lengthy, Gwen commented, "That's right, no fooling around." Nancy encouraged the CCVs to call their participants once with each lesson. Originally, she had planned to notify the CCVs each time their participants progressed to the next lesson, but the three CCVs assured her this was not necessary. The written updates she mailed monthly and her telephone calls were sufficient. Besides, they found out what lesson the participant was on when they called.

A general area of frustration for all of the CCVs was contacting their participants. Each mentioned how difficult it was to telephone their participants and find that person at home. They called participants numerous times before making contact. In Pat's words, it's "catch if catch can." The CCVs were surprised that the participants were as mobile as they were. Many were employed. They were not as debilitated with arthritis and dependent, on the whole, as the CCVs expected. One of Sybil's searches was especially difficult, in part because she did not know the participant's gender. After telephoning the household several times, she was told repeatedly that Willie did not live there. When Sybil tried one last time, the person answering said a woman lived there that he did not know. After asking her name, she turned out to be the missing participant—Willie.

Once the CCV contacted a participant, it was sometimes difficult to establish rapport with the person over the telephone. Some participants did not want to talk for long, whereas others did not want to stop. Sybil took notes when talking with her participants in an effort to connect the voice with a person, because she was afraid she might confuse her participants: "It's not going to be any good for anybody if I can't keep them straight." Although Sybil had contacted her participants only once because she had been on vacation, she liked volunteering for the ASHC better, because she preferred the face-to-face contact with the participants. For example, when trying to assure one of her participants who was severely debilitated with arthritis that she understood her pain because she had arthritis as well, Sybil did not think the participant trusted her. She felt unsuccessful trying to share her experiences effectively over the telephone; it was easier to do this face-to-face. Sybil recognized that the ASHC participants benefited from the social contact they received, which was not present to the same degree in the BUOA program. Elaine, on the other hand, liked volunteering for BUOA better than the ASHC. With her mobility hampered by rheumatoid arthritis, she did not have to travel to any class sites but could talk with participants over the telephone. And the participant could have the BUOA booklet "in front of them so they can see what I'm talking about."

Although Pat was the only CCV who had received any phone calls that were initiated by her participants, she expressed a concern similar to Sybil's. It was difficult establishing rapport. She explained:

I feel like I'm just a total stranger to all of these people. I'm just a name with a phone number . . . and they don't really feel—*confident* is not the word I want—but maybe [they do not] feel like they can just pick up the phone and call me.

Two participants called Pat for assistance. One participant wanted Pat's opinion about a book that claimed to cure arthritis. The other participant's problem was more challenging, however. This person had a rare type of arthritis and wanted more information about the disease. Little information existed. A week after calling Pat, the participant called her again because she had not received any information. Pat explained she had been in bed with a cold and had not been able to find the information yet.

Besides feeling frustrated with the seeming inability to establish rapport with some of her participants, Pat also found it difficult to identify and set boundaries as a helping person. She found it frustrating not to be able to provide ready help to the participants yet also did not want to become overinvolved with their problems. She explained that many of her participants have a multitude of problems.

The CCVs expressed concern at the meeting about an issue related to establishing rapport with BUOA participants. It was difficult to assess how the participants were actually doing, and some CCVs suspected that the participants were not using the lessons. For example, Gwen asserted, "Sometimes I don't even think they listen" to the tapes. Nancy also agreed, commenting that some tapes "look virginal when they come back [and] I'm a little skeptical whether it [the tape] just comes and they hang on to it for a week and then send it back." Sybil and Elaine admitted not feeling certain that the participants were listening to the tapes and using the accompanying booklets at the same time. But Gwen was more emphatic in her opinion: "You know from the way they are answering you that they are not really, they haven't really paid that much attention. Some of them, others have, you can tell by the answers . . . they are not paying attention."

To resolve how to deal with this concern that the participants were lying, or not telling the whole truth, the group decided that their role was to encourage and to be role models. Sybil reminded the volunteers that BUOA was part of a "buffet" where the participants can "take what they want."

A VIEW FROM THE PARTICIPANTS

Overall, the response by five participants interviewed was very favorable toward the BUOA program. Several people commented that the exercises were very helpful. One person's pain was eased by a suggestion she learned about the timing of pain medications. Another person felt she was better able to cope with her disease. Penny explained that the program "makes you aware that you are still living and there is still life even though you do have the pain, and you'll be able to survive by taking care of yourself." Furthermore, the program "helped me probably more than the doctor. I will say the doctor's shots seem to help, but I think without them I could get along just as well with this information."

Two participants explained why they were not progressing through the lessons very quickly. After a full day of jury duty, it was too exhausting for Penny to listen to tapes. Violet wanted a quiet environment so she could hear the tapes well and wanted to listen to the tapes only when she felt well, which was not very often. Arthritis has affected most of her joints and she describes her pain as "unbearable" most of the time. Her primary concern focused on why she had the disease. She wanted her arthritis cured rather than acquiring information about how to care for it. Her anger with the disease and the accompanying depression overwhelmed her coping abilities or desire to learn to cope. However, she did recognize that her "outlook" toward the disease differed from the outlook expressed by her CCV toward arthritis.

None of the participants objected to receiving the lessons in the mail. Vanessa, a participant who had recently undergone surgery for a hip replacement, said she could not participate if she had to drive somewhere to pick up the lessons. One participant commented about receiving the lessons one at a time. Penny preferred this method:

This way, if you've got one lesson you can keep it and go through it two or three times, if you want. Or if there are parts that you are dubious about you can listen to that over again. Whereas if you've got it all, I think you might slight it even—just sort of put it over on the side. Whereas this week I think, oh, a new tape is coming! I've got to listen to what it is. It's like getting a new toy!

Four of the five participants mentioned that someone had called to see how they were doing with the program. Rachel recognized how difficult it would be to reach her at home, because she was accompanying her husband to a hospital 60 miles away every day for his radiology treatments. The other four participants could not identify the person calling about BUOA by name or title. For example, one person knew that the caller was from the Great Lakes AF chapter but did not know her name. Another person

knew that the "follow-up person" had arthritis herself, but she did not know what to call this person. Nora mentioned that several people had called to see how she was doing almost every week. She explained, "I'm not any good at names. I think it's the same person, but I'm not sure. They ask if I understand or need any special help with it." Vanessa referred to the person who called as the "follow-up person." She described her role as a monitor or someone she could call if she had a question. None of the participants interviewed had ever called their volunteer or felt the need to do that yet.

REFLECTIONS ON THE PROCESS

NANCY'S PERSPECTIVE

As volunteer coordinator, Nancy described the implementation process as occurring smoothly on the whole: "Far beyond my expectations, and to my great relief! It took a lot of work getting the program off the ground." The work was worthwhile, however, because "It's a great program."

By the beginning of November, Nancy described her job responsibilities as "Pretty well calmed down. It's just a matter of record keeping and making sure that the lessons get out . . . just basically more or less of maintenance." In her opinion, the initial process of implementing BUOA occurred in two major spurts: recruiting the CCVs and then recruiting the participants. She admitted feeling "really frustrated trying to get the PR [going] and making umpteen zillion calls back to people who we sent questionnaires to and getting no response." After the volunteers and participants were recruited and the delivery system developed, the program "just rolls along. . . . It seems to build its own momentum as it goes along." In November, a new volunteer was trained to help with the BUOA mailing system. At the end of December, Nancy was hired for another program within the Great Lakes chapter, but she explained that her commitment as volunteer coordinator for BUOA would continue until all 50 participants completed the program.

When reflecting on the BUOA program in retrospect, Nancy thought "the positive atmosphere" at the chapter office facilitated the implementation process. She explained, "Everyone works hard and laughs and has a common goal, which is to get whatever the job that you're doing done." Furthermore, "It's a very positive, can-do approach that you have here. It's not hard to live up to expectations when you're in an environment like that. Which is the same thing we're trying to have the contact volunteers instill in the participants."

Other factors facilitating the implementation process from Nancy's perspective included "being organized" and being supported by experienced people like "Joan, Kate, Tara, and Lee." Tara agreed that the implementation went smoothly because "we have a large enough branch that's well organized; people are responsible for various aspects of the branch operation. I could not have done this without Kate. . . . She knows the volunteers better than I do."

JOAN'S PERSPECTIVE

By mid-December, when the pilot enrollment officially ended, 4 persons had completed the lessons and 45 people were using the program. Another 7 or 8 people were almost finished with the enrollment requirements. Joan felt "bad" that she and Nancy had not made any plans for persons who expressed an interest in participating in BUOA but did not complete the enrollment process by the December 15 deadline. They decided that anyone who started the enrollment papers would have the opportunity to use the lessons, but they would just not be part of the research study.

By the end of December, the CCVs had received few questions from their participants and had turned to Nancy or Joan to discuss only a couple of questions. One CCV called Nancy when she was having difficulty contacting a participant. Another volunteer wondered how to respond to a participant who did not want to work on the lessons until after the Christmas holidays. Joan assured her that this was "a natural thing" to expect and to just call again after the holidays. The chapter staff had not made any home visits; participants had not asked any questions that required a health professional's expertise. Joan had not recruited an advisory group, other than a rheumatologist who agreed to help if needed, although this expectation was stated clearly in the initial memo to chapters from the national office. So far, she had not had adequate amount of time for this task. With the scant number of

questions asked by participants, she wondered if an advisory group was necessary.

Because the current budget for the chapter was facing cutbacks, Joan feared that no matter how successful BUOA might be, the program would not continue if there were not enough funds to support it. With budget cuts, new programs were usually "the first to go" before the more established programs. Joan described her apprehension:

We didn't need a lot of budget for it [BUOA] right now and I think we're going to hit the crunch after the first of the year. The budget's not going to be there and all of a sudden it's going to be, 'it was real nice, but shove it in the closet and we'll get back to it when there's money.' . . . I would feel really bad if we've got the mechanism and we've got the interested volunteers and we can't do it. If the budget's not there, the budget's not there.

Although Joan knew the members of the board would carefully examine next year's budget, other programs besides BUOA might be curtailed. Securing grant money to support the BUOA program was crucial. Joan identified seven potential granting sources by late summer. One grant application she submitted was approved by a local foundation if matching funds by another agency were located. Joan explained that chapter members would "assume BUOA will continue. This is the only way to function, otherwise there would be a gap between programs and budget."

Although there had been a lack of information and time during the initial implementation process, Joan felt that the BUOA program had worked well. In her opinion, the main reason behind its success was an "excellent volunteer coordinator who actually coordinated the program. . . . We had a coordinator that was a coordinator." Their weekly meetings decreased in time gradually as Nancy handled more of the daily implementation concerns. Joan appreciated Nancy's conscientious reports, which kept her well-informed of the program's progress:

I knew what she was doing, not only at the beginning of the day, but as she left, samples of everything that went out ended up in here with her little note that I got these done, I didn't get to this but I'm going to do that next week. I knew exactly where things were and to me, if you have a coordinator that can do that for a program, it goes smooth. It just goes smooth."

REFERENCES

Arthritis Foundation. (1986). *The Arthritis Foundation in 1986*. Atlanta, GA: Author.

Boutaugh, M., & McDuffie, F. C. (1984). The arthritis self-help course. *Clinical Rheumatology in Practice, 2,* 17-20.

Goeppinger, J., Arthur, M. W., Baglioni, A. J., Brunk, S. E., & Brunner, C. M. (1989). A re-examination of the effectiveness of self-care education for persons with arthritis. *Arthritis and Rheumatism, 32,* 706-716.

Goodwin, R. M. (1986). The role of voluntary health organizations in the community phase of cardiac rehabilitation throughout the world. *Bibliotheca Cardiologica, 40,* 20-29.

Hamlin, R. H. (1965). The role of voluntary agencies in meeting the health needs of Americans. In A. H. Katz & J. S. Felton (Eds.), *Health and the community: Readings in the philosophy and sciences of public health* (pp. 374-384). New York: Free Press.

REFERENCES

Bandura, A. (1977). *Social learning theory.* Englewood Cliffs, NJ: Prentice Hall.

Bandura, A. (1986). *Social foundations of thought and action.* Englewood Cliffs, NJ: Prentice Hall.

Basch, C. E. (1984). Research on disseminating and implementing health-education programs in schools. *Journal of School Health, 54,* 57-66.

Berman, P. (1978). Study of the macro-implementation and micro-implementation. *Public Policy, 26,* 157-184.

Bloom, P. N., & Norvelli, W. D. (1981). Problems and challenges in social marketing. *Journal of Marketing, 45,* 79-88.

Connell, P. B., Turner, R. R., & Mason, E. F. (1985). Summary of the findings of the school health education evaluation: Health promotion effectiveness, implementation, and cost. *Journal of School Health, 55,* 316-323.

Goodman, R., & Steckler, A. (1989). A model for the institutionalization of health promotion programs. *Family and Community Health, 11*(4), 63-78.

Green, L. W., Gottlieb, N., & Parcel, G. (1987). Diffusion theory extended and applied. In W. B. Ward (Ed.), *Advances in health education and promotion.* Greenwich, CT: JAI.

Havelock, R. (1971). *Planning for innovation through dissemination and utilization of knowledge.* Ann Arbor, MI: Institute for Social Research.

Helvie, C. (1991). *Community health nursing: Theory and practice.* New York: Springer.

Huberman, A. M., & Miles, M. B. (1984). *Innovation up close.* New York: Plenum.

Kanter, R. (1983). *The change masters.* New York: Simon & Schuster.

Kolbe, L. J., & Iverson, D. C. (1981). Implementing comprehensive school health education: Educational innovations and social change. *Health Education Quarterly, 8,* 57-80.

Kotler, P., & Andreasen, A. R. (1987). *Strategic marketing for non-profit organizations* (3rd ed.). Englewood Cliffs, NJ: Prentice Hall.

Lefebvre, R. C. (1990). Strategies to maintain and institutionalize successful programs. In N. Bracht (Ed.), *Health promotion at the community level.* Newbury Park, CA: Sage.

Norvelli, W. D. (1990). Applying social marketing to health promotion and disease prevention. In K. Glanz, F. Lewis, & B. Rimer (Eds.), *Health behavior and health education.* San Francisco: Jossey-Bass.

Oppewal, S. R. (1992). Implementing a community-based innovation: Organizational challenges and strategies. *Family and Community Health, 15*(3), 70-79.

Orlandi, M. A. (1986). The diffusion and adoption of worksite health promotion innovations: An analysis of the barriers. *Preventive Medicine, 15,* 522-536.

Orlandi, M. A. (1987). Promoting health and preventing disease in health care settings: An analysis of barriers. *Preventive Medicine, 16,* 119-130.

Orlandi, M. A., Landers, C., Weston, R., & Haley, N. (1990). Diffusion of health promotion innovations. In K. Glanz, F. M. Lewis, & B. Rimer (Eds.), *Health behavior and health education.* San Francisco: Jossey-Bass.

Parcel, G., Perry, C., & Taylor, W. (1989). Translating theory into practice: Intervention strategies for the diffusion of a health promotion innovation. *Family and Community Health, 12*(3), 1-13.

Parcel, G., Perry, C., & Taylor, W. (1990). Beyond demonstration: Diffusion of health promotion innovations. In N. Bracht (Ed.), *Health promotion at the community level.* Newbury Park, CA: Sage.

Patton, M. (1978). *Utilization-focused evaluation.* Newbury Park, CA: Sage.

Paul, B. (1955). *Health, culture and community.* New York: Russell Sage.

Puska, P., Koskela, K., McAlister, A., Mayranen, A., Smolander, A., Moisio, S., Viri, L., Korpelainen, V., & Rogers, E. (1986). Use of lay opinion leaders to promote diffusion of health innovations in a community programme: Lessons learned from the North Karelia project. *Bulletin of the World Health Organization, 64,* 437-446.

Rogers, E. M. (1983). *Diffusion of innovations* (3rd ed.). New York: Free Press.

Rogers, E. M., & Shoemaker, F. (1973). *Communication of innovation: A cross-cultural approach.* New York: Free Press.

Shea, S., Basch, D., Lantigua, R., & Wechster, H. (1992). The Washington Heights-Inwood healthy heart program: A third generation community-based cardiovascular disease prevention program in a disadvantaged urban setting. *Preventive Medicine, 21,* 203-217.

CHAPTER 10

COMMUNITY INTERVENTIONS
Using Mass Media and the Political Process

OBJECTIVES: INTERVENTIONS AND MASS MEDIA

1. Discuss the energy theory and interventions.
2. Identify the nurse's role in interventions.
3. Discuss use of mass media as a community-focused intervention.
4. Use a variety of models for mass media education.
5. Use planning steps for mass media presentations.
6. Use guidelines to make media presentations effective.
7. Plan effectively with media sources for presentations.
8. Discuss the advantage of multiple approaches over single approaches in changing behavior.
9. Discuss media advocacy as a behavioral change technique.

OBJECTIVES: THE POLITICAL PROCESS

1. Define concepts used in politics.
2. Discuss the influence of politics on nursing.
3. Relate the concept of power to politics.
4. Discuss conflict and conflict management.
5. Discuss negotiation as a political concept.
6. Relate networking to politics.
7. Evaluate the influence of nursing on politics.

The focus of this book is on aggregates and the community for the advanced community health nurse. Thus, interventions should be community or aggregate focused. In this chapter, a discussion of intervention in general is followed by discussions of interventions that use mass media and the political process. Chapter 11 covers interventions to promote community empowerment, build coalitions, and involve professional and lay community leaders as well as industry. Chapter 12 covers interventions such as the establishment and marketing of mass screenings, practice clinics, and nursing centers, as well as working with subsystems such as schools and industry on behalf of the community.

INTERVENTIONS AND THE ENERGY THEORY

Implementation or intervention is the organization and carrying out of activities identified in the plan. This involves mobilizing appropriate people and resources to carry out the identified activities.

The purpose of interventions are to regain or maintain the balanced energies. From the community point of view, this may be accomplished when the population or aggregate has increased its energies or increased or decreased certain identified environmental energies that influence health, whether by learning new concepts and behaviors (e.g., through mass media presentations) that are more conducive to health; by developing new skills (e.g., through empowerment and coalition-building interventions) that will assist them in bringing about community change toward health, or by instigating certain changes in the laws (through the political process) that will influence the health of the population.

Nurses use a variety of energies to establish or reestablish the energy balance of a community. Although one energy may dominate the activity, usually, interrelated energies are present. For example, when nurses assist communities in building coalitions or recruiting professionals to assist with interventions, they employ both social and mental energies, but the social energy is probably the most important.

THE NURSE'S ROLE IN INTERVENTIONS

The nurse's role in interventions varies depending on the program, community, and extent of community involvement. In some instances, the community will already be actively involved and the nurse's role may be merely that of facilitator, collaborator, and coordinator. In others, the nurse may carry out the plan and manage the program relatively independently.

Interventions may be directed toward (a) strengthening the ability of community aggregates to prevent environmental assaults (by mass media or group presentations, immunizations, or preventive activities in nursing centers), (b) identifying and treating the effects of environmental assaults early to reduce complications (by providing nursing center primary care and screening), (c) building community competence (through empowerment projects), (d) making the environment more conducive to health for aggregates or the total community (by using the political process), and (e) strengthening the probability that an aggregate of the community can bring about desired changes for health (through coalition building). These interventions will be discussed in this section of the book.

INTERVENTION TASKS

There are several tasks during the implementation stage. First the nurse must identify the knowledge and skills needed to carry out the planned activity. For example, if the nurse plans to discuss preparation for a hurricane on the radio with residents of Rudyville, he or she must prepare for this activity. This may involve reading about hurricane preparation, talking with disaster coordinators, talking with residents to see what information would be most helpful, or talking with other nurses who have participated in aiding a community during a disaster.

A second task involves identifying who will carry out the specific activities in the plan. In the social planning approach to the community, the nurse will often carry out the activities or share them with others who are qualified. For example, the task of providing health education on radio or television might be shared by the nurse and the health educator, or that of teaching nutrition to obese adolescents could be shared by the nurse and a nutritionist. In a community development approach, the interventions may be carried out by community laypeople as well as by professionals in community subsystems or others identified by community-based committees.

A third task involves making everyone involved in the interventions aware of which actions he or she is responsible for carrying out. For example, if a health educator is to assist with health education, this should be planned and implemented jointly, and both the nurse and health educator should be aware of their responsibilities.

A last task of implementation is serving as a resource or providing resources. The nurse serves as a resource especially in the locality development approach to community change. The nurse also ensures that resources are available to community committees or others carrying out the intervention. For example, if a health educator is presenting information to a group of obese adolescents at school, a room should be scheduled, and if appropriate, handouts should be prepared.

USE OF MASS MEDIA AS A COMMUNITY INTERVENTION

The term *media* refers to the paths taken by health information to reach the intended audience. This information may arrive visually (TV), in auditory form (radio & TV), or in printed form (newspaper, magazines). Mass media are media channels that reach large segments of the target population (aggregate or total community), such as national or local TV or radio stations and national or local newspapers or magazines.

Some factors to consider in doing mass media interventions are these: (a) how many specific community subgroups are targeted, (b) which senses are affected (visual, auditory), (c) the magnitude and demographics of the audience, (d) whether messages are repeated or presented one time, (e) the length of the message, (f) the opportunity for feedback, (g) the amount of control by the receiver, (h) the message coding type, and (i) the power of message preservation (McGuire, 1981; Schramm, 1982).

HEALTH EDUCATION MODELS

One aspect of planning a health education program is to base it on an appropriate model for how and why people change their behavior. Models discussed here include the health belief model, the fear drive model, the dual-process self-regulatory model, the Ajzen-Fishbein model, the behavioral decision-making theory, and the staged social cognitive model. Some of these are single-stage models, whereas others are multiple-stage behavior change models. For some programs, the nurse may wish to use one model, and at other times, he or she may wish to combine components of several models for maximum effectiveness.

HEALTH BELIEF MODEL

The health belief model, although basically an individual model, has implications for teaching groups. According to Rosenstock (1974) and Becker (1974), people's decisions to take action to avoid diseases are motivated by (a) their perceived susceptibility to the disease, (b) the perceived disease severity, (c) the perceived benefits of complying with proposed actions, and (d) their perception of barriers to taking action, which may include fear, pain, cost, embarrassment, and inconvenience.

These factors are further modified by (a) demographic factors such as age, sex, race, and ethnicity; (c) sociopsychological factors such as social class, peer pressure, and attitudes toward health care personnel; and (c) structural factors such as personal experience with the disease and knowledge of the disease. Cues to action may also modify behavior; these may be internal, such as identifying symptoms of illness, or external, such as mass media information or advice from friends.

Using this model in a health education program would require emphasizing susceptibility and the other motivating factors in the model. For example, the practitioner might discuss smoking consequences with a target group of teenage smokers. The program might include (a) a film on the consequences of smoking, such as lung cancer, surgery, or death; (b) a discussion of the statistics on the relationship between smoking and health problems; (c) a discussion of the length of time one may smoke before developing the disease; (d) presentational tables of cancer rates for smokers and nonsmokers; and (e) a discussion of resources and ways to quit.

FEAR DRIVE MODEL

According to the fear drive model (Leventhal, Safer, & Panagis, 1983), behavioral changes do not follow knowledge and understanding alone. In addition, fear is necessary. A series of steps in this model leads to a behavioral change. Initially, the individual receives a fear-inducing message such as pain. The individual usually responds with fear. A subjective discomfort, usually worry, follows and leads to a change in behavior.

This model proposes fear as a stimulus for behavior changes. A mass media intervention using this model might show pictures of automobile accidents, AIDS patients, or cancer patients to elicit this reaction. A review of the literature on this model can be found in Hale and Dillard (1995).

DUAL-PROCESS SELF-REGULATORY MODEL

This model (Leventhal et al., 1983) postulates that behavioral changes result from an integration of cognitive and emotional factors. At the cognitive level, the person plans ways to cope with health threats, using past and current information and experiences. At the same time, the individual reacts emotionally to the threat. The type of threat and perceived susceptibility will determine the force of the reaction and the change in behavior. When cognitive and emotional processes do not operate together, a behavioral change does not take place. Thus, a person may realize, at the cognitive level, that smoking causes cancer but persist in smoking because, at the emotional level, fear of smoking-caused cancer is a weaker force than the gratification provided by smoking. In this situation, it would be necessary to deal with the driving and restraining forces discussed by Lewin (1958) to increase the person's fear by increasing the perceived risk of cancer or to reduce the emotional gratification of smoking (e.g., by reducing the number of places where smoking is acceptable behavior).

AJZEN-FISHBEIN MODEL

This model (Fishbein & Ajzen, 1975) identifies four factors that must be changed in a sequence to change behavior. New health *beliefs,* must lead to changes in *attitudes,* which in turn must trigger changes in *intentions,* which in turn can lead to changes in *behaviors.* The performance of a new behavior can then reinforce the new beliefs, attitudes, and intentions, thereby leading to the permanent establishment of the new behavior. But new beliefs in themselves are not sufficient to instigate behavioral change. For example, someone exposed to information on the relationship between smoking and disease might come to believe that this relationship exists but still have the attitude that he or she is immune or in good health and not likely to get ill and thus might feel that smoking cessation is unnecessary for him or her.

BEHAVIORAL DECISION-MAKING MODEL

According to Holtgrave, Tinsley, and Kay (1995), the behavioral decision-making model is mainly concerned with the cognitive processes of evaluating alternative courses of action and goes beyond the "relatively simplistic cost benefit components in the health belief model, the theory of reasoned action and protective motivation theory" (p. 25). It looks at risk perceptions, problem structuring, valuation of consequence or outcome, judgment based on probability, and biases. Although there is no one universally accepted descriptive theory on how people make decisions, the behavioral decision-making model is based on extensive testing and literature review and is useful in planning mass media programs.

People make incremental moves toward behavioral changes and a stages-of-change framework is therefore important because different health education messages are appropriate at different stages of change. In addition, a consideration of developmental levels are important because decision making in children and adolescents differs from adults.

STAGE MODEL OF BEHAVIOR CHANGE

In contrast to the health belief model, stage models see behavioral change as a series of actions over time. According to this theory, people at different stages behave in ways that can be qualified and, thus, interventions needed to move people toward behavioral change, such as health education messages, will vary by the stage of change (Weinstein, 1988).

There are five stages in the stages of change model:

1. *Precontemplative:* There is no recognition of the problem or need for change because the person either is unaware of the risk or refuses to acknowledge the risk.
2. *Contemplative:* There is recognition of the problem and the need for change is seriously considered. This stage usually lasts a long time because there is difficulty evaluating costs and benefits of the behavioral changes.
3. *Preparation:* There is a commitment to and steps taken for change.
4. *Action:* There is a successful change in behavior lasting from 1 day to 6 months.
5. *Maintenance:* The change initiated lasts for an indefinite period.

This model has been modified from a linear to a spiraling model because it has been found that people have relapses and recycling periods. The factors and processes that help people move from stage to stage vary by the stage and will be discussed following this section.

Stage-appropriate processes facilitate movement through the stages, and when processes are used excessively at inappropriate stages they may cause a relapse to an earlier stage. Audience segmentation (Slader, 1995) by placing the audience in the five stages allows the practitioner to know how many people are at each stage for planning purposes. The reader is referred to Prochaska and

DiClementi (1986) for additional information on the process of change and to Baranowski (1989-1990) for additional information on moving individuals through the stages of change using individual- and environmental-level strategies.

Moving From the Precontemplative Stage to the Contemplative Stage. One of the change processes needed for this change is consciousness-raising, or helping people increase their perception of the personal risks involved in risky behavior, including the absence of preventive behaviors.

It has been found that the lay public have a different way of conceptualizing risks than do professionals. The following dimensions have been identified related to their concept of risk: voluntariness, dread, control, knowledge, catastrophic potential, novelty, and equity (Kraus & Slovic, 1988). The National Research Council (1989) says involuntariness of the assumption of risk, high levels of dread concerning it, lack of control, low levels of knowledge, high catastrophic potential, a high level of novelty, and a low level of equity lead to perceptions of higher risk.

When communicating with the lay public, the practitioner should use risks with similar dimension profiles because people reject as inappropriate comparisons of risks that they perceive as having different profiles. For example, if the practitioner compares AIDS risk with the risk of other sexually transmitted diseases, the message may be rejected because of dissimilarities in dimensions of dread, control, catastrophic potential, and novelty. Because AIDS is a fatal disease whereas other STDs usually are not, it is a more dreaded risk. Likewise, although both can be prevented by avoiding specific risk behaviors, other STDs can be cured, whereas AIDS cannot. Thus, there is less control over AIDS. Finally, AIDS is relatively new as a health problem, whereas STDs have been around for years. Thus, AIDS is considered novel.

On the basis of this comparison, it would not be a good idea to compare the risk of contracting AIDS with the risk of contracting other STDs. Holtgrave et al. suggest that drunk driving might be a better comparison in terms of dread and control.

According to Holtgrave et al. (1995), another consideration in presenting risk information is that people generally have trouble processing probability information and either overweight small probabilities or underweight large ones. They also have difficulty revising probability judgments when new information is presented.

One source of estimation error is that people tend to overestimate the probability of events that are easy to imagine. In addition, although they may accept the probability of an event's occurrence from one risk exposure, they have difficulty estimating the cumulative probability; thus, they may correctly estimate the probability of acquiring HIV from one exposure to an infected HIV contact but then underestimate the probability of acquiring it from multiple contacts with the same person. That is, they tend to underestimate cumulative risks. The practitioner who is interested in moving the audience from the precontemplative to the contempletative stage of behavioral change should emphasize cumulative as opposed to one-shot probabilities. Instead of emphasizing the low risk of contacting HIV infection from one exposure, the practitioner should stress the probability of contacting HIV infection from repeated exposures and the need for condoms as a preventive measure.

The practitioner who is attempting to transmit risk information must also deal with the imprecision of the qualitative terms for probabilities that people generally use. People tend to talk about probabilities in words rather than in numbers, saying, for example, "It is unlikely that I will get the job" rather than "There is a 10% chance that I will get the job" (Holtgrave et al., 1995, p. 30). Because there is no agreement among people about what numerical values should be attached to a qualitative term such as *probably,* the practitioner should review qualitative literature to find the range of quantitative values found from research. In addition, the practitioner can present both probabilities in qualitative and quantitative terms to get his or her message across.

Finally, presenting the same information in different ways has been found to alter results, the so-called framing effect. For example, if one is discussing the success of using condoms in preventing HIV infections, one may say either that condom use is 95% successful or that it has a 5% failure rate. The two statements are the same in factual content but will receive different responses from people in terms of condom use. From research it was found that the "95% successful" statement was more effective in changing behavior related to condom use than the "5% failure rate" statement. Thus, practitioners should evaluate responses to statements and plan accordingly.

Moving From the Contemplative Stage to the Preparation Stage. Moving from the contemplative to the preparation stage of behavioral change involves developing and committing to an action plan and selecting from alternatives.

According to Holtgrave et al., the practitioner who is attempting to move an audience to the preparation stage must remember that the audience's decision-making perspective may vary from that of the practitioner. For example, cigarette smoking may be a hazard to the practitioner but a comfort to the recipient of the message. Thus, the practitioner should address the decision making of the audience from the audience's perspective.

Another thing to keep in mind is that research has found that all decisions are made considering the time over which the consequences of the actions will extend. For example, people from stable environments may consider the long-term consequences of HIV infections when deciding whether to use condoms with a new sex partner, but people who live in high-homicide areas where life is viewed in terms of years instead of decades may view condom use differently. Thus, the recipient's time frame should be considered when planning programs that attempt to move audiences from the contemplative to the preparation stage of behavioral change.

Still another consideration is that people weigh various factors in decision making differently and this may influence outcomes. For example, when considering four factors—disease protection, comfort, cost, and the partner's reaction—in a decision to use or not to use condoms with a casual sex partner, one person might weight disease protection highly and thus use condoms, whereas another might weight comfort highly and thus choose not to use them. There are several well-developed theories of how people make decisions when considering multiple factors, among which the multiple-attribute utility theory (von Winterfeldt & Edwards, 1986) is the most famous. Thus, practitioners should determine the factors that are given the most weight in the targeted population and address these factors in planned programs.

Additional information on aspects of moving through other stages of behavioral change can be found in Coombs, Dawes, and Tversky (1981); Ford, Schmitt, Schechtman, Hults, and Doherty (1989); and Hutchinson (1986), who research the process by which people make decisions, including the use of feedback in decision making (Hammond, Stewart, Brehmer, & Steinmann, 1986).

STAGED SOCIAL COGNITIVE MODEL

Maibach and Cotton (1995) base their theory on the five stages of behavioral change that Holtgrave et al. (1995) used in their model, but they draw on social cognitive theory to explain health behavior changes. In this theory, internal personal factors and the environment are viewed as reciprocally determining human behavior. Thus, people and their behavior are shaped by the environment, which is also shaped by people. From this perspective, health behavior can be changed by modifying either personal factors or environmental factors. Research has shown the predictive and explanatory value of social cognitive theory in relation to health behaviors such as diet and nutrition, weight loss, exercise, controlling use of addictive substances such as tobacco and alcohol, contraception and STD/HIV reduction, and stress management. Reviews of this research will be found in Bandura (1997) and Strecher, DeVellis, Becker, and Rosenstock (1986). In addition, Bandura (1997) reviews the literature on the positive effects of interventions that enhance the effects of relevant social cognitive factors on health behaviors.

Personal factors identified in the staged social cognitive model include knowledge, skills, self-efficacy, outcome expectations, and personal goals; environmental factors include social, institutional, and physical; and behavior determinants include frequency, consistency, and other relevant aspects.

Role of Personal Factors in Health Behavior Change. Knowledge is necessary for behavior changes, and people need information on risk factors or conditions that place them at risk and on ways they can reduce their risk. However, knowledge is not sufficient to bring about behavioral changes. Information on effective presentations will be presented later in this chapter.

Skill is another important personal factor, and a lack of skill can hamper behavioral changes. According to Bandura (1986), new health behaviors depend on complex cognitive, social, behavioral, and self-regulatory skills. For example, practicing safe sex requires recognizing situations that lead to sexual coercion (a cognitive skill), negotiating safe sex with a partner (a social skill), using a condom properly (a behavioral skill), and adhering to a decision made previously to engage only in safe sex (a self-regulatory skill). Skill messages should break the skills down into component parts and demonstrate how to reconstruct the behavior from the parts. Such programs usually present a model of the behavior and then break the behavior into its parts for demonstration. Each of the components (cognitive, social, etc.) should be identified and modeled individually, and then the behavior should be modeled as a whole. Skill behaviors are maximized if the audience is allowed to practice the modeled behavior.

Self-efficacy is a third personal factor in the model. This facilitates or hampers behavioral changes and is related to a person's belief that he or she can or cannot successfully complete the actions necessary to perform the behavior (Bandura, 1997). Self-efficacy beliefs include confidence in one's ability to regulate motivation, thought processes, emotional states, and physical and social environments to accomplish a behavioral goal and confidence in one's ability to overcome difficulties involved in changing and maintaining specific behaviors when these are efficacious. Four mechanisms related to efficacy judgment that affect adoption and maintenance of a new health behavior are (a) choice of behaviors, (b) effort expenditure and persistence, (c) thought patterns, and (d) emotional reactions.

People choose to avoid tasks they believe are beyond their capabilities and to pursue those that they believe they can perform (Bandura, 1986). Thus, low-efficacy smokers attempt to quit smoking less often than do high-efficacy smokers. In addition, effort and persistence are required in mastering a new behavior, and high efficacy motivates people to engage more completely in a behavior change and to persist longer in the change. High-efficacy people meet obstacles to behavior change with increased intensity of efforts to reach the goal, whereas low-efficacy people may give up or decrease the effort. Efficacy beliefs affect thought patterns such as goals, aspirations, visualization of success or failure, and the ability to deal with setbacks, any of which can facilitate or hamper behavioral changes. Finally, efficacy beliefs affect emotions, and those who have low efficacy react to taxing situations more often with stress and depression.

Self-efficacy can be heightened by four types of influence: (a) provision of performance mastery experience, (b) provision of vicarious mastery experience, (c) verbal persuasion, and (d) inferences from physiological and affective states (Bandura, 1986). *Performance mastery* is the most direct method to enhance self-efficacy. This involves having the target audience attempt and succeed with the selected health behaviors. Repeated success in safe practice areas increases self-efficacy. *Vicarious mastery experience* is provided by models who have been successful with the behavior. Models who are most useful are those who are similar in demographic or behavioral variables to those of the target group. Effective modeling is also enhanced by making observable the unobservable aspects of the behavior, such as the thought processes involved in it, and by discussing the strong and weak elements of the modeling performance for the target audience. *Verbal persuasion* that may increase self-efficacy includes the assessment of credible others and accounts of positive arousals such as excitement resulting from the successful accomplishment of a behavior.

Outcome expectancies are the beliefs people have about the results of a behavior. They may involve physical effects (increased or decreased health), social effects (approval or disapproval of friends), and self-evaluation effects (self-approval or self-disapproval). Behaviors believed to have a desirable outcome will motivate one to perform them. Outcome expectations are related to self-efficacy: The greater one's perceived self-efficacy, the greater the likelihood of a positive outcome expectation of performance. Likewise, one may expect a positive outcome but not be motivated to try it because of perceived low self-efficacy.

The practitioner can influence outcome expectancies by communicating through direct experience, allowing an audience to learn by observation, transmitting persuasive messages, or any combination of the above. A positive influence on trying the new behavior may be obtained by presenting a new positive health outcome expectancy, or reducing a negative outcome expectancy can motivate people to try a new behavior.

Personal goals are major motivators for behavior changes and, when reached, give a strong sense of satisfaction. Practitioners who communicate with the public should encourage short-term goal setting. This will motivate behavior and allow monitoring of progress.

Stages of Change. Social cognitive theorists advocate providing different health messages to people at different stages of the behavior change model to facilitate movement to the next stage. In addition, the order in which personal factors are addressed will vary by these stages.

During the *precontemplation* stage, there is no intention of or motivation for changing behavior. Therefore, to facilitate a shift to the contemplation stage, information should focus on self-examination instead of on behavioral change, with an emphasis on increasing the audience's knowledge of risks and outcome expectations and personalizing the health message. The messages may include information such as the consequences of the behavior on self, family, and friends and may be personalized by reminders of recent personal exposures, if these are known.

In addition, because people at this stage view the disadvantages and barriers of the new behavior as outweighing the advantages, the practitioner should emphasize the positive aspects of the new behavior and encourage use of this new positive information to reevaluate the outcome. This reevaluation is an important part of making the new behavior more desirable.

At the *contemplation* stage, people know the value of a behavioral change but are not ready to take action. They may ask for information from a variety of sources but will take no action due to the distress experienced over acknowledging the problem and a lack of emotional, cognitive, or behavioral abilities to make the change or a failure to change beliefs about a valued behavior that must be given up if the new behavior is to be adopted. Encouraging a person to try the behavior one time or to try substituting the new behavior for the risky behavior may help movement to the preparation stage. Outcome expectations are still a consideration also. A weighing of the costs versus the benefits of the risky behavior that includes a consideration of physical (health vs. enjoyment), social (family and friend approval), and self-evaluation (self-esteem) factors may be useful. Positive outcomes that outweigh the risks are a motivating factor. Thus, information should focus on the positive outcomes of the new behavior and dispute commonly believed negative but untrue consequences of the new behavior. In addition, presenting ways to minimize the negative consequences of the new behavior may be motivating. People at this stage also need to see themselves as capable of performing the new behavior (self-efficacy), so programs should seek to remove any identified barriers.

People in the *preparation* stage have had some experience with the new behavior and are attempting to change. Movement to the action stage requires restructuring the environment to emphasize important cues for practicing the new behavior that are socially supported. Another important step is identifying and planning solutions to obstacles that may be met. Still another step involves setting appropriate behavioral goals. Setting and reaching short-term goals is a strong motivating factor. Self-efficacy is also important at this stage, and messages should strengthen self-efficacy to deal with the obstacles to the change process. People at this stage need reinforcement for changing, whether this is external (such as social approval) or internal. Thus, social reinforcement of the appropriate behavior should be a goal of media messages.

At the *action* stage, people have practiced the new behavior for a long time, and relapse is a threat. Communications to people at this stage should facilitate movement to the maintenance stage by refinement of skills to prevent relapses or to cope with setbacks that might lead to full relapses. In addition, the practitioner using mass media should help people feel good about the new behavior and their progression toward their goals. He or she should also make the long-range positive consequences of the new behavior concrete.

OTHER HEALTH EDUCATION MODELS

Monahan (1995) suggests using positive affect to increase success when communicating about health. Literature is reviewed to support the contention that positive feeling may influence social behavior and cognitive processes, and a theoretical framework is presented.

Pfau (1995) presents data on the inoculation approach in prevention. This approach seeks to strengthen existing attitudes so that they are less susceptible to change. For example, it could be used to assist children who hold negative attitudes about smoking, drinking alcohol, and other risky behaviors to maintain those attitudes and to be more resistant to later pressures to participate in the risky behaviors.

PLANNING FOR EDUCATIONAL PROGRAMS

PLANNING PROCESS

Before offering an educational program to a targeted community or aggregate, the practitioner should assess the educational needs and determine the best channel of and time for media presentation so as to ensure the best returns for the resources expended. Most of the information to answer these questions should be in the community assessment data, but it may need to be supplemented by surveys or other methods. It might include factors such as age, race, sex, educational level, income, stage of behavioral change (see above), and other educational programs requested.

Another planning task involves obtaining administrative support for the program. Without this, the program could fail for a variety of reasons (see discussion of horizontal and vertical ties in Chapter 2). Next, the planner should establish a community advisory committee made up of health care providers and members of the target population. This committee should evaluate the content and the teaching strategies for appropriateness to the particular group (social class, cultural group, age group, stage of change). Different groups may require different content and teaching methods.

Next, the practitioner should write a rationale for the program detailing why it is being presented. He or she should also write goals and objectives for the audience (see discussion on planning presented in Chapter 8).

An important aspect of planning is determining and judging the fit of program material to the educational level of the target population. This can be done using Gunning's Fog Index (see Laubach & Koschnick, 1977, pp. 12-15), which rates the reading level of the material.

To use the fog index, take a sample of 100 words from the material to be presented and divide it by the total number of sentences to arrive at the average number of words per sentence. Next, add the average number of words per sentence to the number of words in the sample with three or more syllables (excluding capitalized words, compound words, and syllables made by using *es* or *ed*). This total sum is multiplied by 0.4 to obtain the fog index score. The following scores correlate with the noted levels: 17 = college graduate; 15 = college junior; 13 = college freshman; 11 = high school junior; 9 = high school freshman; and 7 = seventh grade. The practitioner should aim for a fog score of 10 or less.

After completing a program for mass media, it is important to pilot it on a sample of the target group for appropriateness, understandability, and other factors that may motivate change.

GUIDELINES FOR EFFECTIVE PROGRAMS

Flay and Burton (1990) offer several suggestions for effective mass communication.

Acceptability. First, the message, source, and channel used must be acceptable to the target audience and from a believable source if the audience is to change behavior. For example, "Eat less saturated fat" (message), says "the American Heart Association," (source) and presented on television (channel) must be accepted and acted on by the audience.

Message Dissemination. Another factor in effective mass media health education involves the dissemination of the information. The information should reach the target audience and should be repeated often and consistently over a long time. It should also include some novelty at times to attract attention. Influences on message dissemination include media gatekeepers, political and social support, financial support, target audience characteristics, and message characteristics. Those in control of media sources determine what information can be printed or aired, how much of what type of information will be accepted, and the timeliness and duration of the information. Thus, the practitioner should be familiar with the media's interests.

Dissemination of a health message is easier if the message has support from other sources (social and political) and more difficult if there is opposition or the area is controversial (as in the case of abortion). Financial support aids dissemination by making it more possible to obtain desirable time slots on media sources. A knowledge of audience characteristics can also facilitate the dissemination of the message. Finally, the content of the message must appeal to the gatekeeper and public and not be too controversial.

Gaining Attention of Audience. Another requirement of successful mass media health education is that it helps the audience to attend to, process, and remember the information presented. Factors that influence audience attention are audience characteristics, the message, and channel characteristics; the match between audience and message; and the interpersonal communication stimulated by the information.

Audience factors have been discussed previously. Messages can appeal to the intellect or emotions, be persuasive or educational, elicit fear or be positive. Information messages are reported to be better than emotional messages, but eliciting empathy is desirable. Action messages are good because they make clear what the desired behavior changes are. In addition, messages should be simple.

Stimulating Interpersonal Communication. Stimulation of interpersonal communication is important because the more that people discuss an issue, the more likely it is that the public will do something about it.

Stimulation of communication depends on audience, message, source, and channel characteristics and the level of attention of the audience. Audience characteristics that are important include involvement in the issue and readiness for change. Those who are more involved in the issue and who are ready to change will be more likely to discuss the issue with others. The involvement of opinion leaders is also important in stimulating discussions. Factors related to the message that improve the probability of interpersonal communication include increasing the salience of the issue, promoting debate, monopolizing the issue, and supplementing the media message with other efforts involving the issue. Combining media efforts with face-to-face interaction has been found to increase effectiveness in changing behavior and will be discussed later in this chapter.

Instigating Behavioral Change. Finally, effective health education through the mass media must change knowledge, skill, and behavior. Such change depends on audience characteristics, attentiveness, interpersonal communication, and broader social changes. In relation to the last factor, it is known that the more society changes, the more individuals within society change. Thus, communications should "attempt to modify the social environment or influence social policy in ways that encourage and reinforce the desired change once individuals make them" (Flay & Burton, 1990, p. 132). For example, people are more likely to quit smoking if they have support of significant others and if smoking is discouraged in the workplace.

Factors that Flay and Burton cite as effective in behavioral changes include (a) modeling the desired behavior, (b) showing the behavior as achieving desirable goals such as feeling good and looking better, (c) showing the behavior as pertinent to real-life situations, (d) nurturing the motive to avoid harm or improve well-being and instilling the belief that the behavior will lessen the risk, (e) portraying the behavior as being approved and supported by the community, (f) mobilizing public support for the behavior, (g) providing self-guidance for self-management of the behavior change and for coping with relapses, (h) encouraging interpersonal social support for the behavioral change, (i) providing the infrastructure to support behavioral changes by encouraging enforcement of existing laws or proactive behavior by the audience to pressure legislators to provide new ones, and (j) encouraging activism against parts of the system tending to resist the desired behavior.

PLANNING WITH MASS MEDIA SOURCES

The power of mass media as a health tool is seen in the following quote: "The media's most obvious strength lies in the number of people they can reach. A story covered by the three morning [television] shows will reach 10 million homes and almost 17 million people" (Ulene, 1987, p. 3).

Although mass media can serve educational purposes, those controlling mass media are not required to perform this service. It is up to public health practitioners to convince editors and producers of the value of disseminating health information. Part of planning a mass media educational program involves selecting and working with mass media sources. Arkin (1990) reports on strategies to increase health coverage on mass media from data collected at a meeting of public health service agencies, foundations, and research institutions. Ways to increase collaboration include the following:

- Working within the priorities of the mass media by doing periodic surveys of what would interest them, by converting health information into human interest stories, and by shortening and clarifying health information

- Establishing long-term contacts with multimedia sources and involving them in program planning to gain their interest in health problems

- Establishing contacts with minority media policymakers and convincing them of the health information needs and interests of their audience

- Planning for multiple facets of coverage of an issue over time by using media departments such as public service announcements, news, public affairs, and entertainment so that the issue has continuity for the public

- Considering paid advertising for health messages, which allows some choice in time placement and can thus reach a larger audience

- Lobbying for nontraditional measures to support media health coverage financially, such as Proposition 99 in California, which proposed an excise tax on unhealthy products to finance mass media efforts to promote health, or by lobbying for the transfer of funds from one area into mass media efforts

- Advocating with the media for public health efforts by monitoring and providing feedback on public health coverage

- Increasing clout with media over specific issues by forming coalitions

- Educating the public about health information on media sources

- Improving communication skills of public health representatives dealing with the media so they can be more effective

- Increasing understanding of public health issues among media personnel by working with professional associations and schools of journalism, editors, producers, and writers

- Increasing media personnel access to background information on issues, policies, and people who can speak to the health topics

- Considering an awards program for media gatekeepers

- Establishing guidelines for partnerships between media personnel and health practitioners to ensure mutual benefits and encouraging cooperation by identifying mutual benefits

- Establishing guidelines for health claims made on specific issues

- Researching the effects of health claims

- Monitoring content of advertising to ensure that informal guidelines are adhered to

- Researching the health image of television

MULTIPLE VERSUS SINGLE APPROACHES

Research on health education has found that multiple approaches are better than single approaches for changing behavior. Early research demonstrated that mass media can be effective in disseminating health education information but that this does not always lead to changes in behavior. Current research has identified some mediators of effective behavioral changes to assist in improving mass media communication. One of the most important mediators, which was mentioned earlier, is the use of interpersonal communication such as discussions by teachers or other role models. This approach increases the likelihood of behavioral changes. A second mediator is the degree to which the mass media presentation is supplemented by additional written or other follow-up activities. A third mediator is the degree to which the program models the desired behavior. For example, a demonstration of how to engage in the new behavior is more effective than a description.

Bracht (1990) identifies four roles of the media in health interventions: (a) as sole change agent, (b) as a method supplementing other methods, (c) as a source of recruitment for and promotion of services and programs, and (d) as a way to provide support for the behavioral change. The role of the media as the only change agent is frequently used but has been questioned as to its effectiveness. Bracht reviewed one study comparing the use of media alone with the use of media in combination with face-to-face interactions and found that some behaviors such as diet may be changed by media alone but that more addictive behaviors such as smoking required supplementation of media efforts with programs involving face-to-face interaction such as workshops or support groups in addition to media presentations (multiple approaches). The combination was also found to be more effective in reducing cardiovascular risks over a 3-year period.

Media have also been used to increase audiences' awareness of health behaviors, products, and programs and to encourage them to participate. In one study, researchers evaluated how most people found out about a quitting smoking contest and found that television was mentioned more often than newspaper ads or fliers distributed at schools, libraries, the workplace, and physician's offices.

Finally, media may be used to reinforce health messages, to keep issues before the audience, or to support behavioral changes over the long term. One study of smokers who had quit and restarted smoking showed that their fear of relapse kept them from stopping again. Public service announcements of testimonies by local citizens who had quit were used in which the citizens discussed their urges to smoke, the lessening of the urges over time, and their methods of coping with the urges.

MEDIA ADVOCACY

Media advocacy is a new concept involving the use of mass media to advance a social or policy initiative. It uses several community organization concepts, including empowerment, citizen participation, and involvement in issue selection.

The focus of media advocacy is on the social conditions that led to the behavior instead of individual risk behavior. For example, instead of focusing on alcohol as an individual risk problem, one focuses on those who shape the environment in which individuals make decisions about health-related behavior. In this instance, media would cover the ethical and legal issues of alcohol companies' promotion of deadly products for teenagers. The goal is to redefine what have been seen as individual problems into public health or social problems. Additional information and case studies on this approach can be found in Wallach (1990) and Wallach, Dorfman, Jernigan, and Themba (1993).

SELECTED STUDIES ON HEALTH BEHAVIOR CHANGE THROUGH MEDIA INTERVENTIONS

Several studies have evaluated the effectiveness of mass media and other educational methods in changing health behavior. Farquhar et al. (1990) discuss the Stanford Five-City Project, the purpose of which was to determine if communitywide health education could reduce stroke and coronary disease. Two treatment cities ($N = 122,800$) and two control cities ($N = 197,500$) were compared for changes in knowledge of risk factors, smoking rate, blood pressure, and other factors. The treatment cities received a 5-year, low-cost, comprehensive program. Social learning theory, a communication-behavior change model, community organization principles, and social marketing methods were used in 25 hours of exposure on multichannel and multifactor education. Risk factors were assessed at the beginning and at three later times. After 30 to 64 months of education, the community's average reductions in plasma cholesterol (2%), blood pressure (4%), resting pulse rate (3%), and smoking rate (13%) favored the treatment cities. In addition, there was an important decrease in the composite total mortality risk scores (15%) and coronary risk scores (16%). The authors concluded that low-cost programs can influence risk factors in broad population groups.

Jason et al. (1989) report on a study at 38 workplaces that focused on assisting smokers to stop or reduce their smoking levels. The study used television programs, support groups, incentives, and self-help manuals in various combinations. Of employees provided with group support plus incentives, 42% were not smoking compared with 15% of the group provided with self-help manuals only. At a 12-month follow-up, 26% of the support-and-incentive group were not smoking compared with 16% of the self-help manual group.

Warnecke et al. (1989) evaluated smoking cessation for a 1-year period following a televised, self-help smoking cessation program. Readiness to quit, degree to which self-help materials were used, amount of exposure to the television program, and environmental support for behavior change were evaluated. Fewer than half of the smokers who quit following the intervention continued abstinence at 1 year. A major factor that differentiated the successful from the unsuccessful over the year was social support during the smoking cessation. The authors concluded that a combination of television and self-help was effective for smoking cessation for a substantial number of smokers.

The case study by Bethany Hall-Long at the end of this chapter on the use of mass media for community health demonstrates how these concepts can be applied in practice.

THE POLITICAL PROCESS AS A COMMUNITY INTERVENTION

Working to change laws, alone or in combination with other interventions, may be effective in changing health behavior of the community or aggregates. For example, seat belt laws have reduced injuries from accidents, and laws prohibiting smoking in restaurants and public buildings have reduced the health threats of secondary smoke. Both have influenced individual health behavior as a result. Most of the research discussed previously demonstrates that multiple approaches are more effective than single approaches in changing behavior. Thus, using the political process is an approach that can be used in combination with other interventions to influence behavior.

Because of the focus of the advanced practice nurse, the emphasis on working with the political process is on political changes that will affect aggregates or the community. Community changes may be directed toward local, state, or national targets. A knowledge of concepts and processes of influencing the political process should assist the nurse who is interested in improving community health behavior.

DEFINITIONS

Politics has been defined as "the authorative allocation of scarce resources" (Mason, 1985, p. 38), "influencing the allocation of scarce resources" (Talbott & Vance, 1981, p. 592), and "a process by which one influences the decisions of others and exerts control over situations and events" (Mason & Talbott, 1985, p. 7). The political system is defined as "any persistent pattern of human relations that involves, to a significant extent, control, influence, power or authority" (Dahl, 1984, p. 10). Together, these definitions suggest that politics is about competition for scarce resources. Groups and individuals compete for resources, and some people or groups have power and others do not.

Political action has been defined as "a form of human behavior that involves the negotiation, alteration, or entrenchment of social values and resources" (Abrahams, 1992, p. 329) or as "purposeful, planned interventions devised to influence . . . policy" (Burgess, 1983, p. 208). These definitions suggest that there are planned efforts by some groups and individuals to maintain resource allocation and values and by others to shift resource allocation and change values. Implicit in the definitions are concepts of power, conflict, and negotiation, all of which will be discussed in this section of the book.

SPHERE OF POLITICAL INFLUENCE ON NURSING

Politics takes place in most situations where there are limited resources and interest groups vying for them. It occurs in the workplace in the form of efforts to obtain resources for patient care or teaching of students. It also occurs in employee maneuvers to obtain salary increases from those who make decisions. Politics also takes place within professional organizations, the community, and local, state, and national governments. The major focus of this section is on politics at the community and governmental levels. Those who are interested in other aspects of politics are referred to Mason, Talbott, and Leavitt (1993).

Politics at the governmental level (local, state, or national) provides a legal definition of nursing, influences reimbursement systems of health care, and determines what types of health care are available to which people, what health problems are funded for research, and other aspects of the nurse's work.

Some of these same influences will be experienced at the community level. For example, in the case study of Rudyville in Chapter 6, the local city council allocated less than 1% of the city budget for health. Because of limited resources, only selected programs could be offered by the community, and consequently, some people with health problems received community care, whereas others did not.

MAINTAINING OBJECTIVITY IN THE POLITICAL ENVIRONMENT

Nurses should be aware of the competition for scarce resources (conflicting goals and interests) and the ensuing power struggles to avoid becoming a part of them during community work. For example, defining a problem in different ways will produce different solutions. If a large number of students fail a course, one can view this problem as due to poor teaching or due to a lack of student motivation. Depending on the definition of the problem, the strategies to correct it will vary. The next logical step might be to evaluate and clarify the problem further. When looking at problem clarification as a lack of information (structural view of the world), it would seem that more information would lead to a better idea of what the problem is. This rational and logical approach is typical of the structural view, which also says that organizations exist to further identified goals and the needs of these organizations are best met by adhering to rational and impersonal rules (Riger, 1989).

A different viewpoint is that organizations are made up of different individuals and interest groups who jockey for positions and power in view of scarce resources (political). This concept of the world is quite different from that of an organization governed by rationality (structural view).

For example, following a needs assessment for and establishment of a battered spouse shelter, nurses might expect entrance requirements to be followed (structural view) and be surprised to see clients in the shelter who do not meet admission requirements. However, the situation should be viewed using political rather than structural concepts (strict following the rules). In a political view, information from the needs assessment was used in the struggle over resources and after obtaining a shelter, the group fights to keep control (Riger, 1989).

Nurses should remember that in the political view of the world, individuals, groups, and organizations have competing goals, and they struggle with one another for control of resources. When one group is empowered, another may lose power, and the powerful do not give up power easily (Riger, 1989). Nurses may innocently become involved in these community struggles and should view them using political rather than structural concepts.

CONCEPT OF POWER IN POLITICS

Power is an important concept in politics. According to Hewison (1994), political power is the "ability to influence or persuade an individual holding a governmental office to exert the power of that office to affect a desired change" (p. 1171). He goes on to say that power is more than governmental influence and policy formation, and he proposes a framework of political activities with three levels: interpersonal, organizational, and external. Activities and forms of power at each level are identified, although from a community perspective, external political activities or political action to influence governmental policies is the most appropriate.

BASES AND SOURCES OF POWER

What allows some people to influence others? What is the basis for this power? French and Raven (1959) identify five power bases:

1. *Coercive power,* which involves using force to gain compliance and in which compliance results from real or perceived fear
2. *Reward power,* which involves providing something of value for compliance and in which compliance results from the perceived potential for reward or favor of someone in power

3. *Expert power,* which results from special knowledge or skills and is person instead of position oriented

4. *Legitimate power,* which results from a position or title and is position instead of person oriented

5. *Referent power,* which results from admiration of and identification with one believed to be a leader

Hersey, Blanchard, and Natemeyer (1979) added two additional categories:

6. *Information power,* resulting from the desire of one for information held or perceived to be held by another

7. *Connection power,* resulting from the perception that a certain person has a special connection to a person or organization believed to be powerful

Bacharach and Lawler (1980) say these categories are useful but that they fail to clearly distinguish the bases of power from sources of power.

For Robbins (1993), power comes from position, personal qualities, expertise, and opportunities (power sources). On the other hand, a *power base* refers to what one controls and is a result of the knowledge and skills of the power holder. Thus, the power holder obtains the power base from power sources. Four types of power are useful in maintaining a power base: information power, persuasive power, reward power, and coercive power.

ACHIEVING POWER

Nurses may achieve power in a variety of ways. One source of power is knowledge. Nurses can gain knowledge about their profession, the problems and concerns of nursing, and the clients of nursing, as well as knowledge of the political and change process. Using this background, they may meet with legislators or with community clients to introduce change favoring health. Additional information on the political process follows later in this chapter.

A second way to achieve power is through affiliation with others on behalf of community problems. There is strength is numbers when proposing change to those in power positions. Groups of consumers or coalitions of people and organizations can be effective in bringing about change. Strategies for coalition building will be discussed in the next chapter.

CONFLICT AND CONFLICT RESOLUTION IN POLITICS

PHILOSOPHY OF CONFLICT

If we accept the concept of opposing groups competing for limited resources in the political arena, conflict is inevitable. Conflict is the internal discord that results from differences between two or more people. Robbins (1974) outlines three philosophies of conflict in the social sciences. Until the 1940s, conflict was viewed as negative and destructive by the *traditionalists.* Between the 1940s and 1960s, it was viewed as inevitable but should be minimized or suppressed—*behaviorists'* view. Currently, the *interactionalists* have a more positive view of conflict and say it is both functional and dysfunctional and must be stimulated and resolved. Stagnation results from the absence of conflict. Robbins (1974) sums up the interactionalist view this way: "[We] should stimulate conflict to achieve the full benefits from its functional properties, yet reduce its level when it becomes a disruptive force" (p. 42).

CATEGORIES OF CONFLICT

Lewis (1976) outlines three categories of conflict: intrapersonal, interpersonal, and intergroup. Intergroup conflict occurs between two or more groups or organizations and results from conflicting beliefs, values, or wants. This category of conflict is most common in politics and will be encountered by the nurse in the process of coalition building or other interventions in this chapter.

STAGES OF CONFLICT

Factors such as scarce resources, unclear roles, and different values and interests precede conflict. According to Kast and Rosenzweig (1970), there are five stages in conflict:

1. *Latent conflict,* in which the conditions are right for conflict, as in the case of important valued differences that have not yet manifested
2. *Perceived conflict,* in which the conflict is intellectualized because people know about the conflict situation but have not reacted to it
3. *Felt conflict,* in which the conflict is emotionalized in feelings of anxiety, stress, fear, or hostility
4. *Manifest or overt conflict,* involving actions such as withdrawing, competing, debating, or seeking resolution
5. *Conflict aftermath,* or the period following the resolution when all people involved know the outcome

CONFLICT MANAGEMENT AND RESOLUTION

Various techniques may resolve conflict. The particular technique used will depend on the situation, the time needed to reach a decision, the power and maturity of the involved people, and the importance of the issue. One beneficial resolution mode is *problem solving,* in which there is open discussion and investigation of the problem and its dimensions until an outcome is reached that is considered to be a win situation for all parties involved.

A second technique is *negotiation,* which will be discussed later. *Avoidance* is a third mode of resolution but is usually not effective in the long run because the problem will resurface. However, avoidance may offer the opportunity to "cool off" or to gather additional information for a more effective solution.

Another technique is *compromise,* in which each party gives up something to resolve the conflict. To avoid later antagonism about who gave up the most, both parties must agree to give up something of equal worth. Still another approach is *competition,* in which one party wins and another loses. The winning person or group uses a power position or influence to force the resolution, and losers, who feel powerless to challenge, are left angry, frustrated, and wanting to get even.

In *cooperation* or *accommodation,* one party wants the other to win and is willing to sacrifice its own beliefs in exchange for later payback. This is often used in the political arena and in effect is "I'll support you today if you support me tomorrow." This is effective when the conflict involves an issue that is of minor value to the one who is accommodating.

A final technique is *collaboration,* which results in a win-win situation. In this approach, all people discard their original goals and establish a priority common goal through problem solving. This is considered one of the better solutions for complex problems. Some of these techniques were discussed in Chapter 2 as part of the theory for the book.

NEGOTIATION AND THE POLITICAL PROCESS

Negotiation is an important aspect of the political process, especially coalition building and other interventions that deal with one or more groups. Bagwell and Clements (1985) define negotiating as "the effort to resolve disagreements on specific issues" (p. 8). By this definition, *effort* means work or energy expended, *resolved* means a decision or end to the disagreement, *disagreements* are differences, and *issues* are the areas of disagreement. Negotiation usually involves accommodating to the differences of the other group so that each party gives up something. In negotiations, each party should feel satisfied.

NEGOTIATION PROCESS

Bagwell and Clements (1985) identify eight steps involved in informal or formal negotiating. Step 1, *preparation,* involves (a) collecting information to learn the facts, (b) seeking advice and consulting experts, (c) gaining an understanding of the other person's or group's view of the situation, (d) determining the priorities of your group, and (e) planning your group strategy.

Step 2, *entrance,* involves (a) learning the scope of authority of the other negotiators; (b) starting the proceedings in a positive way by developing trust, credibility, and distance from the issue; (c) seeking common interests and offering to host the meeting or write the agenda; and (d) agreeing on the rules and procedures for negotiating such as the size of groups, frequency of meetings, and scope and duration of negotiations.

Step 3, *working with people,* means being courteous and confidently presenting your position. Step 4, *exploration,* involves (a) identifying issues to be resolved and related factors; (b) asking questions such as Why? How? What? and Where? (c) seeking agreement on minor issues such as ground rules or alternative presentations of points; and (d) looking for common interests and areas of mutual agreement.

Step 5, *inventing,* involves (a) reviewing Steps 1 to 4; (b) brainstorming, evaluating, and selecting appropriate actions to solve the problem; (c) considering beliefs, facts, forecasts, interests, cost, benefits, objectives, and priorities of both sides; and (d) developing an informal or formal agreement from the joint choices.

Step 6, *bargaining,* involves (a) making legitimate, rational, and routine requests that are rewarding for all; (b) listening for offers or opportunities to make or change your offer; and (c) using tactics such as beginning with large demands that are precise and limiting negotiators' authority so that recesses, consultation time to reassess position, and other strategies are possible.

Step 7, *agreeing and closing,* involves (a) delaying if there is inappropriate pressure to settle; (b) ensuring that the agreed-on terms are operational and that it is known who will do what by when, including incentives for sticking to the agreement; (c) considering ways to settle disputes; and (d) celebrating and publicizing the agreement.

Step 8, *implementing,* involves carrying out the agreement and using dispute settlement if needed.

NEGOTIATING TACTICS

Bakker and Bakker-Rabdan (1973) identify 14 negotiating tactics that are competitive rather than collaborative and that may lead to unsatisfactory resolution. The negotiator should be aware of these in order to deal effectively with the negotiation process. They include ridicule, "smoke screen," "over the barrel," seduction, flattery, sex, illness-helplessness, guilt induction, definition, self-definition, paternalism, gifts, aggressive takeover, and pacifism. Some of these that may not be self-explanatory are discussed here. *Ridicule* invades the psychological space of others and should be countered by maintaining a relaxed body posture, steady gaze, and patient smile to prevent the psychological *takeover. Over the barrel* takes advantage of known vulnerable areas in another such as anger or crying to force concession and should be countered by hiding weak areas or desensitizing them. *Seduction* involves promise of future rewards and desired gratifications. *Definition* involves defining another person in terms of a pleasant quality—for example, saying that he or she is a "reasonable person," which limits the other's freedom to be otherwise—that is, unreasonable. *Self-definition* is a similar technique applied to one's self to hide the truth and to justify unacceptable behavior, such as calling oneself "temperamental." Negotiators should point out that they do not accept the self-definition as an excuse for the behavior. *Aggressive takeover* occurs when one party assumes authority and rapidly resolves the conflict in a manner benefiting himself or herself before others realize it. This should be countered by suggesting a break in the negotiations, using a simple "I need time to think this over."

NETWORKING IN POLITICS

Another important concept in political action is *networking*. Networking has been defined as "the establishing and maintaining of relationships with other professionals and community leaders for the purpose of solving common problems, creating new projects or programs, identifying experts for future consultation, maintaining mutual support, or enrolling others to work toward common ground" (Smith & Maurer, 1995, p. 20).

According to Black (1992), networks can (a) increase contacts that may be useful in one's development, (b) improve care of clients by contact and interaction with other caregivers, (c) advance nursing concepts and theories and improve practice in a supportive environment, and (d) through pressure groups, effect policy changes to benefit nursing care.

There are several ways to establish networks. These include (a) being active in professional organizations, (b) contacting others by phone or in person to discuss common concerns or problems, (c) seeking and accepting appointments to health and community boards, (d) remembering others with congratulations or thank-you notes, (e) joining a speakers bureau and speaking to community groups, (f) maintaining a list of community clients and directors in community resources, (g) being involved in political campaigns, and (h) maintaining contact with elected officials on issues of importance to nursing.

TEAM BUILDING FOR COMMUNITY WORK

Team building is important for involvement in the political process, coalition building, empowerment strategies, and other community interventions. This is discussed in Helvie (1981) and in Rubin, Plovnick, and Fry (1975).

NURSING INFLUENCE ON POLITICAL ACTION

Nurses may get involved in political action by providing information to clients or consumers and to other health care professionals on important upcoming health and health-related issues and on ways to influence decisions about these issues. Mass media can be used to provide information on pending legislation and to inform the public about how the issue affects health. Nurses can also discuss health issues with legislators in person or by letter or telephone. A further option is running for political office. Donley (1981) suggests several ways to become involved in political action, including (a) volunteering for political activities, (b) becoming assertive, (c) developing a network of contacts, (d) learning to compromise, and (e) understanding various points of view.

CONTACT WITH POLITICIANS

Nurses can contact politicians by telephone, letter, personal visit, or telegram. Prior to contact, one should learn about the background, current status, and ways to keep informed about a specific piece of legislation. Contacting organizations involved with the issue may be helpful. In addition, the League of Women Voters and Planned Parenthood may have information on the structure, the political process, and elected local or state officials. Nurses also need the following background information before contacting a politician: political party, tenure in office, date of reelection, favorite issues, committee assignments, views on health and nursing issues, and whether the politician has been supported by a nurses' political action group. Data can be obtained from the local legislator's office or the nurses' organization.

When writing a legislator, type letters on personal stationery using your own words unless you represent an organization. A personal letter is better than a form letter, and either is better than a postcard or telegram. Include a return address, and identify your residence within the legislator's district. Also include your profession and position, place of employment, and other relevant data. Identify clearly the issue you are addressing, such as the House or Senate bill number and name of legislator, your position on the bill and why you favor or oppose it, and how the bill could affect you, your profession, your clients, and so forth. Also indicate what you would like your legislator to do about the issue, and offer your services if additional information is needed. The best time to contact a legislator is while a bill is in committee. The president (U.S.) or the governor (state) should be contacted after a bill has been passed by the House and Senate and before it is signed into law.

The format for addressing officials is as follows:

- The president is addressed as "Mr. President," and the letter is mailed to "The White House, 1600 Pennsylvania Avenue, Washington, DC 20500"
- A senator is addressed as "Dear Senator _____," and the letter is mailed to "The Honorable _____, Senate Office Building, Washington, DC 20510"
- A member of Congress is addressed as "Dear Representative _____," and the letter is mailed to "The Honorable _____, House Office Bldg., Washington, DC 20510"
- A governor is addressed as "Dear Sir or Madam," and the letter is mailed to "The Honorable _____ of _____"
- A state senator is addressed as "Dear Senator," and the letter is mailed to "The Honorable _____"
- A state representative is addressed as "Dear Mr., Ms., or Mrs. _____," and the letter is mailed to "The Honorable _____."

When visiting a legislator, additional preparation is necessary. While making an appointment, it is appropriate to identify yourself and the bill or issue you wish to discuss. Preparation before the visit includes knowing the senator and the issue, as discussed earlier. During the visit, you introduce yourself to the legislator or his or her staff person and identify the issue of concern. Identify the legislator's position on the issue and explain yours. In addition, present facts on nursing in your state or district; determine if there have been contacts from other supporters or opponents; determine who they are and what they are saying. Offer to send additional information if needed and follow up the visit with a thank-you note.

A case study by a nurse leader involving political action follows. This will show what has been accomplished by nurses and should serve as a stimulus for further action.

Case Study 5
Mass Media as a Community Health Intervention

BETHANY HALL-LONG

THE EAST SIDE

BACKGROUND AND ASSESSMENT

Buried in the heart of the quaint city of Charleston, South Carolina, are three census tracts known as the "East Side." The East Side is located on the borders of the city's historic district as well as its major seaport. Despite the charm of the South, one cannot help but notice the rundown housing, high population density, and general "lack of luster" in the East Side compared with the rest of Charleston.

Sue, a community health nurse new to Charleston and a graduate student at an area nursing school, recently heard about the East Side's many health needs and decided to work with this at-risk population. She started with a comprehensive assessment of the East Side and found important health, economic, and social needs.

OBJECTIVE AND SUBJECTIVE DATA

Demographic findings include the following: Of a population of 6,783, (a) 88% are black, (b) 30% are on public assistance, (c) 60% are high school graduates, (d) 2% are college graduates, (e) 66% are employed in technical labor, and (f) 44% have a household income at or below 200% of the federal poverty level. In addition, 47% of households are headed by females, the unemployment rate is 13%, and the median age of the population is 34.

Health and human services are vital to the residents, but as is true of other inner-city areas, there are a number of barriers: lack of transportation, long waiting lists and waiting times at clinics, understaffed clinics, insufficient numbers of primary care providers, a 65% rate of uninsured residents, and a huge need for health promotion and disease prevention services.

In the region, there are 3 large private hospitals, 1 large public hospital, 1 Veteran's Administration hospital, 9 long-term care facilities, 11 home health agencies, 3 freestanding drug and counseling centers, and the Charleston County Health Department. A neighborhood clinic, Franklin C. Fetter Clinic, provides general care but has very long waiting lists and minimal health promotion services. For the most needy, 2 homeless shelters provide mental health counseling as well as job counseling and referrals.

Residents can receive basic health services from the local health department but often lack transportation to health care facilities and, once there, face long waits. The neighborhood Fetter clinic has a sliding scale fee that many cannot afford. There is one practitioner in the census tracts other than the community clinic. Thus, the East Side is known as a medically underserved area.

The leading causes of mortality in the East Side parallel the nation's major killers: cardiovascular disease, cancer, and accidents. The leading causes of morbidity are cardiovascular disease, diabetes, and accidents. The community suffers from a variety of communicable diseases as well as broader social and mental health issues, including a high rate of teen pregnancy (21%) and a significant rate of substance abuse among all residents (35%).

Sue soon discovered that hypertension was an urgent problem. One in every 3 residents was estimated to have high blood pressure, with 90% of the deaths from hypertension in Charleston County among blacks. Some of the resident's predisposing risks are age (45% > 40 years), genetics (88% black), lifestyle (diets high in fat and sodium, minimal exercise), and deficient availability of health resources.

Sue also explored recreation and cultural services for the East Side. She found several playgrounds for youths but limited adult recreation opportunities. There are a variety of small parks throughout the East Side, but these are poorly maintained and often serve as hangouts for unsavory characters. The East Side's Community Center offers a variety of cultural outings but only a few aerobics and weight training sessions. Residents report that most of their exercise comes from walking, but few exercise on a regular basis. The city's recreation department offers youth sports, a city gym, a tennis center, and a large park. However, because of limited funds and poor transportation, many East Side residents do not use the recreation facilities. A number of cultural events, such as concerts and art exhibits, are available in the downtown area if residents can afford to attend them.

Sue immediately recognized the importance of religion to this population. In the city and surrounding region, there are 330 churches and synagogues of 30 different denominations and 9 that are nondenominational. Residents of the East Side often turn to churches for assistance and direction with their personal needs, including health care. Ecumenical groups are key partners in many community service programs for the city.

When Sue assessed the transportation services, she went to the state and city Departments of Transportation and to census data for objective information. She also interviewed area residents and observed their use of transportation. Only 50% of the residents own a car. The remainder rely on the public bus service or private taxi services. The bus service operates frequently during the workday but provides limited evening and weekend hours. Many residents walk to work, school, church, the market, and other areas of need.

The official local government is an elected city council. The East Side also has an informal

neighborhood council (the East Side Neighborhood Council), made up of nine elected residents, that follows community issues such as safety, recreation, health and human services, and economic development. These community leaders, as well as formal policymakers, were very supportive of Sue and her initiatives to establish a health promotion and disease prevention program for the East Side.

Sue interviewed more than 35 city residents, including politicians, informal leaders, clergypeople, businesspeople, police officers, health care providers, and educators about the overall needs of the East Side. The recurring major concerns had to do with the need for (a) access to affordable comprehensive health care, (b) primary and secondary public health resources, (c) adequate transportation, (d) child care, (e) job training, (f) recreation for youth, (g) increased public works services, and (h) environmental cleanup. All 35 interviewees remarked on the East Side's sense of pride, support for others in the community, and informal networks.

More than three fourths of those interviewed suggested that a health education and screening program on hypertension was needed. In particular, residents and health care providers felt that free blood pressure screenings and related health education classes for all ages would be most valuable. Broader issues of child care, transportation, and follow-up also need to be part of the implementation of any program.

HEALTHY HEARTS BLOOD PRESSURE PROGRAM

As a result of the assessment, Sue brought together key players from the East Side whom she felt would be strong board members for a hypertension program. Over an informal luncheon at an area restaurant, she was able to get key leaders and residents to support the idea. Sue knew from past experience that the community must "own" the program even though she would serve as the catalyst and a facilitator. Thus, East Side residents and leaders united to form the Healthy Hearts Blood Pressure Program (HHBPP) board.

Sue and Ruth, a nurse and vice president of the East Side Neighborhood Council, served as co-coordinators of the program. Other board members were William, from the City of Charleston Recreation Department; Sister Jenkins, from Catholic Neighborhood House; Sherry, from the American Heart Association, Charleston Affiliate; and Art, president of the East Side Neighborhood Council. The HHBPP also had a series of teams and committees that included 15 to 20 volunteer members who were educators, health providers, and media experts. Each cosponsor contributed different physical, fiscal, and human resources to fund the program. In addition, the partners had a large network, including several media contacts and resources.

All of the volunteers had the necessary expertise or were trained for their specific roles. For instance, only nurses, paramedics, nursing students, and physicians performed the blood pressure screenings. During a 2-hour volunteer training session, information was provided about the East Side's population so that services were appropriate as well as culturally sensitive. The chair of the volunteer committee oversaw the training and maintenance of client records.

The health promotion and disease prevention program was originally offered twice a month (every other Saturday from 11 a.m. to 2 p.m.) at the East Side Community Center. Because of demand, the program expanded a few weeks later to every weekend (each Saturday from 10 a.m. to 3 p.m.) at the East Side Community Center and once a week (each Wednesday from 5 p.m. to 8 p.m.) at the Neighborhood House, Catholic Charities. HHBPP sponsored special programs in response to requests from throughout the East Side.

Each program started with one-to-one blood pressure screenings and counseling and shifted into 30 minutes of health education and demonstrations on topics such as diet, exercise, and stress management. Objective data (i.e., blood pressure readings, weights) were documented. A variety of teaching strategies and audiovisuals were used, depending on the educational needs and age level of the group.

Measurable program objectives and assigned activities were established. The nation's health objectives were integrated. These objectives were constantly monitored to assess the effectiveness and efficiency of the program. Integral to this process were specific media strategies as well as a media committee. Getting the press, community, and policymakers working together was essential to attaining a collective vision and program objectives.

WORKING WITH THE MEDIA

Media and marketing strategies were the heartbeat of the program. They served as the communication link with the East Side and helped to keep the program active, useful, and successful. All of the program's cosponsors used marketing strategies to sell the product, the HHBPP, backed by an East Side-oriented program promotion at the right place and price (no fee).

Because the HHBPP was made up of residents and leaders of the East Side, the targeted audience was known. The message was kept simple for the at-risk population. The central slogan was "High blood pressure is a silent killer and if you are black, there are some facts you need to know." The lifelong residents and leaders on the board felt that this one sentence would grab residents' attention. Details on the program, such as time, place, and prizes to encourage attendance were given below the slogan. All representatives of the HHBPP had a laminated, pocket-size card fact sheet as a reference in case they needed to "jog" their memory when approached by a member of the press.

Because this was a broad-based program with members of academia, churches, nonprofit groups, government, and community organizations participating, media connections were more readily accessible than many would imagine.

MEDIA STRATEGIES AND OBJECTIVES

Media strategies were ongoing, and objectives were developed to monitor the HHBPP's progress and program needs. The immediate (within 6 months) objectives were as follows:

1. Over 50% of city businesses and public buildings would have received at least one type of media release from the HHBPP.

2. The three large area TV networks would have aired a program on the HHBPP (live or taped) at least once, and information about the HHBPP would be part of their weekly PBS announcements.

3. The six identified radio stations would announce the HHBPP on their regular community service announcement series, and at least three live interviews would occur with HHBPP board members.

THE HEALTHY HEARTS BLOOD PRESSURE PROGRAM (HHBPP)

Date
February 1, 1988
Phone
(803) 555-5400

Release **February 7**

Contacts
Sue Long
Ruth Green

HHPBB: Attacking the "Silent Killer"

High blood pressure, or hypertension, has been identified as one of the top three killers in United States and in South Carolina. In the East Side neighborhood of Charleston, South Carolina, it is the number-one killer. One of every three residents has high blood pressure, and most do not even know it. More than 90% of the state's hypertension deaths occur among Blacks.

Now, the community is attacking this "silent killer" with a free blood pressure program, the Healthy Hearts Blood Pressure Program (HHBPP). This program is for all ages and offers free health education and screening programs by many experts. Its major cosponsors are the Graduate Community Health Nursing Program, Medical University of Charleston; the American Heart Association; Neighborhood House; the City of Charleston Recreation Department, and the East Side Neighborhood Council.

Celebrate Valentine's Day with a healthy heart by attending the first HHBPP program on February 13, 1988, between 11 a.m. and 2 p.m. at the East Side Community Center, 1 Cooper Street. There will be **free** diet, stress management, and exercise sessions as well as coupons for healthy eating. Call about free child care and transportation.

Please see the attached program and background details!

FIGURE CS5.1. Sample Press Release

4. Over 200 press releases would be disseminated throughout the East Side and the city, county, and state.

5. The three major newspapers would print at least one feature article on the HHBPP, three to five short articles, and 20 to 25 ads.

6. Over 800 posters and fliers would be distributed throughout the community at churches, schools, centers, the East Side's main grocery store, and other key locations.

7. Over 100 area public, nonprofit, and private organizations would include HHBPP information in their newsletters.

Sue and members of the board were most pleased when they had attained 80% of the objectives after the first 6 months. This took much planning and synergy on the part of the community-based partnership in the HHBPP.

A press release, to attract media attention and be informative to the layperson, was developed to be used in print, on TV and radio, and in organizational newsletters (see Figure CS5.1). Press releases were distributed a month in advance and follow-up calls occurred 2 weeks and 1 week before the HHBPP's kickoff day, February 13. Ads, fliers, and posters were also developed and widely disseminated throughout the East Side as well as in the broader city.

Financial support for these ads, fliers, and releases came from in-kind contributions. As a marketing strategy, businesses were invited to assist with the media announcements, and in turn, their business would be cited on the bottom of the announcement as a community supporter.

Thus, the HHBPP received free support, and more than 15 businesses were recognized as partners in public service. For example, the Insty-Prints Company devised large, colorful posters for the program and referenced their business along the bottom of the flier as a partner and cosponsor.

HHBPP board members informed the press of the program through face-to-face interactions, calls, and letters. The press releases reached the three key newspapers. As a result, a reporter with the city's most widely circulated newspaper, *News & Courier,* contacted Sue and did a face-to-face interview that was printed as a cover story. Sue and the board members requested that pictures be taken during one of the HHBPP sessions. The article featured two photos of HHBPP participants exercising and board members screening clients. The article attracted more than 30 additional residents and their children to attend the next session. The paper also included the HHBPP in its community calendar and periodically ran free ads. Two leaders on the HHBPP team wrote op-ed responses about the benefits of the program.

Next, the HHBPP media team delivered an article every week for 14 weeks to the grassroots East Side newspaper, *The Chronicle*. This publication was specific to the residents and reached almost 75% of area households and businesses. In addition to the articles, the HHBPP had free weekly ads and an occasional question-and-answer column on blood pressure-related health topics in *The Chronicle* as well as in the *Coastal Times.*

To monitor and perform ongoing program media strategy changes, the media committee added three questions to the HHBPP participant registration form: How did you hear about HHBPP? Have you seen or heard anything about the program in print or on the TV or radio? If so, where and approximately when? This information was helpful in directing the media campaign. For instance, it was learned that the ads placed in *The Chronicle* attracted more residents than those published in the *News & Courier.*

Members of the media committee also followed up on the press releases by calling three local television stations about the program and requesting their support. All of the TV networks included the program in their weekly scheduled PBS announcement times. Each of the networks visited the East Side Community Center on separate occasions and did a 3- to 5-minute taped interview that was shown at least twice to their viewing audiences.

Sue and the board members prepared for meetings with the press by having three key points: (a) knowing facts they wanted to reveal, (b) eliminating jargon from their language, and (c) "prepping" their attitudes and appearance. For instance, members participated in videotaped practice sessions and trained for tough questions, examining their nonverbal communication and monitoring their dress for the TV.

The three TV reporters were very supportive and provided Sue and participants the opportunity to add additional information to the end of their taped sessions. Sue and the members were sure to emphasize the need for the program and to "sell" its value to East Side viewers. Youth participants especially loved the television exposure and were good spokespersons on the importance of starting young with a healthy lifestyle to avoid "high blood." When one of the interviewers asked biased questions, Sue redirected the focus away from stereotypes of the low-income population to the health and program facts. After the program on the HHBPP was aired for the first time, more than five new health volunteers were added to the program and 19 residents enrolled in the program.

Four area radio stations aired the HHBPP PBS announcement at least once during the business hours the week before the program started and every other day after the program was under way. Two of the HHBPP Board members were interviewed separately by different stations for approximately 10 minutes about the HHBPP and its focus. Board members were prepared with fact sheets and again were concerned with getting a simple, clear, and appealing message across the airwaves. These members, Art (president of the East Side Neighborhood Council) and Sister Jenkins (from Neighborhood House), were excellent interviewees because they are contributing members of the East Side community. They are exceptionally articulate and influential with residents as well as with politicians and businesspeople.

HHBPP information and press releases were widely circulated to more than 200 different organizations and agencies in the county through their newsletters and communiques. For instance, the Chamber of Commerce, YMCA, YWCA, Medical University of South Carolina, and American Heart Association placed the information in newsletters to spread the word and to recruit volunteers. A positive and enthusiastic approach was used, and the seriousness of hypertension was a key selling point.

Sue and the board members made it a point to generously thank all members of the press and community for their support. This was an important HHBPP strategy to reciprocate its varied partners, including residents, the business community, and the press. For instance, an evening appreciation reception was held at the East Side Community Center at which time volunteers and partners, including the members of the press,

were recognized for their contributions to the growing success of the HHBPP.

SUMMARY

Sue worked with the HHBPP for 15 months before turning over the program entirely to the community. The program continues to be a success because of the synergy of the community partnership and established East Side ownership of the effort. The media were the heartbeat of the program in the beginning, and it remains vital to the program. Sue, like all community health nurses, values the role of mass media in working with populations in public health.

Case Study 6

The Political Process as a Community Intervention

CLARE HOUSEMAN

Focused political action by professional nurses is essential to achieve many goals important to nursing.

Virginia Trotter Betts (American Nurses Association [ANA], 1996, p. i)

The United States has 2 million nurses providing health care, and more and more these nurses see "the alarming effects of a system that has lost touch with the communities it is supposed to serve" (American Nurses Foundation [ANF], 1992, p. 5). There is no doubt that community health nurses see much that needs changing about the health care system as they go about their daily work. They should consider taking political action. Health policy change is not just for those who specialize in this area. "Every nurse can be an effective agent for policy

change, especially when armed with current information and a firmly supported, well-tested set of political skills" (ANA, 1996, p. i). I hope to explore the truth of this statement in this case study, which describes how a small group of nurses with little previous political experience launched a grassroots effort to successfully pass state legislation to enable psychiatric nurse clinical specialists to be directly reimbursed by insurance companies in the state of Virginia. During this process, we learned what a good reputation nursing has as a professional group and the high esteem in which we are held by legislators. Also, despite feeling powerless at times, we learned that earnest one-to-one contact by nurses with legislators can overcome the opposition of a group of more experienced, highly paid lobbyists.

BACKGROUND

Nursing's Agenda for Health Care Reform (ANF, 1992) specifies that steps to decrease health care costs include "assurance of direct access to a full range of qualified providers" (p. 3). This was certainly not the case in Virginia. In the 1970s, nursing care by clinical nurse specialists (CNSs) was not available to clients in outpatient private practices. Advanced practice nursing for CNSs was not clearly delineated in the state rules and regulations, and the State Board, when questioned, indicated that the conservative approach that is usually upheld in Virginia requires specific legislation to make practice legal (Houseman, Hurt, Smith, & Zimmerman, 1989). Nevertheless, in the early 1980s, a few CNSs began private practices despite the legal, professional, and economic consequences that might ensue. In retrospect, these actions were extremely important because in nursing domains, practice very often must precede law. There must always be people who are willing to push the limits to allow new practices to be legalized.

In 1985, members of the Psychiatric Professional Practice Group of the Virginia Nurses Association (VNA) officially asked for a definitive stand from the State Board regarding this issue. The State Board was unable to provide this. In 1986, nine psychiatric CNSs met to investigate methods of legitimizing independent practice for psychiatric CNSs. The group decided to ask that the VNA seek consultation from the ANA to provide strategy because the ANA had helped nurses in other states to accomplish this. The ANA's recommendation was for the VNA to meet with insurance companies to investigate the procedures for direct reimbursement. These negotiations turned out to be a dead end.

THE PRELIMINARIES

In 1987, an ad hoc group of certified psychiatric CNSs began meeting on a regular monthly basis. This informal group, which would become the VNA task force, began the strategizing that eventually led to the presentation of a bill, HB1024. The decision to include only certified CNSs in the group was an important one, although we did not realize it at the time. This credential would become the crucial issue for the State Board committee on which our success would eventually hinge. Also, the homogeneity of the group eliminated turf battles and competing agendas that can undermine political efforts in nursing. After meeting as an independent group for a brief period, members decided to petition the VNA to allow it task force status. As a task force, the group was able to function autonomously and raise and handle its own money. This was important because frequently the task force had to move quickly and decisively and did not have time to get approval from an executive board. Although not apparent initially, the group's ties to VNA were extremely important because the political task at hand could not have been accomplished without the support of the professional organization, no matter how determined the group was.

Meanwhile, changes in the Nurse Practice Act to allow specialty practice in the state had been drawn up by the Health Regulatory Board after its study of nursing in the state. These were withdrawn when they met with objection from the VNA regarding how specialty practice should be defined. This was quite a challenge to the task force as it pondered strategies to move toward independent practice, knowing that the two major players crucial to success were unable to negotiate a resolution to their conflict. The task force drew up a compromise paragraph and submitted it to both parties, but this was to no avail. The group voted to press on, whatever the outcome of the conflict, believing that perhaps action could change things.

The strategy the task force used to move forward was one that had already been used by psychologists, social workers, and licensed professional counselors to obtain direct reimbursement in the state. The task force hoped that the legislature would see this amendment to the insurance legislation as familiar ground and treat the group as it had the other professional groups. The fact that it was not clear that CNSs could legally practice in the state was a problem the group pushed into the background as it pressed on. It is clear that the use of denial as a coping strategy as well as a little magical thinking was involved here.

GETTING ORGANIZED

The task force interviewed a lobbyist in 1987. He stated that the cost of changing the law would range from $8,000 to $12,000, depending on the amount and degree of opposition. About 15 attendees at this late summer meeting agreed to hire the lobbyist and raise the money. Although money is often an obstacle to nursing political action, there was enough "fire in the belly" of this group that its members were not deterred by the enormity of the commitment. Looking back, it seems like an incredible risk, but at the time, it was just something that had to be done.

Once the decision was made, the task force needed to have some kind of organization beyond its ad hoc beginnings. Perhaps nurses who prefer to work outside of hospital settings have a natural distrust for heirarchial organizations. This was certainly the case in the task force, which had thrived on a consensus approach to decision making and a flattened hierarchy. Individuals volunteered to do whatever short- or long-term tasks were needed. This model was continued; however, certain task force members volunteered to take responsibility for specific roles. Specific individuals were to be the main contacts with the lobbyist, and one person was to handle the money.

A network of regional contact persons was set up to facilitate communication and recruitment. This network was invaluable because it became the basis of a telephone tree that enabled the contact persons to relay information throughout the state and poll grassroots membership for their responses and opinions. The regional contact persons also stimulated fund-raising in their areas and organized constituents to contact their legislators so that a coordinated effort was made. It was to the credit of the group that people did what they could do, and if they couldn't do something, someone else stepped in to take the responsibility. There was little pathologizing as sometimes occurs in organizations, with people saying, "Well, if everyone isn't going to participate, I'm not going to." If a person couldn't do something at one time, the group counted on a contribution later. If someone couldn't contribute time and energy to strategizing or lobbying, perhaps he or she could donate money to the cause.

GETTING STARTED

To change the insurance law, a bill would have to be passed in both houses of the general assembly. Our lobbyist, who was a lawyer, drafted the language of the bill. As the January 1988 session approached, the task force had difficulty finding a chief patron. Immediately prior to the deadline for legislative initiatives, a regional contact person announced that a sponsor had been tapped. The fact that this chief patron was a member of the minority party in the general assembly caused some consternation for the lobbyist, but this was soon overcome as others were recruited to cosponsor the bill. A group with more political experience probably would have sought a member of the majority party to sponsor their bill, but in our naïveté, we were just happy to have someone on our side.

The bill was first slated for the House of Delegates Corporations Insurance and Banking Committee, and regional contact persons recruited nurse constituents of each committee member to influence their legislator in favor of the bill. Many nurses for the first time found out who their representatives were and arranged meetings with them or their aides. Fact sheets with bulleted information related to HB1024 were developed to provide nurses and legislators with facts regarding the bill. At the hearing in which the committee would determine whether the bill would go to the house floor, the lobbyist and selected VNA representatives testified on behalf of the bill. HB1024 passed both the committee and the house of delegates by comfortable margins. This passage surprised groups who might have opposed the bill. A representative of one of those groups indicated that it was counting on the usual divisiveness among diverse interest groups of nurses to scuttle their own bill. When this didn't happen, lobbyists from groups representing medicine, psychology, and insurance interests became involved, and from that time forward, all of our efforts were counteracted by the opposition's paid lobbyists.

CONTINUING THE FIGHT

HB1024 was to be heard next by the Commerce and Labor Committee of the state senate. It had been labeled as a controversial bill and was therefore sent to a subcommittee for preliminary decision. Nurse constituents of members of the committee who were convinced that this was a good bill for all nursing began contacting their legislators. Although some were disgruntled because a few advanced practice nurses would not benefit directly from the legislation, this problem was managed expertly by task force members and the VNA, who explained the importance of limiting the opposition concerned with the bill. For if nurse midwives, nurse anesthetists, and nurse practitioners were included, so much opposition would have been aroused, there would have been no chance of success. The group used the example of getting the camel's nose in the tent before trying to get the whole camel in. Nurse practitioners supported the group in this legislation, and several years later, the group supported them in a bid for prescriptive privileges. As it was, almost a dozen lobbyists from opposing groups faced off against the task force in the subcommittee hearing. CNSs and VNA representatives came to tell the "whole truth and nothing but the truth" about their services to clients over many years. They were amazed to discover that opposing lobbyists were "either seriously uninformed or deliberately chose to ignore both the current practice of nursing in the state, and the educational preparation and credentialing process of Clinical Nurse Specialists" (Houseman et al., 1989, p. 33). After much testimony and debate, some of it quite heated, the bill passed the subcommittee by a 2 to 1 vote.

The intensity of the discussion continued late when the bill went for hearing before the full committee. CNS qualifications were explicated along with the importance of the service to clients with limited access. Cost benefits of using CNS services were also discussed as well as the fact that nurses did not require medical supervision to practice. Lobbyists for opposing groups insisted that nurses must be supervised by physicians and pointed out that there was no mechanism for legally recognizing clinical nurse specialist practice in the state. This was, of course, the major stumbling block that the Task Force had decided to ignore and just hope for the best outcome. The senate committee then asked the director of the Department of Health Regulatory Boards to study the issue of advanced nursing practice and report back the next year.

EXPERIENCING DISAPPOINTMENT

Although the bill's being held over was a favorable outcome as opposed to its being "killed," some members of the task force were disappointed that the goal had not been achieved after so much hard work. Lacking experience in the political arena, they did the unthinkable and publicly expressed their frustration toward key political figures after the hearing. This is not "the way the game is played" in the legislature; someone may have voted against you today, but you might need her or his help tomorrow. Phone calls were made and letters of apology were sent for these breaches of political etiquette. Patience and politeness are, indeed, important values in the political process.

The task force held a debriefing session to handle these feelings. Participants cursed at one another, complained about people who weren't there, and ranted at the unfairness of the world in general. "The task force experienced this as its lowest point, and anxieties were expressed as to whether it would be able to recreate the emotional commitment necessary to see the bill through" (Houseman et al., 1989, p. 34).

Meanwhile, the Health Regulatory Board, as directed, began to study the issue of legal mechanisms for advanced practice, and task force members regrouped to recruit appropriate testimony. Not knowing what the results of the study would be, the group decided to press on as if there would be a favorable outcome. Plans for the 1989 general assembly had to be made. The most significant issue was money.

FUND-RAISING

The bill for the lobbyist the previous year totaled $10,000. The task force had sent letters to psychiatric CNSs in the state asking each one to contribute $125. Regional contact persons organized local fund-raising efforts both inside and outside of district VNA meetings. A raffle was held at a regional conference for CNSs, and donations were collected at the state nurses convention in the fall and on Legislative Day in the spring. The sum total of all of these CNS fund-raising endeavors was $8,000. VNA had loaned the group $2,000 and generously offered to forgive the loan. The task force was therefore not burdened with debt as the next session began.

To prepare for lobbyist fees in the upcoming legislative session, CNSs came up with a variety of strategies. CNSs across the state were again asked to contribute $125 each. Member organizations of the Alliance, a consortium of nursing organizations in the state, were challenged to raise $1 for each member of each organization. District nurses associations were again asked to contribute. Because this was seen as a good cause for nursing in general and it was supported by VNA, many nurses contributed, even though they had little to gain personally from this legislation. It was wonderful to see nurses working together toward a common cause rather than splitting off into their separate interest groups. The task force had nurtured these sentiments by appointing individual members to market the cause to the nursing organizations of their choice. Eventually, most nursing organizations were visited by task force members who told them about the effort and answered their questions.

Preparatory fund-raising efforts also included a continuing education program, organized and presented by task force members. The November workshop raised $2,000, precisely what the lobbyist billed for services that month. As the legislative session approached, task force members decided to postpone financial concerns until after the session so as to concentrate all efforts on lobbying. In December, members of the Senate Commerce and Labor Committee were lobbied by nurse constituents all over the state regarding what was interpreted as a consumer-oriented bill, backed fully by the VNA.

When the bill was again heard by the Commerce and Labor Committee, task force members testified. The executive director of the Health Regulatory Board presented its report, which included a statement that "certain nursing functions are legally performed independent of physician supervision in the State of Virginia" (Houseman et al., 1989, p. 35). The task force lobbyist presented the amendments added to the bill that would allow for the regulation of advanced practice nurses. Task force members testified along with VNA representatives, and the bill's patron strongly argued in its defense. The medical lobby withdrew its opposition, their concerns regarding regulation of practitioners having been addressed. The insurance lobby remained opposed, viewing the legislation as an economic threat.

Even though the Commerce and Labor Committee voted in favor of HB1024, certain powerful members of the committee who remained opposed to the bill decided to pass it along to a second senate committee, Health and Education, whose membership consisted of many senators who were believed to view the bill negatively. Although this seemed like an obstacle at the time, it did allow task force members and other nurses across the state to use their influence to convert more senators to a favorable view. Ultimately, this resulted in less opposition when the bill finally reached the floor. After more discussion at this hearing, during which many of the same people said the same things for and against the bill (patience is indeed a virtue in the political process), HB1024 narrowly passed the committee, thereby guaranteeing a floor fight when it reached the full senate, because there was still enough opposition to label the bill "controversial" and prevent the senate from "rubber stamping" the work of the committee. The one-to-one contacts by nurses with senators continued because each senator's vote was important.

COMPLETING THE TASK

Ordinarily, the bill would have gone to the senate floor by the end of that week, but because many state politicians were traveling to Washington to participate in the presidential inauguration that weekend, the schedule had been limited. This allowed an extra weekend for nurses across the state to convince their senators who had voted against the bill in committee to vote for the bill when it came to the floor. After a heated discussion, HB1024 passed the senate by a 23 to 15 vote. Seasoned legislative observers were surprised by the outcome, indicating that "anyone who was anyone in the assembly was opposed to the bill." It seemed that the relentless one-to-one contact of senators by their nurse constituents changed the usual political pattern to allow for passage of this particular bill.

HB1024 was returned to the house of delegates for reconsideration because it had been amended to include the State Board's regulation of advanced practice nursing. It passed again without controversy, obtaining a 99 to 1 vote.

The Board of Nursing later approved a mechanism for regulating advanced practice in the state. This also did not occur without controversy because this had been a problem even before the beginning of the legislative process. Nevertheless, the issue was eventually resolved with input from task force members, the VNA, and representatives from the Health Regulatory Board.

After much jubilation, the task force turned with some trepidation to look at the financial situation. Over the 2-year period, approximately $14,000 had been billed by the lobbyist, and this had been paid by the fund-raising efforts of all concerned. The VNA decided that having a lobbyist would be useful in the future and hired our lobbyist's partner to represent professional nursing in the state.

LESSONS LEARNED

The following summarizes advice about the political process described in this case study:

1. Have a particular goal and want it badly.
2. Assemble a reasonably homogeneous group and organize it in a way in which power can be shared and communication can be rapid.
3. Don't be afraid to take risks.
4. Involve other nursing organizations and interest groups and help them to understand that a victory for one group of nurses is a victory for all nurses.
5. Don't take on more opposition than can be managed at one time.

6. Be persistent. Don't give up even when obstacles and losses come your way. Find a way to process these as a group and move on.
7. Keep things in perspective and maintain established protocol. Although this may be a life-and-death issue to you, it is one of many other issues for legislators or even other nurses. It is more important to lose graciously and maintain a relationship than to close doors with anger.
8. Stay involved with your legislators after the bill is passed. There will always be a "next time."

With these ideas in mind, there is no reason why every nurse can't "ensure that policy makers support and initiate health care delivery system change for the better" (ANA, 1996, p. i). The process is invigorating, frustrating, rewarding, humbling, and, above all, addictive. So embrace the political process, leave the world your legacy, and "go for it!"

REFERENCES

American Nurses Association. (1996). *104th Congress 1st Session directory.* Washington, DC: Author.

American Nurses Foundation. (1992). *Nursing's agenda for health care reform.* Kansas City, MO: American Nurses Publishing.

Houseman, C., Hurt, L., Smith, L., & Zimmerman, M. (1989). House Bill 1024: A chronology. *Virginia Nurse, 57,* 32-36.

REFERENCES

Abrahams, N. (1992). Toward reconceptualizing political action. *Sociological Inquiry, 62,* 327-347.

Arkin, E. (1990). Opportunity for improving the nation's health through collaboration with the mass media. *Public Health Reports, 105,* 219-223.

Bacharach, S. B., & Lawler, E. J. (1980). *Power and politics in organizations.* San Francisco: Jossey-Bass.

Bagwell, M., & Clements, S. (1985). *The art of negotiating: A political handbook for health professionals.* Boston: Little, Brown.

Bakker, B. B., & Bakker-Rabdan, M. K. (1973). *No trespassing.* San Francisco: Chandler & Sharp.

Bandura, A. (1986). *Social foundations of thought and action.* Englewood Cliffs, NJ: Prentice Hall.

Bandura, A. (1997). *Self-efficacy: An exercise of control.* New York: Freeman.

Baranowski, T. (1989-1990). Reciprocal determinism at the stages of behavior change: An integration of community, personal, and behavioral perspectives. *International Quarterly of Health Education, 10,* 297-327.

Becker, M. (1974). *The health belief model and personal health behavior.* Thorofare, NJ: Charles B. Slack.

Black, F. (1992). Network for change. *Nursing Times, 88*(1), 58-59.

Bracht, N. (Ed.). (1990). *Health promotion at the community level.* Newbury Park, CA: Sage.

Burgess, W. (1983). *Community health nursing.* Norwalk, CT: Appleton-Century-Crofts.

Coombs, C., Dawes, R., & Tversky, A. (1981). *Mathematical psychology. An elementary introduction.* Ann Arbor, MI: Mathesis.

Dahl, R. (1984). *Modern political analysis.* Englewood Cliffs, NJ: Prentice Hall.

Donley, R. (1981). How can I get a job on Capitol Hill? *American Journal of Nursing, 81,* 112-116.

Farquhar, J., Fortmann, S., Flora, J., Taylor, C., Haskell, W., Williams, P., Maccoby, N., & Wood, P. (1990). Effects of communitywide education on cardiovascular disease risk factors: The Stanford five-city project. *Journal of the American Medical Association, 264,* 359-365.

Fishbein, M., & Ajzen, I. (1975). *Belief, attitude, intention and behavior: An introduction to theory and research.* Reading, MA: Addison-Wesley.

Flay, B., & Burton, D. (1990). Effective mass communication strategies for health campaigns. In C. Atkins & L. Wallach (Eds.), *Mass communication and public health* (pp. 129-146). Newbury Park, CA: Sage.

Ford, J., Schmitt, N., Schechtman, S., Hults, B., & Doherty, M. (1989). Process tracking methods: Contributions, problems and neglected research questions. *Organizational Behavior and Human Decision Processes, 43,* 75-117.

French, J. R., & Raven, B. (1959). The basis of social power. In D. Cartwright (Ed.), *Studies in social power.* Ann Arbor: University of Michigan Press.

Hale, J., & Dillard, J. P. (1995). Fear appeals in health promotion campaigns. In E. Maibach & R. L. Parrott (Eds.), *Designing health messages* (pp. 65-80). Thousand Oaks, CA: Sage.

Hammond, K., Stewart, T., Brehmer, B., & Steinmann, D. (1986). Social judgement theory. In H. R. Arkes & K. R. Hammond (Eds.), *Judgement and decisionmaking: An interdisciplinary reader* (pp. 56-76). Cambridge, UK: Cambridge University Press.

Helvie, C. O. (1981). *Community health nursing: Theory and process.* New York: Harper & Row.

Hersey, P., Blanchard, K., & Natemeyer, W. (1979). Situational leadership: Perception and impact of power. *Group Organizational Studies, 4,* 418-428.

Hewison, A. (1994). The politics of nursing: A framework for analysis. *Journal of Advanced Nursing, 20,* 1170-1175.

Holtgrave, D. R., Tinsley, B. J., & Kay, L. S. (1995). Encouraging risk-reduction: A decision-making approach to message design. In E. Maibach & R. L. Parrott (Eds.), *Designing health messages* (pp. 24-40). Thousand Oaks, CA: Sage.

Hutchinson, J. (1986). Discrete attribute models of brand switching. *Marketing Science, 5,* 350-371.

Jason, L. A., Lesowitz, T., Michaels, M., Blitz, C., Victors, L., Dean L., Yeager, E., & Kimball, P. (1989). A worksite smoking cessation intervention involving the media and incentives. *American Journal of Community Psychology, 17,* 785-799.

Kast, E. E., & Rosenzweig, J. E. (1970). *Organization of management: A systems approach.* New York: McGraw-Hill.

Kraus, N., & Slovic, P. (1988). Taxonomics analysis of perceived risk: Modeling individual and group perceptions within homogeneous hazard domains. *Risk Analysis, 8,* 435-455.

Laubach, R. S., & Koschnick, K. (1977). *Using readability: Formula for easy adult materials.* Syracuse, NY: New Readers.

Lewin, K. (1958). Group discussion and social change. In T. Newcomb & E. Hathey (Eds.), *Social psychology.* New York: Holt, Rinehart & Winston.

Lewis, J. (1976). Conflict management. *Journal of Nursing Administration, 6*(10), 18-22.

Leventhal, H., Safer, M., & Panagis, D. (1983). The impact of communications on the self-regulation of health beliefs, decisions, and behavior. *Health Education Quarterly, 10*(1), 7.

Maibach, E., & Cotton, D. (1995). Moving people to behavior change: A staged social cognitive approach to message design. In E. Maibach & R. L. Parrott (Eds.), *Designing health messages* (pp. 41-64). Thousand Oaks, CA: Sage.

Mason, D. (1985). The politics of patient care. In D. Mason & S. Talbott (Eds.), *Political action handbook for nurses.* Menlo Park, CA: Addison-Wesley.

Mason, D., & Talbott, S. (1985). *Political action handbook for nurses.* Menlo Park, CA: Addison-Wesley.

Mason, D., Talbott, S., & Leavitt, J. (1993). *Policy and politics for nurses.* Philadelphia: W. B. Saunders.

McGuire, W. J. (1981). Theoretical foundation of campaigns. In R. Rice & W. Paisley (Eds.), *Public communication campaigns* (pp. 41-70). Beverly Hills, CA: Sage.

Monahan, J. (1995). Thinking positively: Using positive affect when designing health messages. In E. Maibach & R. Parrott (Eds.), *Designing health messages* (pp. 81-98). Thousand Oaks, CA: Sage.

National Research Council. (1989). *Improving risk communication.* Washington, DC: National Academy Press.

Pfau, M. (1995). Designing messages for behavioral inoculation. In E. Maibach & R. Parrott (Eds.), *Designing health messages* (pp. 99-113). Thousand Oaks, CA: Sage.

Prochaska, J. O., & DiClementi, C. C. (1986). *The transtheoretical approach: Crossing the traditional boundaries of therapy* (2nd ed.). Homewood, IL: Dow Jones/Irwin.

Riger, S. (1989). The politics of community intervention. *American Journal of Community Psychology, 17,* 379-383.

Robbins, S. P. (1974). *Managing organizational conflict.* Englewood Cliffs, NJ: Prentice Hall.

Robbins, S. P. (1993). *Organizational behavior* (6th ed.). Englewood Cliffs, NJ: Prentice Hall.

Rosenstock, I. (1974). The health belief model and preventive health behavior. *Health Education Monographs, 2,* 354-385.

Schramm, W. (1982). Channels and audiences. In G. Gumpert & R. Cathcart (Eds.), *Inter/media: Interpersonal communication in a media world* (pp. 78-92). New York: Oxford University Press.

Rubin, I., Plovnick, M., & Fry, R. (1975). *Improving the coordination of care: A program for health team development.* Cambridge, MA: Ballinger.

Slader, M. (1995). Choosing audience segmentation strategies and methods for health communication. In E. Maibach & R. Parrott (Eds.), *Designing health messages* (pp. 186-198). Thousand Oaks, CA: Sage.

Smith, C. M., & Maurer, F. A. (1995). *Community health nursing.* Philadelphia: W. B. Saunders.

Strecher, V., DeVellis, B., Becker, M., & Rosenstock, I. (1986). The role of self-efficacy in achieving health behavior change. *Health Education Quarterly, 13,* 73-91.

Talbott, S. W., & Vance, C. (1981). Involving nursing in a feminist group—NOW. *Nursing Outlook, 29,* 592-595.

Ulene, A. (1987, July). National education for health: Health in the media. *Healthlink,* pp. 3-4.

von Winterfeldt, D., & Edwards, W. (1986). *Decision analysis and behavioral research.* New York: Cambridge University Press.

Wallach, L. (1990). Mass media and health promotion: Promises, problems, challenges. In C. Watkins & L. Wallach (Eds.), *Mass communication and public health* (pp. 41-51). Newbury Park, CA: Sage.

Wallach, L., Dorfman, L., Jernigan, D., & Themba, M. (1993). *Media advocacy and public health.* Newbury Park, CA: Sage.

Warnecke, R., Langenberg, P., Gruder, C., Flay, B., Phil, D., & Jason, L. (1989). Factors in smoking cessation among participants in a televised intervention. *Preventive Medicine, 18,* 833-846.

Weinstein, N. D. (1988). The precaution adoption process. *Health Psychology, 7,* 355-386.

CHAPTER 11

COMMUNITY INTERVENTIONS
Empowerment, Coalition Building, and Involving Citizens, Organizations, and Professionals

---

OBJECTIVES: EMPOWERMENT

1. Define empowerment and community empowerment.
2. Discuss community competence.
3. Evaluate multilevel models of community empowerment.
4. Identify barriers to community empowerment.

OBJECTIVES: COALITION BUILDING

1. Define coalitions.
2. Discuss the purposes and advantages of coalitions.
3. Discuss the steps in forming coalitions.

OBJECTIVES: INVOLVING CITIZENS, ORGANIZATIONS, AND PROFESSIONALS

1. Define and discuss the purposes of citizen participation.
2. Discuss factors influencing the participation of citizens, industries, and professionals.

EMPOWERMENT

Health professionals have found that the community development social planning model in which the planner identifies problems, plans services, and intervenes has not been the most effective approach to solving community problems. At the same time, budget constraints have forced planners to consider different approaches to solving community problems (see Case Study 1 in Chapter 3). One approach is the empowerment process in which the planner assists community aggregates to develop the knowledge and skills necessary to assess and provide for their own needs. Zerwekh (1992) says empowering people in a community means helping them develop competence to control their lives and meet their own needs. Although empowerment has been discussed in relation to individuals, organizations, and communities in the literature, the major emphasis of this chapter will be on community empowerment.

DEFINITIONS

Kreisberg (1992) defines empowerment as a process of developing knowledge and skills that increase one's mastery over the decisions that affect one's life. A second definition, proposed by Rappaport (1987), is this: "a mechanism by which people, organizations and communities gain mastery over their affairs" (p. 122). Another definition developed by Rappaport (1984) is: "a process by which individuals and communities are enabled to predict, control and participate in their own environment" (p. 2).

POWER, POLITICS, AND EMPOWERMENT

According to Kent (1970), power is the ability to predict, control, and participate in one's environment. This definition is closely related to the definitions of empowerment just mentioned and also to the concepts of political power discussed in Chapter 10. In addition, many other nursing interventions are directed toward increasing power of community aggregates when viewed from the perspective of controlling and participating in one's environment. These include interventions such as coalition building and teaching small or large groups (mass media).

COMMUNITY EMPOWERMENT

According to Wallerstein (1992), community empowerment is a "social action process that promotes participation of people, organizations, and communities toward the goals of increased individual and community control, political efficacy, improved quality of community life, and social justice" (p. 197).

COMMUNITY EMPOWERMENT AS COMPETENCE

Community empowerment has been operationalized as community competence, and having community competence is defined as being a community in which the parts can (a) identify problems and needs of the community by effective collaboration, (b) achieve agreement on goals and priorities, (c) agree on how to implement goals, and (d) collaborate effectively in implementing plans to achieve goals (Cottrell, 1976). Eight dimensions of community competence were also identified. Eng and Parker (1994) used these dimensions in a study but combined two dimensions, communication and articulation, and added social support. These follow.

DIMENSIONS OF COMMUNITY COMPETENCE

Dimensions of community competence used by Eng and Parker (1994) include the following:

1. *Participation,* defined as the process of committing to the community and contributing to setting goals and planning interventions: Questions identified to measure this dimension have to do with issues such as staying in the community or leaving for entertainment; involvement in governmental, civic, or private organizations; past or future plans for involvement in neighborhood activities; decision-making involvement; and identifying who carries out plans in the community.

2. *Commitment,* defined as a relationship worthy of enhancing and maintaining: Questions to measure this dimension concern the amount of time spent volunteering for community activities, the extent of caring about the community or feeling actively involved, and the extent of feeling the influence of community change on one's own life.

3. *Self-other awareness and clarity of a situational definition,* defined as how well each part of the community perceives its identity and position on issues related to other parts of the community: Questions to measure this are concerned with whether or not there are strong opinions about how things are done in the county, about how much the county considers the opinions of the community, and how often it tries to influence the community.

4. *Articulateness,* defined as the ability to articulate involvement in the collective views, attitudes, needs, and intentions of the community; the process of exchanging information; and how well the community derives a common meaning from the different parts of the community: Questions to measure this dimension have to do with the number of people who will express unpopular opinions; number who could speak to community issues in front of a group, and number who could interpret the needs of the community to outsiders.

5. Conflict containment and accommodation, which relates to the establishment of procedures to accommodate open conflict and continued interaction between different parts of the community: Questions to measure

this dimension concern ways to work out differences and questions about which ways are used in the particular community.

6. *Management of relations with wider society,* which involves using resources and support offered by the larger society and reducing the threats of larger social pressures on community life: Questions related to this dimension are about the number of people owning their own homes, the number who are knowledgeable about services in the community, and the amount of influence the community exerts on the county.

7. *Machinery for facilitating participant interaction and decision making,* which relates to ability of the community to establish formal mechanisms for representative input into decision making: Questions to measure this relate to the amount of involvement in the community by letter writing, phone calls, personal interviews, and serving on boards and the extent of involvement compared with other communities.

8. Social support, which involves knowing and caring for others in a neighborhood and the willingness of people to assist by providing support: Questions to measure this dimension have to do with the extent of lending money and objects to others, the extent of offering advice, and the extent of offering support, such as a sympathetic ear.

Eng and Parker (1994) developed a rating scale on these dimensions. Theoretically, communities could be rated at two points in time on the scale to evaluate changes in empowerment.

COMMUNITY EMPOWERMENT: A PROCESS OR AN OUTCOME?

Flynn, Ray, and Rider (1994) and Eng and Parker (1994) refer to action research as a process that leads to empowerment (outcome). Although according to Eng and Parker (1994) this process was first described by Lewis in 1946, the process is similar to the community development process of locality development discussed by Rothman (1970) and presented in Chapter 8.

Flynn et al. (1994) say that community empowerment is not an end product but an ongoing action process that is transforming. The process of action research is a collaborative effort between the researcher and community people and builds capacity to solve problems. Important concepts in this process include a focus on the community, citizen participation, assisting communities to obtain information and problem-solving skills, sharing of power, and improved quality of life. These concepts were used in case studies of two communities presented in the article.

According to Israel, Checkoway, Schulz, and Zimmerman (1994), empowerment can be defined as enabling others or giving them the ability to use their own efforts to gain power. From this point of view, it is a process in which practitioners are involved with the community. However, *empowerment* used as a noun refers to being empowered, and that is an outcome. Viewed as an outcome, empowerment allows measurement of the effects of the interventions. Thus, they agree with Wallerstein (1992), Swift and Levin (1987), and

Gerschick, Israel, and Checkoway (1990) that empowerment is both a process and an outcome.

MULTILEVEL MODELS OF EMPOWERMENT

MULTILEVEL STRESS-HEALTH MODEL

Israel et al. (1994) propose a multilevel model of community empowerment that has a similar focus to the multilevel intervention model discussed in Chapter 8. Their model focuses on the individual, organization, and community. They say that programs can be directed toward individual empowerment but that the failure of professionals to consider the context in which individuals are embedded, such as in an organization or in a community, is less likely to increase an individual's control and influence and may result in failure of health and quality-of-life improvements.

Their model proposes empowerment across the three levels as well as at each level. Freire's (1973) concept of conscientization, discussed in Chapter 8, provides the link between the levels. This concept supports the development of identification with others and a feeling of self- and collective efficacy. Thus, the belief in possible effective action and the necessary skills and resources to develop effective action strategies are fostered.

Concurrently, Israel et al. propose a framework within which empowerment concepts fit (see Figure 11.1). In this model, stress is viewed as causing physiological, psychological, and behavioral outcomes, and psychosocial factors such as control are important in modifying levels of stress, health, and the relationships between them. Stress should be seen within a community context and can affect health and quality of life at the individual, organizational, and community levels.

The five major elements in the stress process model are (a) stressors, or psychosocial-environmental conditions that may produce stress, such as powerlessness or death of a community leader; (b) perception of stressors by individuals and the community; (c) immediate responses to perceptions of stress, such as tension and elevated blood pressure; (d) long-term health outcome of perceptions and short-term affects, such as cardiovascular disease and alcoholism, and (e) conditioning variables that influence the relationships between the previous four aspects of the model. Conditioning variables may include factors such as community control, supportive relationships, and the presence or absence of community problem-solving capabilities.

Five categories of psychosocial-environmental conditions are conducive to stress in the model. Major life events, the first category, are discrete disruptive events that often require adaptation and can be experienced by communities as well as by individuals. Major life events for a community might be the death of a community leader or the closing of a factory. Daily hassles are the second category and refer to minor frustrating events in daily life, such as a disagreement with a governmental official over contaminated water. Chronic stressors, the third condition, are long-term challenges or problems, such as poverty, lack

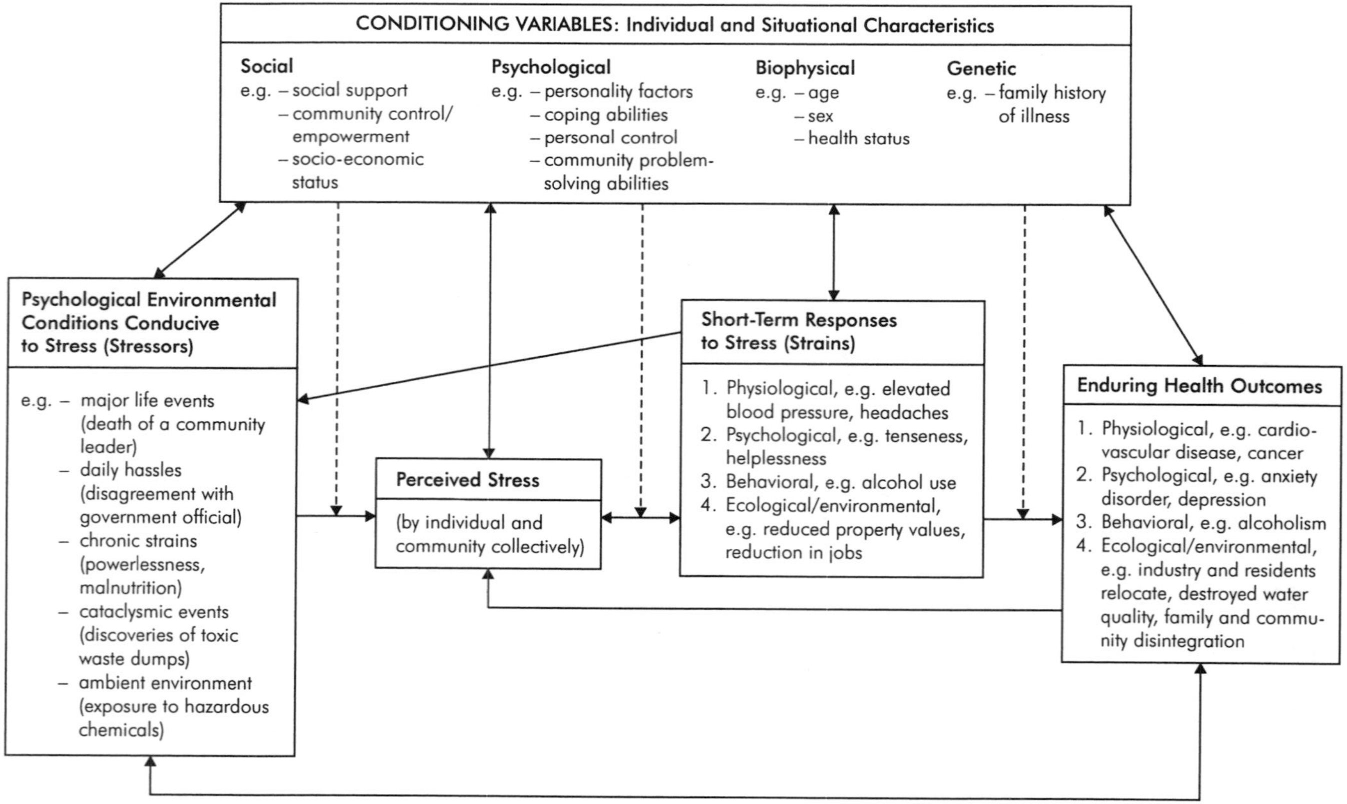
CONDITIONING VARIABLES: Individual and Situational Characteristics
Social
e.g. – social support
– community control/ empowerment
– socio-economic status
Psychological
e.g. – personality factors
– coping abilities
– personal control
– community problem-solving abilities
Biophysical
e.g. – age
– sex
– health status
Genetic
e.g. – family history of illness
Psychological Environmental Conditions Conducive to Stress (Stressors)
e.g. – major life events (death of a community leader)
– daily hassles (disagreement with government official)
– chronic strains (powerlessness, malnutrition)
– cataclysmic events (discoveries of toxic waste dumps)
– ambient environment (exposure to hazardous chemicals)
Perceived Stress
(by individual and community collectively)
Short-Term Responses to Stress (Strains)
1. Physiological, e.g. elevated blood pressure, headaches
2. Psychological, e.g. tenseness, helplessness
3. Behavioral, e.g. alcohol use
4. Ecological/environmental, e.g. reduced property values, reduction in jobs
Enduring Health Outcomes
1. Physiological, e.g. cardio-vascular disease, cancer
2. Psychological, e.g. anxiety disorder, depression
3. Behavioral, e.g. alcoholism
4. Ecological/environmental, e.g. industry and residents relocate, destroyed water quality, family and community disintegration

FIGURE 11.1. Conceptual Framework of the Stress Process: Individual and Community Level

SOURCE: Israel, B. A., Checkoway, B., Schulz, A., & Zimmerman, M. (1994) Health education and community empowerment: Conceptualizing and measuring perceptions of individuals, organizations, and community control. *Health Education Quarterly, 21,*(2) 160. Reproduced with permission.

NOTE: Solid lines between boxes indicate a presumed direct relationship between variables. Dotted lines indicate the hypothesized buffering effects of the conditioning variables on the relationship between stressors and perceived stress, between perceived stress and short-term responses, and between short-term responses and enduring health outcomes.

of influence or control over community decisions, and high crime rates. A fourth condition, cataclysmic events, has to do with sudden disasters, such as hurricanes, earthquakes, or discovery of toxic waste dumps, that require major adaptive responses. The last condition is ambient stressors, or continuous environmental (physical) conditions, such as long-term toxic chemicals or high levels of noise.

In the model, four kinds of variables—social, psychological, biophysical, and genetic—mediate between the stressors and health outcomes and influence how an individual or community experiences the stress process. For example, an empowered community or one with social support is better equipped to deal with stressful situations than one that is not empowered or that lacks social support.

The authors (Israel et al., 1994) developed a tool, reproduced in Table 11.1, to measure empowerment at the three levels. They discuss the limitations of the tool but say that the perceived control indicators are useful and should be used and refined in a community empowerment intervention.

Israel et al. use an action research approach to community empowerment that facilitates viewing the intervention as both a process and outcome. When viewed as an outcome, evaluation of a measurement tool is possible. In the model, the purpose of the empowerment process is to modify the influence of stress on the health outcome by assisting communities to feel in control. The effects of empowerment should be reflected in the health statistics and quality-of-life measures. Empowerment may also help community aggregates to acquire the knowledge and skills necessary to form coalitions or participate in political action to bring pressure on governmental and other officials to deal with problems such as violence, inadequate housing, or environmental hazards.

MULTILEVEL COMMUNITY COMPETENCE MODEL

Eng, Salmon, and Mullan (1992) propose a multilevel empowerment model with three levels of change: (a) the individual's perceptions and behavior, (b) the social support functions of social networks, and (c) institutional services and policies. They believe multilevel interventions will lead to optimum improvement in health and community competence.

At the individual level, increased community competence encourages greater individual participation in the community through group interaction, and this influences the individuals' health perceptions and practices. This is a result of learning about the perceptions and experiences of self and others in these interactions and moves people to greater shared commonalities in a process similar to the looking-glass self described by Cooley (1902). Thus, community competence leads to increased interaction with community groups and through a socialization process leads to improved health (a behavioral change).

Commenting on social support, Eng et al. say that increased specialization has produced barriers to accessing professional services and people have turned to social ties for assistance. This may take the form of material assistance and services, emotional support or counseling, problem solving, referral, or advocacy.

TABLE 11.1 Perceived Control Scale Items: Multiple Levels of Empowerment Indices

For the first five items, the interviewer asked the participants to "please answer the following questions thinking about the organization that you identified as most important to you. Do you agree strongly, agree somewhat, disagree somewhat, or disagree strongly?"

  1. I can influence the decisions that this organization makes.
  2. This organization has influence over decisions that affect my life.
  3. This organization is effective in achieving its goals.
  4. This organization can influence decisions that affect the community.
  5. I am satisfied with the amount of influence I have over decisions that this organization makes.

The interviewer then commented that "I have been asking about your participation in specific organizations. I am also interested in how much influence you think you have in your life and in your community. I am going to read you a list of statements. For each one, please tell me how strongly you agree or disagree."

  6. I have control over the decisions that affect my life.
  7. My community has influence over decisions that affect my life.
  8. I am satisfied with the amount of control I have over decisions that affect my life.
  9. I can influence decisions that affect my community.
  10. By working together, people in my community can influence decisions that affect the community.
  11. People in my community work together to influence decisions on the state or national level.
  12. I am satisfied with the amount of influence I have over decisions that affect my community.

INDICES

Perceived control at the individual level includes Items 6 and 8 above (alpha = .66).

Perceived control at the organizational level includes Items 1 through 5 above (alpha = .61).

Perceived control at the community level includes Items 7, 9, 10, 11, and 12 above (alpha = .63).

Perceived control at multiple levels includes all 12 items above (alpha = .71).

SOURCE: Israel, B. A., Checkoway, B., Schulz, A., & Zimmerman, M. (1994). Health education and community empowerment: Conceptualizing and measuring perceptions of individuals, organizations, and community control. *Health Education Quarterly, 21*(2), 149-170. Reproduced with permission.

They suggest that practitioners should mobilize interactions across these networks as a strategy to increase community competence and to influence health.

Regarding the last area of the model, services and policies of institutions, the authors say that community competence results from the collective mediation of families, churches, and organizations in relation to the larger community. These mediation systems interpret the larger institutions to individuals and may help alleviate alienation and feelings of a lack of control. This empowers individuals to do things that the more affluent have always been able to do. Building the competence of members of a neighborhood or church in negotiating for community resources for one type of problem will increase their coping ability with other problems. Thus, as community competence increases in dealing with a problem, the group is better able to deal with other problems.

PARTICIPATION AND EMPOWERMENT

Zimmerman and Rappaport (1988) studied psychological empowerment and used 11 indicators in the areas of (a) personality, including indicators of control ideology, change ideology, internal control, influence of powerful others (internal vs. external locus of control), and beliefs that people (but not necessarily self) can influence the social and political systems (control ideology); (b) cognitive functions with indicators of internal and external political efficacy and self-efficacy (evaluated by one's ability to achieve goals and influence the political process and community decision making). In addition, one's sense of competence and mastery was measured. (c) Motivation indicators had to do with desire for control and sense of civic duty, or the belief that one ought to participate in the political process.

Three studies examined the relationship between empowerment measured on these 11 indicators and participation in the community. The first study evaluated differences between groups who were willing to participate in personally or community-relevant situations, whereas Study 2 looked at groups who either were or were not involved in community activities and organizations. Study 3 replicated Study 2 but with a different population. In each study, those reporting a greater amount of community involvement scored higher on the empowerment indicators. The authors concluded that psychological empowerment is the connection between personal competence and a desire for and willingness to take action in the community.

BARRIERS TO A COMMUNITY EMPOWERMENT PERSPECTIVE

Israel et al. (1994) summarize the barriers to a community empowerment perspective:

- The influence of past experiences and normative beliefs of not being influential in community efforts, which hinders current efforts at empowerment interventions

- Community members and practitioner differences in social class, race, or ethnicity that hinder trust, communication, and collaboration

- Role-related tensions and differences arising between community members and the practitioner related to values and interests, resources, skills, politics, control, rewards, and costs

- Problems in measuring and showing change in community empowerment

- Lack of value in the approach by the practitioner

- Resistance encountered when considering change from the community members', organizations', and practitioner's perspectives

- Discrepancy between short-time-frame expectations of practitioners, their employers, and community members and the sustained long-term commitment of financial and personal resources needed in this approach

- Perceived slowing of the process when collecting the large amount of qualitative and quantitative data needed for analysis, action, and evaluation
- A belief that a focus on the local community may be ineffective in the context of today's global world

COMMUNITY EMPOWERMENT CASE STUDIES

Two community empowerment case studies by nursing leaders appear at the end of this chapter. One takes place in an urban area (Case Study 7), and the other takes place in a rural community (Case Study 8). These studies demonstrate some of the concepts of this section.

COMMUNITY COALITION BUILDING

Coalitions may be made up of loosely organized, informal groups of individuals or composed of formal, official groups of individuals and organizations. The goals and issues around which coalitions come together may also vary. Thus, coalitions may be short term or long term in nature, for legislative or nonlegislative purposes, public or private, or local, national, or international in composition. With a range in types of coalitions, resources needed to carry out the goals will also vary. These variations preclude specificity, but certain guidelines and concepts are useful and will be presented in this section. In addition, a case study of coalition building by a nursing leader appears at the end of this chapter (Case Study 9).

DEFINITIONS

According to Flynn and Rains (1990), community coalitions are "diverse groups and individuals who join together to accomplish goals they are unable or unlikely to achieve individually" (p. 395). Cohen, Baer, and O'Keefe (1991) say that a coalition is "a union of people and organizations working to influence outcomes on a specific problem" (p. 1). According to the American Association of University Women (AAUW, 1981), a coalition is "an alliance of individuals and or/organizations working together to gain specific goals or mutual advantage" (p. 207). Thus, coalitions are composed of individuals and organizations working on a specific problem and having goals and plans to influence an outcome.

THEORETICAL BASIS

A void exists in the literature regarding a theory for coalitions. However, Nelson (1994) suggests resource mobilization theory as a way of looking at the functioning and outcomes of coalitions. This theory states that a coalition's outcomes are a result of its activities and processes and of two contextual factors: support from organizations and the "political climate" in which the coalition exists. Outcome successes include changes in "(a) public policy, (b) the politics of decision making (i.e., who is included and how decisions are made)" (p. 229), (c) how resources are allocated, (d) collective consciousness changes resulting from diffusion of a different ideology, and (e) resource development permitting further mobilization.

Coalition activities and processes that influence successful outcomes include focused and sustained advocacy, organizational support for coalition activities, and political climate changes suggesting that change is possible. Success involves support from the elite and established organizations and changes in public sentiment that favor the coalition's position. It is also more effective to recruit organizational groups with established networks, which usually have group solidarity and commitment to goals, than to recruit individuals. In addition, a closely divided electorate may favor successful coalition outcomes because politicians will support the coalition in exchange for votes.

Nelson (1994) relates this theory of coalition activities, support from organizations, and changes in politics to accomplishing goals in mental health such as increasing community funding over institutional funding (see scarce resources in Chapter 9) or increasing participation of consumers in policy and program decisions. Examples of success using this approach were included in the article.

PURPOSES

Purposes of a coalition include (a) preventing duplication of effort, (b) pooling and maximizing resources, and (c) engendering greater publicity than might be possible by individuals acting alone (Cohen et al., 1991). From a different point of view, Dluhy (1990) says coalitions have two functions: task oriented and interpersonal. The task-oriented function relates to change and may include political goals, such as policy changes or obtaining governmental resources, or may have nonpolitical goals, such as community education or social networking for exchange of ideas and support. The interpersonal function relates to increasing and maintaining membership in the coalition.

BASIC TENETS

Leavitt and Herbert-Davis (1993) identify five basic tenets of collectives:

1. The whole is greater than the sum of the parts, or there is strength in numbers and diversity and in the empowerment of the process.
2. The process of forming and using coalitions is the same despite different goals and strategies.
3. All political action is local, and action at that level is the most effective for politics at any level.

4. Coalitions challenge the power structure and lead to an effort to take or share power.

5. The goal of coalitions involves both a change in a particular policy and the empowerment of people to actively participate in politics.

ADVANTAGES

Cohen et al. (1991) identify several advantages of coalitions: (a) conserving resources, such as involving teachers in efforts to educate children about bicycle helmet safety and laws; (b) increasing influence within a community and reaching more people by combining mailing lists of member organizations for needed activities; (c) accomplishing more objectives than would be possible in single organizations, such as lobbying efforts by coalition members; (d) increased credibility over single organizations due to a broader purpose and greater breadth of interest, which reduces self-interest suspicions; (e) increased opportunities for sharing of information, such as reporting on upcoming events and conferences attended related to the topic of interest; (f) a greater range of advice to the lead organization from member organizations; (g) increased satisfaction and a broadened perspective for members on their jobs, such as showing a traffic engineer the impact of his work on pedestrian safety; and (h) fostering cooperation among grassroots organizations, diverse organizations, and community members.

STEPS IN BUILDING AN EFFECTIVE COALITION

Cohen et al. (1991) identify eight steps for building effective coalitions: (a) deciding whether or not to form a coalition, (b) recruiting the right members, (c) establishing preliminary objectives and activities, (d) convening the coalition, (e) anticipating resources needed, (f) considering a structure for a successful coalition, (g) maintaining the vitality of the coalition, and (h) improving the functioning of the coalition through evaluation.

DECIDING TO FORM A COALITION

Certain factors determine whether or not an organization should consider forming a coalition: (a) recognizing a community need for a coalition or responding to a request, (b) recognizing that a coalition will facilitate goal fulfillment, and (c) meeting a grant requirement or initiating a conference outcome project.

The initial step in deciding to form a coalition is determining whether a coalition is the appropriate method for meeting the established need. Next, consider what resources are needed from both the lead organization and other members. Last, determine if a coalition is the best use of the resources to be used. Examining objectives and the necessary actions to achieve the objectives will assist in answering these questions.

Further steps useful in determining whether to establish a coalition include (a) clarifying the objectives and coalition actions, (b) assessing the strengths and weaknesses of the community, and (c) determining cost versus benefits to the lead organization. The authors discuss a tool for planning objectives that they call the "spectrum of prevention." This tool lists six types of interventions that are useful to coalitions: (a) to influence policy or legislation, (b) to change the practices of an organization, (c) to foster coalitions and networks, (d) to educate providers, (e) to promote education of the community, and (f) to strengthen the knowledge and skills of individuals. Each of these interventions works best in combination with others on the list, and using a combination of interventions promotes permanent, effective change. For example, a program of injury prevention may require environmental changes as a result of planned changes in the practices in organizations and of policy and legislation changes in the community in addition to public education. For example, education is often used for child safety around water. However, children drown quickly even when an informed caretaker is nearby. A fence around a pool resulting from a city ordinance may be more effective and a better use of the resources of the coalition to meet the objective of childhood safety.

Questions to be considered when deciding to establish a coalition include the breadth of what the coalition can accomplish and the extent of coalition activities—for example, whether the focus be narrow, such as getting parents to use car seats, or broad, such as preventing all childhood injuries. The direction of the coalition depends on both the interest of the lead organization and the composition and interest of other members.

Community strengths and weaknesses should also be assessed. The community can be viewed in terms of potential barriers and supports. Organizations or coalitions with similar or related objectives and the successes and failures of the community in dealing with similar problems should be assessed. Organizations within and outside the community that could provide support or help overcome barriers should be assessed and invited to participate. In addition, organizations that would oppose the proposed coalition objectives should be identified.

Last, the cost and benefits of a coalition should be assessed. Determine the extent of drain on agency resources, decide whether or not the resources are available, and estimate the returns to the agency program. A lack of resources and an estimated minimal return may mean an end to the idea of a coalition.

RECRUITING THE RIGHT MEMBERS

There are important questions to answer when recruiting membership in the coalition. Although most coalitions have diverse membership, the goals of the coalition should determine the type of membership. Initially, organizations that currently work on the identified issue and others who might be interested should be identified. Potential members include influential organizations, supportive organizations, and those who may be considered obstacles. Planners should also identify representatives from each organization who will best represent the organization on the coalition. Directors may be more credible, but staff may be more committed, enthusiastic, and available. Agency directors should appoint representatives, but input may be given by directors. Next, identify individuals such as community leaders, community members, and those who have experienced the problem under consideration by the coalition. Decisions should also be made about the inclusion or exclusion of potential adversaries and competitors based on their acceptance of coalition goals and on whether they will be more of an impediment if included or excluded.

Membership size may be influenced by the tasks involved. The diversity and desired number of organizations should be determined before approaching organizations. When a group is larger than 12 to 18 members, additional resources are needed and group identity and common purpose take longer to establish.

ESTABLISHING PRELIMINARY OBJECTIVES AND ACTIVITIES

Objectives of the lead organization established in the first step should be blended with those of other group members. All members should be involved in the objective and activity development process. In addition to long-term goals, short-term ones that are reachable in a reasonable time should be established. Activities that meet the needs of participating organizations should also be established. Short-term success in these is important, and activities such as press releases about the formation and purposes of the coalition or its initial findings may assist motivation by increasing visibility and credibility.

CONVENING THE COALITION

A meeting of potential members is held, and the lead agency defines the purposes of the coalition and members specify their expectations. All people introduce themselves, state their perceived role in the coalition, and consider their organization's interest in participation. Members may also recommend others whom they think might be interested.

Lead agency members should present a proposal for the structure, mission, and potential membership of the coalition. After coalition activities are clarified, membership may be reconsidered, and some organizations may decide not to participate. Determinants of participation may include the specific activities of the coalition and the worth of the coalition from the viewpoint of the management of member organizations.

ANTICIPATING NEEDED RESOURCES

Although coalitions may require minimal financial resources for supplies, the need for human resources in terms of time commitment may be large. Thus, staffing by leadership organizations is an important consideration, and the lead agency usually provides most of the human resources. Agenda preparation as well as written and telephone contact with members before meetings is necessary. Although coalition members may be expected to fulfill some responsibilities, members of the lead agency should anticipate that others will not always fulfill their commitments.

Staffing demands on the lead agency include (a) clerical time to prepare mailings, type minutes and agendas, make photocopies, and make reminder calls; (b) staff time before and during meetings, including planning the agenda, arranging for the meeting site, providing refreshments, taking minutes, and coordinating with the coalition's chair or steering committee; (c) membership duties, including recruitment, orientation, regular contact, and support and encouragement; (d) research and fact-collecting duties, including data collection and evaluation (process and outcome); (e) public relations and information duties, including developing informational material, preparing press releases, and interacting with local reporters; (f) coordination activities for media campaigns, special events, and joint projects; and (g) fund-raising activities, including obtaining resources in addition to money.

Financial resources from the lead agency may be decreased by evaluating outside sources. Five potential sources of supplemental resources include (a) media, which may provide media coverage; (b) foundations, which may provide seed money for coalition activities; (c) local service clubs, which may provide assistance; (d) students and trainees, such as university students who may contribute time for learning purposes; and (e) volunteers, who often contribute in return for learning about coalitions.

CONSIDERING A STRUCTURE FOR A SUCCESSFUL COALITION

Structural issues to consider include (a) life expectancy of the coalition; (b) location, frequency, and length of meetings; (c) parameters of membership; (d) processes for decision making; (e) agenda for meetings; and (f) how to participate between meetings. Additional information on some of these factors follows. The goals of the coalition should determine its life expectancy, and this should be decided after two or three meetings when objectives are established. A majority rule decision-making approach is usually more manageable than consensus.

MAINTAINING THE VITALITY OF THE COALITION

The vitality of a coalition can be maintained by dealing with problems as they occur. In addition, identifying and addressing coalition difficulties, sharing power and leadership, recruiting and involving new members, providing training, bringing challenging new ideas, and celebrating successes are all ways to revitalize the coalition.

CONSENSUS VERSUS CONFLICT STRATEGIES

The methods by which a coalition makes decisions is important to its functioning. The AAUW (1981) identifies situations in which consensus or conflict strategies should be used. Consensus strategies should be used to (a) gain cooperation when planning action, (b) obtain broad-based support, (c) obtain win-win issue resolution, (d) resolve differences with opponents who have equal power, (e) continue talking until agreement is reached by all parties, and

(f) confront hostility and continue talks until problems are resolved. Conflict strategies should be used to (a) focus official attention on an issue following the failure of an opponent to respond to repeated inquiries, (b) force negotiation by an opponent, (c) resolve win-lose issues, (d) equalize the dynamics of differences in power when the coalition is in a weaker position, (e) hasten a faltering process, and (f) talk with opponents whose views differ from those of the coalition. Conflict management was discussed further in Chapter 10.

IMPROVING THE COALITION THROUGH EVALUATION

Formative and summative evaluations should be carried out, and evaluation should be ongoing throughout the life of the coalition. When this leads to positive changes, the coalition is improved.

COALITIONS: TEMPORARY OR LONG TERM?

Many authors consider coalitions as temporary groups formed to carry out some goal. For example, according to Leavitt and Herbert-Davis (1993), a coalition is a "temporary alliance of diverse members who come together for joint action in support of a defined goal" (p. 167). According to Chavis (1995), however, studies of coalitions usually show that their focus is on a singular and immediate outcome, such as starting a program or passing legislation, rather than on larger long-term outcomes. Once the immediate outcome is reached, the coalition ends. However, the focus, currently, is more often on coalition building, community capacity, and other long-term outcomes.

COALITION FUNCTIONS

From a review of the literature, Chavis (1995) concludes that coalitions have 10 primary functions: (a) broadening the member organization's mission and developing more comprehensive strategies, (b) developing more extensive issue support from the public, (c) increasing influence over community policies and practices by the community's institutions, (d) reducing duplication of services, (e) increasing financial and human resources, (f) exploiting new resources, (g) increasing accountability, (h) improving planning and evaluation capacity, and (i) improving the responses by local organizations and institutions to the needs and aspirations of their constituents.

SELECTED COALITIONS PRESENTED IN THE LITERATURE

Dahl, Gustafson, and McCullagh (1993) discuss a coalition that focused on providing health care for homeless people in a rural setting. Public health nursing leaders developed a health services center for homeless people who were without health care. With scarce resources for care (see Chapter 3 on economics), they established a coalition of multidisciplinary and multi-institutional resources to meet the established need. The process of coalition building and support was also discussed in the article.

Mayster, Waitzkin, Hubbell, and Rucker (1993) also looked at the void in health care for the medically indigent and discussed strategies used by coalition advocates to improve their access to care. Strategies included (a) using researchers to investigate barriers to care, (b) using political action to increase financial support for services and to improve the administrative procedures of the local government, and (c) using legal services to represent and advise clients who lacked health care. The authors conclude that although these strategies may not guarantee access to care, they have improved services for this population.

Davidson et al. (1994) evaluated coalition effectiveness in preventing severe childhood injuries. The outcome measure was a decrease in injuries during the intervention compared with the rate of injuries before the intervention. Although the decreased incidence of injuries was consistent with a favorable outcome of the program, the authors identify a need for further investigation to ensure that the results are not contaminated by secular trends or spillover effects.

Rosenthal and Harper (1994) discuss the Cleveland Health Quality Choice Coalition established in 1989 as a voluntary, collaborative effort between hospitals, physicians, and consumers. This coalition assesses the quality and efficiency of the hospital care provided to clients. Outcome measures included patient satisfaction, in-hospital mortality, length of patient stay, hospital-acquired complications, cesarean section rates, intensive care outcomes, and specific outcomes of patients in medical, surgical, and other units. Successful results of the coalition were reported.

CITIZEN PARTICIPATION

The importance of involving citizens in assessing, planning, and implementing community care as a community development strategy was discussed in Chapter 8. Citizen involvement was also discussed as an empowering process earlier in this chapter. According to Bracht (1990), studies suggest that citizen participation improves community health outcomes and long-term maintenance of programs. Likewise, the Declaration of Alma-Alta of the World Health Organization (1978) says health care is delivered most effectively by community health workers who have the confidence of the people, who understand the community's health needs, and who can be trained in a short time to perform basic preventive and curative functions. Florin and Wandersman (1990) say that citizen participation has produced benefits at the national, community, interpersonal, and individual levels and has resulted in neighborhood and community improvement and feelings of personal and political efficacy. Citizen participation in community interventions will be briefly reemphasized here.

DEFINITIONS

Zimmerman (1990) defines citizen participation as " non-professional involvement in health care service delivery, policy decisions, and program development" (p. 324). According to Bracht (1990), citizen participation is the "social process of taking part (voluntarily) in formal or informal activities, programs, and/or discussions to bring about planned change or improvement in community life, services, and resources" (p. 110).

PURPOSES IN INTERVENTION

According to Zimmerman (1990), citizens in rural areas assist in health care by (a) providing emergency medical services, such as caring for disabled people, carrying out screening and detection services, and helping others, such as new mothers, which helps to remedy personnel shortages, and (b) improving community acceptance of programs by assisting to tailor the programs to the particular community. He says citizen participation can vary from control of the decision-making process to simply delivering services with no authority for decisions. He discusses the history of citizen participation and several studies that demonstrate citizen effectiveness in health service delivery.

FACTORS INFLUENCING CITIZEN PARTICIPATION

Bracht (1990) identifies the following as factors that influence citizen participation: (a) concern about one's neighborhood; (b) previous experience in community leadership positions; (c) perceived confidence in recruiting competent colleagues to support the project; (d) resource availability for the project; (e) good faith by the sponsoring group; (f) clearly defined citizen authority; (g) the ability of citizens to create, sustain, and control an effective organization; (h) early and broad knowledge of community history, including past successes and failures at change, organizational resources, influence structures, and networks between organizations; (i) early identification and discussion of community change barriers; (j) clearly stated volunteer roles and time commitments; (k) project staff commitment to locality ownership or a partnership; (l) reinforcement of citizen participation by recognition and/or tangible benefits during the planning process; and (m) timely use of conflict resolution when needed.

ORGANIZATIONAL STRUCTURE

In addition, the structure selected may facilitate citizen involvement. Bracht (1990) identifies the following structures involving lay community members: (a) leadership board or council, (b) coalitions, (c) lead or official agency, (d) grassroots groups, (e) citizen panels, and (f) networks and consortia. Each of these structures are discussed, and the author says that successful programs usually use parts from several of these structures.

TASK FORCES

Task forces made up of lay and professional volunteers who report to the community advisory board may also be used. Task forces focus on specific assignments, but these members may move from a task force to the community advisory board over time. Using people on task forces increases the number of community participants involved and broadens the influence of the project.

IDENTIFICATION OF COMMUNITY LAY LEADERS

Michielutte and Beal (1990) discuss a method for identifying lay leaders for community health programs. In their study of cervical cancer among blacks, leaders were identified to help plan and implement an educational program directed at reducing the number of cases of the disease. The method used to identify leaders was a modified snowball technique in which 10 recognized black leaders were contacted and asked to name five additional social, political, religious, business, or less visible black leaders. This process continued until no new names were generated. From this list, leaders for the study were identified.

SELECTED CITIZEN PARTICIPATION STUDIES

Ross, Loening, and Mbele (1987) looked at prolonging unsupplemented breast-feeding behaviors of three groups of mothers who were supported by three types of health workers, including lay workers. A fourth group received limited support, and the fifth group received no support. Significant differences were found between some groups, with the group receiving visits by lay workers being the most effective. The authors concluded that programs offering home visit support by lay workers could be effective in promoting breast-feeding.

Sung et al. (1992) used lay health workers to conduct in-home educational interventions to increase participation of low-income, inner-city black women in screening for breast cancer. Interventions were directed toward increasing their knowledge and changing their attitudes about breast cancer. The authors discussed the purposes, hypothesis, and design of the study; recruitment of subjects; interventions; and an evaluation of the project. Participants were randomly assigned to an intervention or a control group. Intervention group women were visited at home and provided education on cancer and reproductive health by the lay worker. An evaluation plan, but no results, was provided in the article.

Lacey, Turkes, Manfredi, and Warnecke (1991) used lay health educators for a community-based smoking cessation program for young black women in several urban public housing developments. Interventions were either televised smoking cessation classes or reminders of smoking cessation by lay workers. The lay workers successfully organized the hard-to-reach group that responded by being more knowledgeable about the dangers of smoking and more interested in participating in a structured program for smoking cessation. Results showed that lay health educators may assist in mobilizing a population to participate in health programs, but new methods should be developed to sustain the involvement reached by the public.

Meister, Warrick, deZapien, and Wood (1992) developed a program for low-income Hispanic women in migrant and seasonal farm work communities. The program included a prenatal curriculum in Spanish, a group of lay workers recruited from the target communities and trained as health promoters, and the organization of a local health professionals social support network. Rationale for and interventions of the program were discussed, including the restraints and facilitators of the program and guidelines for starting a comparable program. The authors concluded that the program exceeded their expectations in terms of the extent and enthusiasm of response and in its ability to deliver an educational and social support program.

Poland, Giblin, Waller, and Hankin (1992) studied the efficacy of using paraprofessionals (women who had received public assistance) to provide support services on prenatal care received by low-income women and the birth weight of their children. Six weeks of training allowed the paraprofessionals to assist pregnant women with areas of concern, such as housing, food, health, transportation, and other necessities. Women were assigned to a paraprofessional who made intensive home visits or to a control group. Results showed that women seen by a paraprofessional kept significantly more prenatal appointments and had infants with higher birth weights.

INVOLVING INDUSTRY AND OTHER ORGANIZATIONS

The need for multiple community interventions to increase the effectiveness of community change programs was discussed in Chapter 8. One of the intervention targets identified in the model by Simons-Morten, Simons-Morten, Parcel, and Bunker (1988) was organizations. Organizations such as industrial settings, schools, churches, fraternal and civic organizations, and recreational clubs are ideal sites for aggregate interventions. Some of these sites may be interested in health programs that coincide with part of their mission and may provide access to hard-to-reach groups such as low-income or minority people.

In addition, some sites may consent to initiate structural or cultural changes that support long-term changes in health. For example, environmental changes such as nonsmoking policies and removal of cigarette machines, the provision of fitness facilities, and modifications in food offered in cafeterias or vending machines reinforce messages communicated through education. Changes in organizational social norms will also support long-term maintenance of the change.

ACCESSIBLE POPULATION

At least a third of the average adult's life is spent at work. There are 127 million people (46% women) in the workforce in the United States (*Statistical Abstracts,* 1994); thus, the workplace offers a significant opportunity to influence the health of a large segment of the population.

The 10 leading work-related health problems include occupational lung disease, musculoskeletal injuries, occupational cancers, severe traumatic injuries, cardiovascular disease, reproductive problems, neurotoxic illness, noise-induced hearing loss, dermatological problems, and psychological disorders (Millar, 1988; National Institute of Occupational Safety and Health, 1989). An estimated 17 million work-related injuries and illnesses and 99,000 work-related deaths occur annually in the United States (*Statistical Abstracts,* 1994). Environmental factors responsible for many of these deaths and illnesses were discussed in Chapter 4.

ENCOURAGING PARTICIPATION

Like citizen participation, organizational participation should begin early in the community change process, preferably during the assessment and planning stages. During the assessment stage, community, leaders including those in businesses and other organizations, should be identified. Following identification, they may be actively involved in further community assessment and in planning by serving on community boards. They may also be involved in assessing and planning programs in their own facilities to identify employee concerns and ways to tailor the interventions to specific worker needs.

Some organizations may be more willing to participate than others and should be targeted for early inclusion. These include those that are first to adopt new ideas and programs and that may then serve as models for others (Rogers & Shoemaker, 1971). See Chapter 9 on diffusion theory for additional information on pacesetters. In addition, those organizations that have a history of promoting health and environmental change or that are high-profile organizations, such as large worksites, should also be targeted for initial consideration. When these organizations become involved, they serve as models for other, more reluctant organizations to become involved and to commit resources.

According to Bracht (1990), two things are necessary to encourage participation of worksites in health programs: (a) grasping opportunities to point out advantages that assist in the adoption of the program and policies and (b) identifying and removing or diminishing existing or potential barriers to the program. From the employer point of view, advantages may include (a) improved morale and productivity of employees, (b) possible decreases in health care cost, and (c) improved ability to recruit and retain employees; barriers may include (a) resistance to change, (b) concerns about the cost, and (c) concerns about the consequence of participating. From the employee point of view, the advantages may include (a) access to care and convenience, (b) a decreased cost of care, and (c) support (environmental and social) for changing behavior; disadvantages may include (a) factors of confidentiality, (b) perceptions of interference of the company with personal life of the employee, and (c) the company's diverting attention from other important issues. Advantages for the health care provider include (a) access to a large aggregate of people, (b) access to underserved groups, (c) social support for interventions, (d) long-term repeat intervention opportunities, and (e) possible social-environmental changes. A barrier for the health care provider is the program delivery logistics. Success results from addressing any of these factors.

WORKSITE INTERVENTIONS

Worksite interventions are the same as those suggested in Chapter 8 (planning) and in Chapter 10 (mass media). Successful programs use multiple interventions directed toward employees at various stages of change (see multilevel interventions and stage model of behavior change in Chapters 8 and 10). For continuity, these concepts will be reviewed briefly.

The three basic interventions are (a) motivation and incentive, (b) education, and (c) environmental change and social support. Motivation and incentive interventions are directed toward motivating employees to attempt behavioral changes, such as trying a new diet or exercise regime, or to maintain behaviors newly started. Motivators have included incentives or awards, contests within an organization, and contests between organizations. These have been used for change behaviors such as smoking cessation, weight loss, and participation in exercise (see the discussion below of weight loss competition at the worksite). Education gives employees the tools for changing the behavior and should include a variety of methods, such as television or movie presentations and pamphlets or booklets. Counseling and social support used in conjunction with education has been found to increase success. For a further discussion of teaching, see Chapter 10 (mass media).

Environmental changes restructure the physical environment with modifications such as requiring a smoke-free environment, removing junk food and cigarettes from machines, and changing the foods offered in cafeterias. Social support changes the social environment by arranging support for employees while they change their health behavior. Support may be offered by family members, coworkers, or superiors.

Long-term behavior changes necessitate educational programs and incentives that are repeated periodically to help members maintain the new behavior and to assist other employees wishing to begin behavior changes. For a further discussion of long-term maintenance of behaviors, see Chapter 9 (diffusion theory).

The strategies identified above for worksites are also appropriate for other community organizations. Some of the examples below take place in these organizations.

SELECTED ORGANIZATIONAL HEALTH INTERVENTIONS

Stunkard, Cohen, and Felix (1989) discuss the results of weight loss competition at worksites from three studies. In the first study, team competition was more effective than cooperation or individual competition for men, and more effective than individual competition for women. In the second study, 10 worksites were used to replicate this study in relation to four influencing variables (age, sex, employment type—blue collar vs. white collar—and method of assignment to team) on outcomes (recruiting, attrition, weight loss, and cost-effectiveness). In this study, recruitment was high, there was low attrition, there was a large weight loss, and there was favorable cost-effectiveness. The third study was a follow-up of the second study and found only limited maintenance of weight loss over time.

Shipley, Orleans, Wilbur, Piserchia, and McFadden (1988) reported the results of a 2-year smoking cessation program at seven worksites. Four companies offered the Live for Life program to employees and three comparison companies offered only annual health-screening assessments. At the Live for Life companies, 22.6% of the smokers quit, compared with 17.4% of smokers at the companies offering only health screening. The authors concluded that a smoking cessation program can produce significant changes in smoking behavior.

Elder, Sallis, Mayer, Hammond, and Peplinski (1989) reported on a telephone survey of a random sample of churches, labor unions, supermarkets, and restaurants to identify the level of health promotion activities available to customers and members. About two thirds of the churches reported offering single health promotion educational programs; the same amount of labor unions offered single-session group meetings on health with pamphlets distributed; one third of the supermarkets reported distributing brochures on health; and about one third of the restaurants reported programs consisting of enforcement of no-smoking policies. Very few organization in the sample evaluated their programs or wanted assistance with them.

Smith (1989) reported on a study that evaluated the effectiveness and specific role of black churches in hypertension compliance. The sample of 63 hypertensives from two black churches in which one church had a screening program and the other did not was evaluated by tests and chart audits. Clients from the church with the screening program did not score higher on compliance on a self-reporting scale, and no relationship was found between support and compliance and hypertension control. The church with the screening program was viewed as less supportive than the other church.

INVOLVING PROFESSIONALS

Involvement of health professionals throughout the community is important in multilevel community-based interventions (see multilevel models in Chapter 8). Health professionals assist in communitywide acceptance of the program, the integration of the program into different health care institutions, and providing information on health care practices and community health care facilities and may be instrumental in introducing structural changes in health care settings similar to those discussed for organizations. The various activities and processes are similar to those identified for organizations.

PROFESSIONALS ON COMMUNITY BOARDS OR COMMITTEES

Health professionals should be invited to participate on the board or committee that oversees the program. Professionals should be identified during the initial community assessment and should include professionals from different disciplines, such as nursing, medicine, health education, and social work, as well as from different health care facilities and institutions (acute and long-term care hospitals, outpatient facilities, and private or group practice). Names of representatives can be solicited from different health care organizations and professional societies.

These members can interpret health care practices in the community and organizations, offer advice to committee members on health care matters, and interpret and implement the program in their own institutions and practices.

EDUCATION OF PROFESSIONALS

An important aspect of a new program to introduce behavioral changes into a community population is education of health care professionals. Many states require continuing education of physicians and nurses through a system of continuing education units with a certain number required annually for certification. Information related to content and process of the desired community program (e.g., smoking cessation, diet, exercise) could be presented through an established program that awards continuing education units.

Professional societies offer a second opportunity to present programs to professionals about proposed community changes and potential roles of professionals. For example, in our area, the local district of the state nurses association has meetings every 2 months consisting of a planned program as well as the business meeting.

Many institutions also present continuing education to staff. For example, local hospitals and health care facilities may have ongoing educational programs that present topics that assist staff members in carrying out their roles. These educational programs may also provide an opportunity to discuss the new community program.

INSTITUTIONAL STRUCTURAL CHANGES

An important aspect of multilevel intervention programs is the structural changes that assist individuals in their attempt to begin and maintain the desired behavioral change. For example, a change in smoking behavior should involve smoking cessation classes, literature, social support, and other activities. It should also include structural changes such as a smoke-free environment at work, in restaurants, and in public buildings as well as the removal of cigarette vending machines.

Case Study 7

Empowerment for Neighborhoods

LAUREL S. GARZON

The Fairwood Homes Initiative is an empowerment project submitted by a coalition composed of people from Old Dominion University (ODU), the Portsmouth Interagency Network (PIN), and the Fairwood Homes Civic League (FHCL). The initiative provides an innovative and culturally sensitive approach to empowerment of neighborhoods through education, mentorship, and investments, based on the premise that community empowerment is a process of actions taken within a social environment that promote increased individual and community control over issues affecting neighborhood residents (Wallerstein, 1992). The project was de-

AUTHOR'S NOTE: I would like to acknowledge the contribution of Dr. Richardean Benjamin-Coleman and Mr. Anthony Armstrong.

signed to improve the quality of life within the community and to promote social justice by providing opportunities for individual development and Civic League involvement. It emphasizes the close interaction of regional educational institutions, service agencies, and the Fairwood Homes neighborhood as an entity and with special-interest groups within the neighborhood rather than as individual clients, which had been the traditional relationship. This project strived toward developing a neighborhood empowerment model for the Tidewater Region.

SIGNIFICANCE OF THE PROPOSED PROJECT

Flynn, Ray, and Rider (1994) state that community empowerment is a transforming experience that requires a focus on community, citizen participation, collaborative problem solving, sharing of power, and an improvement in the quality of life. This project was designed to support and facilitate achievement of life goals and assist a disadvantaged community in the process of empowerment through a collaborative effort of the community, human services agencies, and an educational institution in an effort to restore a sense of "community" to the neighborhood. Fairwood Homes, as the largest single, private, low-income housing development in the city of Portsmouth, has a disproportionate number of social problems that has affected its growth.

APPROPRIATENESS OF THE EMPOWERMENT MODEL

Citizen participation is a key factor in community and citizen development. Determining who participates and how to keep residents involved is critical to the success of a community development project. Several terms have been used to describe community activity and community development; however, few previous theoretical frameworks can provide a more extensive history of success than the concept of *empowerment*.

Empowerment is the mechanism by which people, organizations, and communities gain mastery over their affairs. Like citizen participation, empowerment is a concept that has been applied to diverse areas such as the family, business management, and the elderly (Block, 1987; Clark, 1988; Dunst, Trirette, & Deal, 1989; Wilt & Martens, 1988). Empowerment is both multi-level (individual, organizational, community) and multidimensional (intrapersonal, social behavioral, political) in nature (Prestby, Wandersman, Florin, Rich, & Chavis, 1990). Distinctions have been made between *empowering organizations* that facilitate confidence and competencies of individual members and *empowered organizations* that influence the environment or community (Swift & Levin, 1987).

Inherent in the empowerment process is an educational component. Killian (1988) describes empowerment as "people gaining an understanding of and control over social economic and/or political forces in order to improve their standing in society." The assumption is that empowerment is possible through educational activities.

Part of the empowerment process requires the neighborhood to identify its own problems, develop its own intervention strategies, and form a decision-making board to make policy decisions and manage resources around the interventions (Braithwaite, Murphy, Lythcott, & Bluenthal, 1988). The empowerment process involves people who have common concerns and who are taught how to be proactive rather than reactive. The process has several key components, including the use of proactive behaviors, delineating the benefits and costs of participation (Prestby et al., 1990), identifying organizational viability (Prestby et al., 1990), creating organizational efficacy, increasing self-esteem, and recognizing the importance of citizen involvement (Kieffer, 1984; Zimmerman & Rappaport, 1988).

In addition to the process components, there are intrinsic components. These neighborhoods and neighbors serve a number of functions. Unger and Wandersman (1985) say that social supports and emotional and material aid are all related to intrinsic components and thus enhance group participation.

Factors that influence group participation in community organizations are material, social, and purposive motives and incentives (Clark & Wilson, 1961). Material benefits refer to tangible rewards that can be translated into monetary value to include wages, increased property value, and more information. Social benefits are derived largely from social interactions and include socializing, status, group identification, and recognition. Purposive benefits are derived from suprapersonal goals of the organization and include bettering the community, doing one's civic duty, and fulfilling a sense of responsibility.

The most active participants in organizations are primarily motivated by positive benefits, such as working toward the improvement of the neighborhood or community, and to a lesser extent by solidarity benefits. Material motives were found to play a relatively minimal role as motivators for the most active participants. In addition, purposive motives are most important for initiating participation and solidarity; purposive and material benefits are important for sustaining participation.

Community groups assume that every neighborhood, no matter what its problems, contains latent strengths and a network of people ready to help themselves and others. Group action builds confidence, combats passivity, and develops a sense of community that reduces alienation.

The empowerment model was identified as the most appropriate for the proposed project because it provides a mechanism for cooperative participation at all levels of community and neighborhood development (Eng & Parker, 1994). Major components of this empowerment project include (a) providing education to community residents in the form of job training and community development skills to promote feelings of confidence and mastery, (b) defining benefits of neighborhood participation to ensure that benefits outweigh costs to residents, (c) organizing a resident-controlled governing board to foster ownership and commitment of ideas, (d) coordinating existing health and social services involving residents in citywide as well as neighborhood planning and program development, and (e) developing programs based on resident-generated ideas and suggestions.

FAIRWOOD HOMES

The project was developed to meet the needs of the Fairwood Homes neighborhood as a whole, residents with special interests, and individuals. Fairwood Homes is a privately owned, low-income housing neighborhood constituting approximately one tenth of the population of the city of Portsmouth, Virginia. There are 7,800 residents residing in 1,514 units in the target community, which was developed in the 1940s as housing for many of the shipyard workers during World War II. Many of the original families or their descendants remain in the neighborhood, although the most recent group of residents have been African Americans, who make up 74% of the community, with whites making up 25.55%. One third of the residents receive Aid to Families With Dependent Children (AFDC) or some form of federal assistance, 30% are retired and live on Social Security and Navy pensions, and another 30% are employed in modest-wage jobs. Although the neighborhood is bounded by other neighborhoods, it has remained a discreet community.

During the year before the initiative was proposed, the FHCL had become active in the development of a safe neighborhoods program and in an elderly network support group, both of which were resident initiated and designed. In addition, residents had requested and received a public safety unit as well as a Head Start program. The owner of the Fairwood Homes complex provided renovated space for these programs and a paid staff position in the Safe Neighborhood Project office.

COALITION CONCERNS

The following concerns were central to the proposed project:

1. About one third of the residents of the Fairwood Homes community receive AFDC or some form of federal assistance. More than 60% of Fairwood Homes residents are unemployed or underemployed. Fairwood Homes has the highest concentration of households under 150% of poverty level in the city of Portsmouth.

2. Single-parent families are the dominant household grouping in the neighborhood, with 417 female-headed households with related children and 84 such households with no related children. This compares to 286 married couples with related children and 248 with no related children, with 54 male-headed households with related children and 36 female-headed household with no related children.

3. Fairwood Homes is listed as the neighborhood highest in crime rates for the city of Portsmouth. Most of the crime is related to substance abuse, and a large portion of the crime is committed by youths.

4. Alcohol-related and other substance abuse arrests of adults in 1990 represented 73% of all arrests in the city.

5. Portsmouth public schools ranked last among Hampton Roads school districts in the percentage of fourth-grade and eighth-grade students—which includes students from the targeted neighborhood—scoring above the median on a state proficiency test. On the test, students fell below the state median in 41 of 50 categories.

6. In the nation, minority elderly, women, and elderly living below the poverty line make up a significant portion of the population. They have increased need of services yet limited access. For the Fairwood Homes neighborhood, where the majority of residents are African American, women constitute 68% of the total population, and 70% of the 55+ and 82% of the 65+ age groups.

7. In Portsmouth, the adolescent pregnancy rate is 68.8 per 1,000 females, compared with the Commonwealth of Virginia's rate of 48. 8 per thousand. Fairwood Homes had the highest teenage pregnancy rate in the city of Portsmouth.

8. With the high prevalence of adolescent pregnancy in the city of Portsmouth and the high number of arrests related to substance, the likelihood of child abuse exists.

9. The Public Health Department and the Department of Social Services are inaccessible to Fairwood Home neighborhood residents because of location on the other side of the city, inadequate public transportation, and limited hours of operation.

10. The privately owned, low-income rental units were built in the 1940s, and residents there make up approximately one tenth of the city's population. The average assessed value of an occupied unit and its land is $9,961.

PURPOSE OF THE INITIATIVE

The purpose of this project was to raise the level of knowledge and ability of residents of the Fairwood Homes neighborhood to act together for their own benefit, further assess their needs through the FHCL, plan programs that meet those needs, and implement services that are resident designed and directed. A central strategy would be training of Civic League members in needs assessment and community organization.

GOALS AND OBJECTIVES

The goal of the proposed project was to model collaborative community and neighborhood competence as an indicator of successful empowerment (Eng & Parker, 1994). To accomplish these goals, the project would (a) link formal community-based services, informal community resources, volunteer efforts, and academic resources; (b) strengthen the ability of the neighborhood to identify, plan, and effectively implement community-based actions to meet the needs of its residents; and (c) enhance resident's ability to effectively act in a concerted manner.

SPECIFIC OBJECTIVES

The specific objectives were based on the eight dimensions of community competence as outlined by Eng and Parker (1994):

1. Develop new, and strengthen existing, neighborhood resources to promote the well-being of neighborhood citizens and their families through (a) neighborhood education and development; (b) coordination and integration of informal, formal, and volunteer resources; and (c) development of new neighborhood resources.

2. Implement an innovative, culturally sensitive program for empowerment of the residents of Fairwood Homes.

3. Provide development activities for the FHCL.

4. Establish a coalition of neighborhood leaders, community service providers, and representatives of education.

5. Assist the residents of FHCL to develop and implement initiatives related to the needs of elders, young parents, youths, and young children.

6. Develop a neighborhood network for problem resolution and project development in response to the needs of neighborhood residents.

7. Evaluate the project in terms of FHCL development, neighborhood resources, project development, and implementation.

8. Generalize the proposed coalition model to other similar neighborhoods.

Implementation of funding agencies have increasingly emphasized the development of academic and co-op partnerships to ensure the application of academic expertise to human problems. This proposal is the product of a truly integrated partnership of neighborhood residents, service agencies, and academia.

The governing body would be a board of directors composed of representation from the FHCL, ODU School of Nursing, and PIN and would serve to guide the project with consultation and advisement from these three entities on issues related to community services, training, and evaluation.

The plan for project implementation included training of residents under the direction of the board of directors to work in the community to meet the specific needs of the neighborhood. The residents would receive training in the areas of human services, office management, community organization, nursing, health care assistance, management, and leadership. Additional job skills training was to be determined by the board. Residents selected by the board of directors to receive job training would provide the neighborhood with service in return for the training and support during the training period. The Citizens Committee for New York City, Inc., would assist the Civic League in providing training in the areas of social and community organization. ODU School of Nursing would provide training in leadership, management, health care assistance, and nursing. Additional training would be provided by the adult education programs and Tidewater Community College. ODU would evaluate the outcomes of the project in relation to the annual goals established jointly with the board of directors.

The project sought funds for training of neighborhood residents as well as for needed services to residents as indicated by the board of directors. Its primary focus was empowerment of the neighborhood to identify, design, and implement services for its residents. The premise was that the increased capability of residents through training to manipulate and use these services would translate into an increased sense of community, power, and ability to address the needs of residents related to safety, health, and standard of living. Following the training periods in the first year of the project, community focus groups would be established to address needs of elders, young parents, youths, and young children. Projects would be developed and implemented using the empowerment model with each component group.

DESCRIPTION OF PROPOSED METHODS

DESIGN

An evaluation plan described for this project was divided into three phases: assessment and planning, implementation, and evaluation. Data would be collected to aid in accomplishing the specified goals and objectives of the project as outlined above.

POPULATION

The sample population included all residents of the Fairwood Homes neighborhood. Individuals singled out to complete the data collection instruments would include (a) all residents selected to complete specialized training programs, (b) residents elected to leadership positions in the neighborhood organization, (c) a random sample of residents not involved in the neighborhood organization, and (d) residents who receive services associated with special initiatives.

ASSESSMENT MEASURES

Demographic information would be collected for residents from the neighborhood, including information on race, age, sex, income, educational preparation, and occupation. A survey of health needs and problems of the elderly, infants, young adults, and youths was to be developed. Interviews of neighborhood residents would be conducted to determine the effectiveness of strategies to increase Civic League membership and participation in focus group projects. A resource network was to be compiled and analyzed for development opportunities.

DATA MANAGEMENT

Data management and statistical analyses were to be performed using the resources of the ODU Computer Center, which operates the IBM 3090 Processor Complex, with vector facility. The Computer Center maintains a large inventory of state-of-the-art statistical programs and packages. Programming for data entry, verification, scoring, and analysis was to be performed by the project assistant and supervised by the project directors.

DATA ANALYSIS

The first component of the analysis was descriptive, providing the background material for later stages. One set of analyses would include tabulating and summarizing a large amount of information about the residents in a manner that would allow useful comparisons to be made with other projects and that would address the objectives and evaluation components of the project. The eight dimensions of community empowerment (Eng & Parker, 1994) were to be used as a framework for interpreting data from interviews.

Preliminary analyses would therefore take the form of tabulations and cross-tabulations of the data describing the residents, together with the appropriate summary statistics and test statistics for categorical data.

HUMAN SUBJECTS

Written consent was to be obtained from all participants before any interview could begin or screening instrument filled out. The consent form explained the purpose of the project, the content of the interview, the voluntary nature of the study, and the respondent's right not to answer certain questions and to terminate the interview at any time. It also explains that the information would be treated as confidential.

IMPLEMENTATION

During the three months of the project, activities would include recruitment of project personnel, establishment of an on-site project office, and organization of the advisory board. These activities would put into place the structural components necessary for further implementation of the project.

During the next three months, the first training sessions for the FHCL with the Citizens Committee for New York City, Inc., in community organization, resident recruitment, and project development, would take place. Recruitment activities would be initiated to increase participation of all residents in the Civic League activities. Residents who sought additional skills could apply for selection as a coalition project-sponsored trainee in areas such as office skills, bookkeeping, accounting, home health aide nursing, data processing, and leadership through programs with Portsmouth Public Schools—Adult Education, Chesapeake Public Schools—Adult Education, Tidewater Community College, and ODU. Training would continue for Civic League members and officers in implementation of the league's organizational plan.

During Months 6 through 12, residents selected for training would complete training programs. The FHCL would initiate a major recruitment activity and increase its involvement in neighborhood activities and the initiation of a youth-oriented activity.

During the second year, in Months 12 through 18, the results of the recruitment activities during the first year would facilitate identification and formation of focus (interest) groups identified by the Civic League (in areas such as the needs of the elderly, families, young parents, youths, mothers, and daughters). The focus groups would have access to continued consultation by project personnel, advisory board members, and consultants in areas of specialty identified as the needs and purpose of the focus groups develop. Support personnel for the focus group would include the project staff and residents who had been trained in areas such as geriatric home care aide and who could provide knowledge and specialized skills related to the needs of the elderly. Residents trained in accounting and document preparation as well as officers trained in leadership would also serve to support these focus groups.

During Months 18 through 24, the focus groups, with leadership from the FHCL, would determine the needs of the neighborhood and plan projects to address those needs. A critical component of these projects would be identification of private and public opportunities for financial support. Ideally, by the end of the first 2 years of the project, Civic League would have recruited additional members, gained new skills in effective organization of the neighborhood, and trained residents in critical skills as expert sources of support for future neighborhood development and the formation of resident groups organized along common interests.

It was projected that during Year 3, the Civic League and its sponsored focus groups would demonstrate the outcomes of the empowerment model used in Years 1 and 2 by implementing special neighborhood projects using a diverse coalition of support, including private businesses, public agencies, and self-supporting work and business arrangements.

During the final years of the coalition project, the advisory board would continue to advise the FHCL, which would be the primary controlling body and which would seek funding for additional projects.

SUMMARY

Empowerment may be defined most accurately as enabling others to control their own destiny or help them obtain the ability to use their own efforts to gain power (Israel, Checkoway, Schulz, & Zimmerman, 1994). The neighbors in Fairwood Homes would be involved in both the process and outcome of empowerment. They would have opportunities for (a) participation in neighborhood assessment and planning, (b) committing themselves to the worth of the neighborhoods, (c) increased self-awareness within the whole community and neighborhood, (d) articulation of a collective view of the community, (e) learning conflict containment, (f) learning to manage relations beyond the neighborhood, (g) formal representation in decision making, and (h) increased social support and caring for others in the neighborhood (Eng & Parker, 1994).

REFERENCES

Block, P. (1987). *The empowered manager: Positive political skills at work.* San Francisco: Jossey-Bass.

Braithwaite, R. L., Murphy, F., Lythcott, N., & Bluenthal, D. S. (1989). Community organization and development for health promotion within an urban black community: A conceptual model. *Health Education, 20*(5), 56-60.

Clark, P. B., & Wilson, J. Q. (1961). Incentive systems: A theory of organizations. *Administrative Science Quarterly, 6,* 129-166.

Clark, P. G. (1988). Autonomy, personal empowerment, and planning for long-term care. *Journal of Applied Gerontology, 7,* 279-297.

Dunst, C., Trirette, C., & Deal, A. (1989). *Enabling and empowering families: Principles and guidelines for practice.* Cambridge, MA: Brookline.

Eng, E., & Parker, E. (1994). Measuring community competence in the Mississippi Delta: The interface between program evaluation and empowerment. *Health Education Quarterly, 21,* 199-220.

Flynn, B., Ray, D. W., & Rider, M. S. (1994). Empowering communities: Action research through healthy cities. *Health Education Quarterly, 21,* 395-405.

Israel, B. A., Checkoway, B., Schulz, A., & Zimmerman, M. (1994). Health education and community empowerment: Conceptualizing and measuring perceptions of individuals, organizations, and community control. *Health Education Quarterly, 21,* 149-170.

Kieffer, C. H. (1984). Citizen empowerment: A developmental perspective. *Prevention in Human Services, 3,* 9-36.

Killian, A. (1988). Conscientisation: An empowering, nonformal education approach for community health workers. *Community Development Journal, 23,* 117-123.

Prestby, J. E., Wandersman, A., Florin, P., Rich, R., & Chavis, D. (1990). Benefits, costs, incentive management and participation in voluntary organizations: A means of understanding and promoting empowerment. *American Journal of Community Psychology, 18*(1), 117-149.

Swift, C., & Levin, G. (1987). Empowerment: An emerging mental health technology. *Journal of Primary Prevention, 8,* 71-94.

Unger, D., & Wandersman, A. (1985). The importance of neighbors: The social, cognitive, and affective components of neighboring. *American Journal of Community Psychology, 13,* 139-169.

Wallerstein, N. (1992). Powerlessness, empowerment, and health: Implications for health promotion programs. *Health Promotion, 6,* 197-205.

Wilt, J. C., & Martens, B. (1988). Problems with problem solving consultation: A reanalysis of assumptions, methods and goals. *School Psychology Review, 17,* 211-226.

Zimmerman, M., & Rappaport, J. (1988). Citizen participation, perceived control, and psychological empowerment. *American Journal of Community Psychology, 16,* 725-749.

Case Study 8

Community Empowerment

KATHLEEN M. MAY

SANDRA L. FERKETICH

BACKGROUND

In response to a request for applications (RFA) from the Agency for Health Care Policy and Research, the National Institute of Nursing Research, and the Division of Nursing, College of Nursing faculty members at the University of Arizona (UA researchers) and Pinal County Department of Public Health (PCDPH) staff collaborated to design a project testing three components of a community health nursing model in rural communities (Ferketich, Phillips, & Verran, 1990).

PROJECT PLANNING

The plan for the project began with assessment of population health data and community interest by a team of UA researchers. An extensive analysis of population health data for rural communities and surrounding areas in the state of Arizona revealed that five small, rural, underserved communities in one county met the criteria for study inclusion as published in the RFA from the sponsoring groups. The UA researchers contacted PCDPH staff in the county and collaborated for further assessment and planning. Two of the communities had populations of under 1,000 people and were adjacent communities, so these had to be considered as one community, resulting in a total of four communities identified as target communities for the project. The PCDPH had a departmental structure and mission based on a traditional community health nursing model, which included public health nurses' role in providing generalist nursing services, including outreach, case finding, and case management. This was important in that differences in health care delivery systems needed to be controlled for the experimental design of the project.

The selected communities were both underserved and interested in assistance. Because the RFA had a deadline of 1 month, complete community involvement in preparation for the response to the RFA was not possible at that stage. Meetings of the UA researchers with PCDPH staff provided input on current services available to the communities.

The project was planned for the four communities, each of which met criteria for rural areas (U.S. Congress, Office of Technology Assessment, 1990). Each of the four communities had fewer than 2,500 residents and was not included in any standard metropolitan statistical area (SMSA). Each community was at least 40 to 75 miles from any major urban area and was in a county with no urban area with a population of 50,000 or more (U.S. Congress, Office of Technology Assessment, 1990). All communities were medically underserved and had populations with low incomes, substandard housing,

AUTHORS' NOTE: This case study is based on a project funded by Grant #1-R18-HSO6801-01, Agency for Health Care Policy and Research (co-principal investigators: Sandra L. Ferketich, Linda R. Phillips, and Joyce Verran).

elderly subpopulations, and high unemployment. The communities had an economic structure based on copper mining and few, if any, migrant workers.

PROJECT DESIGN

The project design included three interventions:

1. Personalized preventive nursing, providing clinic services and community health nurse home visits by a clinic nurse

2. Organized indigenous caregiving, providing outreach health care by community health nurses and *promotoras* (lay health workers promoting health)

3. Community empowerment, fostering community identification of health problems, resources, and solutions by community members, including community health nurses and *promotoras*

Each of the four communities received randomly assigned interventions. The focal community for this case study received both organized indigenous caregiving and community empowerment. However, this case study addresses only the community empowerment intervention, which was in effect for 18 months. Funding limitations precluded the possibility of a community empowerment intervention of longer duration.

COMMUNITY EMPOWERMENT FRAMEWORK

A community development approach to community organization, formerly called locality development (Rothman, 1970), provided the basis for the community empowerment intervention. Using this framework, the project emphasized involvement in problem solving by community members, including community health nurses from nearby communities and neighborhood workers (Rothman, 1970), who were called *promotoras* in this project.

In this framework for community empowerment, communities were supported in exerting their ownership of problems and solutions (Wallerstein, 1992) related to health. The role of health professionals in community empower-

ment is to listen and help community members to identify problems and strengths, develop plans, and act (Wallerstein, 1992). The community health nurses and *promotoras* implemented the community empowerment intervention by planning strategies to foster community participation and control. In this effort, the UA researchers and PCDPH staff provided consultation and support for the community health nurse and *promotoras*. A description of the community provides background for outlining the intervention.

DESCRIPTION OF THE COMMUNITY

The community is a small town located in a river valley divided by a highway and some hills along the river. Much of the community lives in old housing, with 13% of residents living in trailers. There is an elementary school, a town hall, a small courthouse and municipal building, a small building used for community services, and small stores, mostly located along the highway.

In the community of 532 households, 66% are Mexican American. Most residents are long-term members of the community and have close ties to extended family members. For many years, mining was a primary source of income for community members, but the economy had suffered ill effects in recent years due to decreasing employment opportunities in the mines. Some residents believed the environmental effects of mining on the town included pollution of groundwater and contamination due to residue from mining wastes dropped from trucks traveling through town several times a day. Before the project, the only health services in the town were provided once a week at the small building for community services, used by the PCDPH for a clinic staffed by community health nurses. During the project, clinic was held in the same building once a week, and the community health nurse and *promotoras* used the offices each day to implement the project interventions, including the community empowerment intervention.

THE INTERVENTION

The focus of this case study is the planning, implementation, and evaluation of a community empowerment intervention in one community.

The major goal of the community empowerment intervention was the "redistribution of decision making power" (Ferketich et al., 1990, p. 46). This goal was further specified to be measured in five outcomes: (a) increased cultural sensitivity of organized health care programs, (b) redistribution of health resources, (c) refocusing of existing health programs on health needs identified by the community itself, (d) the creation of new health services and programs that are desired by the community, and (e) increased acceptability and accessibility of the services available (Ferketich et al., 1990, p. 51).

To achieve the desired overall goal and outcomes, strategies were (a) identifying resources in the community, (b) eliciting community support, (c) mobilizing resources for assessment, (d) mobilizing resources for creating interventions, and (e) training community members to continue after the project ended (Ferketich et al., 1990, p. 50).

ROLE OF COMMUNITY HEALTH NURSE AND *PROMOTORAS*

To implement the community empowerment intervention, a community health nurse and two *promotoras,* Mexican American community residents who were high school graduates, were hired. The community health nurse was a Mexican American baccalaureate-prepared RN from a nearby rural community, hired to spend half time on indigenous caregiving (outreach activities aimed at neighbors to improve access to health care) and half on community empowerment. The *promotoras* were hired part time for a total of .50 FTE.

UA researchers met with the community health nurse and *promotoras* for an orientation program, with sessions held at least once a week for the 6 weeks, to give an overview of community empowerment and explore how to apply the philosophy of the project. Researchers explained the role of the health professional in the project and how it reflected a philosophy of community empowerment. Sessions included informal verbal presentations by UA researchers, printed materials, discussion, and presentations by the community health nurse and *promotoras,* in which they gained practice in speaking before a group.

The role of the community health nurse and the *promotoras* was characterized as (a) helping the community to identify, prioritize, and solve problems; (b) encouraging community self-help; (c) advocating community participation in health-related decisions; (d) applying the community's knowledge of the local situation, resources, and networks to develop health programs; and (e) giving support as team members rather than as organizers. The community health nurse was the immediate supervisor of the *promotoras* and guided them in planning and implementing strategies for building partnerships with individuals and groups.

IMPLEMENTATION

Implementation of the community empowerment intervention began with close teamwork by the community health nurse and *promotoras,* with consultation from UA researchers, in identifying community resources, including people active in the community. In the process of talking with community members, describing the intervention, and the ultimate purpose of enhancing the health of the community, they elicited community support.

Further strategies for assessment and implementation included (a) conducting a community survey to obtain baseline data and become familiar with community perceptions, (b) identifying community goals and issues requiring political action, (c) identifying individuals and groups already active in the community, and (d) implementing activities such as a health fair and a legislative hearing, through which partnership of team members with other community members fostered community empowerment.

COMMUNITY SURVEY

With community support, the UA researchers trained survey interviewers to conduct a survey as part of a community assessment. To establish a database for evaluating community needs and strengths and for planning the community empowerment intervention, a door-to-door community survey was done. UA researchers conducted more in-depth interviews with key community informants. The community health nurse and *promotoras,* UA researchers, and PCDPH staff collaborated in using results of the community survey and interviews to formalize a list of identified community goals.

COMMUNITY GOALS

The community health nurse, *promotoras,* UA researchers, and PCDPH staff reviewed survey and key informant interview data to formulate and prioritize community data-based health goals. Eleven community goals derived from the data were worded in terms of what targeted residents would do as a result of the interventions of the project. Any of the three interventions (personalized preventive nursing, organized indigenous caregiving, and community empowerment) could address any of the goals. After establishing relationships with community members and informing them of the project, the community health nurse and *promotoras* planned community empowerment strategies to address the goals.

PLANNING SESSIONS

The community health nurse and *promotoras* met in weekly staff meetings to plan and evaluate strategies for the community empowerment intervention. Although they wholeheartedly supported the philosophy, the question was, "How do we do it?" The UA researchers, at the request of the community health nurse and *promotoras,* provided ongoing assistance with designing strategies to implement the philosophy. They provided this assistance in monthly meetings of the total project staff, and through biweekly on-site consultation. However, true to the community empowerment philosophy, the UA researchers provided consultation while emphasizing that the community, including the community health nurse and *promotoras,* had primary responsibility for identifying problems, resources, and solutions.

PARTNERSHIP WITH COMMUNITY

Gaining community support through the survey and key informant interviews, the project provided a basis for the community health nurse and *promotoras* to further identify individuals and groups already active in the community. The community health nurse and *promotoras* knew many who were community leaders. They made appointments to talk individually with community public officials, describe the project, and discuss community goals and issues. Community leaders expressed verbal support of the project.

By talking informally with other community members, the community health nurse and *promotoras* encountered people who were not in official positions but who were active in supporting community activities. Through informal contacts, they continued to hear community members' perceptions about their health concerns and resources. *Promotoras* conducted informal discussion sessions in their own and other community residents' homes to discuss issues of interest and generate strategies.

The community health nurse and *promotoras* made themselves visible in the community by attending community meetings, talking with community members in public places, and distributing flyers about clinic services. The clinic services were part of another intervention, but by using various avenues of communication, the community health nurse and *promotoras* became recognized and developed relationships that were helpful in implementing community empowerment.

The *promotoras* became more active in community groups, such as a coalition formed to coordinate gleaning for community members. All of these efforts increased the visibility of the community health nurse and the *promotoras,* who, in turn, were contacted more frequently by community members when community issues arose.

A specific example of how the community health nurse and *promotoras* mobilized resources for assessment, mobilized resources for creating an intervention, and trained community members to continue empowerment strategies was with a health fair, described here as the second health fair.

HEALTH FAIR

A community empowerment strategy previously described was the implementation of a community health fair (May, Mendelson, & Ferketich, 1995). In the early planning phase of the project, a committee of UA researchers, community members, and PCDPH staff had sponsored a community health fair. The UA researchers gathered brochures and health appraisal equipment and materials, and played a major role in providing basic ideas, planning, and personnel. This health fair, attended by about 60 community residents, provided health screening and education and gave the community a chance to get to know project staff (May et al., 1995).

For the second health fair, the community health nurse and *promotoras,* with only minimal facilitation by UA researchers, assumed major responsibility for planning, implementing, and evaluating the health fair. The *promotoras* assessed community members' perceptions of types of information and activities that would be desirable at the health fair. They marketed the health fair to the community and elicited support from neighbors, friends, and families, resulting in the attendance of 300 residents. Community members participated in making the health fair happen and learned what went into implementing such an activity. This community empowerment intervention was evaluated as much more successful than the strategy used for the first health fair (May et al., 1995), demonstrating the effect of community ownership of planning and implementing a project.

OTHER EMPOWERMENT STRATEGIES

The community health nurse and *promotoras* became involved in many other activities directed toward community empowerment. On issues of importance to the community, they initiated letter writing to legislators to support continuation of, and increases in, services to the community. They became active in community organizations dealing with community issues, such as a coalition on gleaning to provide food for low-income families. They built partnerships with interested community members in other towns to participate in health fairs. And they elicited support from community members to convey to legislators and community leaders, through a legislative hearing, the need for health services for the community.

LEGISLATIVE HEARING

As the research project neared the end of the funding period, townspeople became concerned about the prospect of the loss of services of the community health nurse and *promotoras.* With the assistance of the UA researchers, the community health nurse and *promotoras* set up a legislative hearing. The *promotoras* talked with community members about the importance of the hearing and the need for community mem-

bers to participate. In consultation with the UA researchers, the *promotoras* set up rehearsals to help community members prepare for the hearing. Most of the townspeople had never attended a hearing, much less presented testimony at one. Many could not understand or speak English; or if English was a second language, some preferred to speak in Spanish because they felt more comfortable with their primary language. It was arranged to have a translator available, and all proceedings were conducted in English and Spanish.

As the time arrived for the hearing, only 5 or 6 people came at the scheduled time. However, within 15 to 20 minutes (the meeting was delayed to allow for additional arrivals), the room filled and reached a total of about 45 townspeople. This exceeded the room's capacity, according to fire regulations. However, the fire chief and mayor were there and decided the size of the crowd was acceptable. In addition to the community residents, there were six county, local, and state representatives present to hear the community members' testimony.

Community members presenting testimony were very nervous in this new endeavor, and several presenters were undocumented residents who were especially nervous over the chance that they were taking. However, they testified that the continued presence of the nursing personnel was essential.

One woman stated that she had brought her infant to the clinic. The infant was not breathing, appeared cyanotic, and was in acute distress. The bilingual community health nurse and *promotora* quickly determined that the infant had inhaled some food. The community health nurse performed the Heimlich maneuver, and the baby recovered. This mother was adamant that if the nurse had not been there and had not spoken Spanish, her baby would have died. Others described less dramatic but equally compelling arguments for the continued presence of the community health nurse and *promotoras.*

EVALUATION

Evaluation of the effect of the community empowerment intervention necessitated examination of achievement of the major goal, redistribution of decision-making power, and the five specific outcomes identified previously in this case study. The evaluation begins with the five specific outcomes identified for the community empowerment intervention: (a) cultural sensitivity, (b) redistribution of health resources, (c) refocusing of existing health programs, (d) new health services, and (e) acceptability and accessibility of services (Ferketich et al., 1990). Evaluation of accomplishment of the major goal follows evaluation of the specific outcomes.

CULTURAL SENSITIVITY

The first outcome of the intervention was to be increased cultural sensitivity of organized health care programs. The major organized health program in the community was the clinic service offered by PCDPH. For the duration of the project, the clinic services were expanded. The community health nurse and *promotoras* for community empowerment were bilingual in English and Spanish. They were successful in soliciting and obtaining many educational materials in Spanish, which were used in the clinic, in health education classes, and at the health fair.

Through interactions with health care professionals in nearby communities, the community health nurse and *promotoras* increased responsiveness to the difficulties of Mexican and Mexican American clients, as evidenced by requests for translation and assistance. The project, community health nurse, and *promotoras,* supported by community members, reinforced the importance of culturally sensitive county health services.

REDISTRIBUTION OF HEALTH RESOURCES

Through the community empowerment intervention, the health department and other agencies increased attention toward the community, as people became aware of the work of the community health nurse and *promotoras.* The community health nurse and *promotoras* initiated community support for, and participation in, mobile screening units, group health education sessions, and support groups (e.g., for weight loss and decrease in family violence). Gaps in services were identified, including difficulty in transportation from the community to services. There was permanent redistribution of services to the community through a new community health center, begun as an outcome of this project.

REFOCUSING OF EXISTING HEALTH PROGRAMS

The health fair booths, support groups, and other strategies reflected a focusing of existing health programs on health needs identified by the community itself. One example of community ownership of health problems and solutions was in the second health fair. The positive response of the community in its involvement in planning and attendance implies a degree of community empowerment. The existing health program of the PCDPH expressed commitment to meeting the health needs of the community, which does not necessarily reflect refocusing but does indicate continued support.

CREATION OF NEW HEALTH SERVICES

Before and during the project, many community members expressed desire for a permanent community clinic. An effect of the project was success in creating a new health service that was desired by the community, in the form of a community health center.

As the research funding was ending, the UA researchers, PCDPH, and residents used their best efforts to negotiate with a health care network with services in Tucson, through nursing administration, to set up a clinic in the rural community. An asset was the fact that the project had prepared a trained group of people in the rural community who could continue with a clinic set up by the health care network. All project staff in the community were hired as the new community health center staff, in roles as community health nurse and *promotoras.*

INCREASED ACCEPTABILITY AND ACCESSIBILITY

Although awareness of transportation difficulties was raised and the topic was the focus of town meetings between project staff and community members, there was no permanent change in accessibility through transportation as a result of the project. However, the community health center did increase acceptability and accessibility of the services available to the community. Staffing by community members enhanced acceptability. The community health center is located centrally in the town, assuring community members access to health care.

REDISTRIBUTION OF DECISION-MAKING POWER

In exit interviews with project staff at the end of the project, the *promotoras* expressed a sense of individual empowerment. They described a change in themselves from the beginning of the project to the end. They remembered initial uncertainty about their ability to do the job or support others' efforts to implement change, and they evaluated themselves as more assertive by the end of the project.

In exit interviews, the community health nurse and *promotoras* described community members as more empowered as they assumed more responsibility for managing their interactions with health care professionals and agencies, compared with their situation at the beginning of the project. Through the legislative hearing and the institution of the community health center, community members were seen as empowered.

The time limit of the project prevented evaluation of long-term evidence of community empowerment. However, there was short-term success in ways already described. The involvement of the community in the health fair and the legislative hearing illustrates the effectiveness of the community empowerment intervention aimed at redistributing power for health care. The hearing proceedings were quite exciting as people demonstrated a newly developed understanding of health promotion and disease prevention and the role that nurses and community members have in that activity. The community health center remains in service 18 months after the phasing out of the project's provision of health care services. The *promotoras* continue with their work, although two have left their employment for other opportunities.

DISCUSSION AND RECOMMENDATIONS

Evaluation of the intervention effect focused on the community as a whole, reflected in participation in decision making affecting health outcomes and health services. However, empowerment of the community health nurse, *promotoras*, and individual community members was an indicator of what was happening at the larger unit of analysis, the community.

Community data-based goals guided the community empowerment intervention. One goal is that community members continue involvement in community health activities after the project. Changes in the *promotoras* and other community members as they increased their sense of empowerment may have long-term implications for the community. The experience with implementing a community empowerment intervention reinforces awareness of the difficulty in measuring and evaluating outcomes at the aggregate level. On the basis of anecdotal reports by community members, the community empowerment intervention can be said to have resulted in individual experiences of empowerment and a perception of change in the community.

The ultimate benefits of community-level environmental change and political change (Wallerstein, 1992) are outcomes best measured longitudinally. The community empowerment intervention produced short-term improvements in the health care environment and political participation by community members. Long-term effects need further evaluation.

REFERENCES

Ferketich, S., Phillips, L., & Verran, J. (1990). *Multi-level practice model for rural Hispanics* (Grant No. 1-R18-HSO6801-01). Rockville, MD: Agency for Health Care Policy and Research.

May, K. M., Mendelson, C., & Ferketich, S. (1995). Community empowerment in a rural community. *Public Health Nursing, 12,* 25-30.

Rothman, J. (1970). Three models of community organization practice, their mixing and phasing. In F. M. Cox, J. L. Erlich, J. Rothman, & J. E. Trotman (Eds.), *Strategies of community organization* (3rd ed., pp. 25-45). Itasca, IL: F. E. Peacock.

U.S. Congress, Office of Technology Assessment. (1990). *Health care in rural America* (OTA-H-434). Washington, DC: Government Printing Office.

Wallerstein, N. (1992). Powerlessness, empowerment, and health: Implications for health promotion programs. *American Journal of Health Promotion, 6,* 197-205.

Case Study 9
Coalition Building

JANIE CANTY-MITCHELL
SHARON GARRETT

This case study describes the temporary alliance of a church, two community health nurses, adult volunteers, and inner-city youths and parents who developed a coalition to implement a youth summer program in a midwestern inner city. This coalition was formed to further the purpose of meeting the inner-city community's need for educational, social, health, and recreational programs for youths during the summer months. The church provided the centering and focal point to bridge relationships between two community health nurses and inner-city youths. The case study includes a 1994 assessment of the involved community, a description of the church, a description of the summer youth program organized by the church, and the role of two community health nurses in the program during the summer of 1995. To protect the anonymity of the key informants and the community, fictitious names are included in the body of the case study.

ASSESSMENT OF THE COMMUNITY

The community assessment is taken from 1990 U.S. census data, information from key informants, and data from educational, social service, health, and religious institutions. The community is located in a large midwestern city, within one of the city's nine townships. The community described in this assessment is considered an inner-city area. Today, the community struggles with aging structures, a population that is largely poor, and an aggravated assault crime rate that is the highest in the city. It was not always that way.

The community was developed in the early part of the 20th century by the county's prominent white citizens. Of the 1,014 housing units in the area, 552 were built before 1939, and another 220 were built between 1940 and 1949. Therefore, approximately 76% of the dwellings are at least 45 years old. One former resident described the pattern that emerged during the middle years of the 20th century: "When blacks began moving into the area in the fifties and sixties, like most urban areas, whites became nervous and moved out. Some residents sold their homes and by the middle of the 1960s, most of the dwellings had become rental properties. Many of the people renting the properties were poor." Thus, the area gradually deteriorated, and like many large, urban areas where there is "white flight," the area decayed because of limited economic growth and poverty. Today, the residents remain economically poor with limited resources.

DEMOGRAPHICS

Of the 2,760 people who currently live in the community, 95.5% reported themselves to be black in the 1990 U.S. census. However, blacks constitute only 21% of the population in the entire county and 41% of the population in the township. Therefore, it is obvious that there is a significantly different population of blacks in this community's census tract compared with the county and the township as a whole. Males and females account for 45% and 55%, respectively, of the community's population. This is comparable to the males (48%) and females (52%) for county. The 1990 census reports 282 youths between 15 and 19 years of age. Male youths make up approximately 46% of that number, compared with 54% females.

HOUSING

There are approximately 1,014 housing units in the community, primarily rental units, compared with largely owner-occupied units for the rest of the county. There is also a 19% vacancy rate in the community, compared with a 10% vacancy rate for the entire county and a 14% vacancy rate for the central township. The houses, many built of brick and stone, are mostly two-story, one- and two-family homes and substantial in size. Even though the houses look intact from the outside, many need maintenance and rehabilitation. Many of the homes have not been preserved and have boarded-up windows, doors, and porches; steps and foundations that need repair, and yards and fences that show signs of neglect and age. Vacant lots are overrun with weeds and debris.

ENVIRONMENT

The neighborhood that once was grand, according to present and former residents, now needs nurturing. During a windshield survey, the physical environment, including streets and sidewalks, was found to be poorly maintained. Broken glass was common on streets and in the parking lot across the street from the church. This area is used by the neighborhood children as their playground.

SOCIOECONOMIC STATUS

The community is economically depressed. There is very little economic development, with few stores and no major grocery chains or shopping malls serving the immediate area. Based on U.S. census data, the black per capita income in the community is $6,028, whereas that of white persons is $11,319. The black per capita income in the community is 66% that of black persons in the county, 37% of whites in the county, and 41% of all persons in the county. Based on the poverty guidelines set by the federal government in 1989, 36% of families in the community have incomes below the poverty guidelines of $12,674 per year for a family of four; 12.4% of black families have income levels that were 100% to 124% of poverty. Census data indicate

that 37% of black families have income levels under $10,000 per year; 29% have incomes between $15,000 and $35,000, and have had incomes between $50,000 and $75,000. This is a sharp contrast to the small percentage of white families living in the community. According to the 1990 U.S. census, five white families have incomes in access of $100,000, and the other 42 white families have incomes under $50,000.

The 1990 U.S. census indicates that 59.7% of the males were employed, as were 53.6% of the females in the community. Single women predominate as heads of family households. Of the 611 family households in the census tract, 232 (38%) were headed by married couples, 334 (54.7%) were headed by a female with no husband present, and 45 (7%) had no wife present.

EDUCATION

To settle a racial integration suit in the 1970s, a federal judge ordered children living in this community to be bused to another township school. The bus trip is approximately 40 minutes each way to the school. As a result of the judge's decision, the area schools were closed. One long-term resident reflected on this decision: "We've always had violence and liquor stores and broken down homes. But our neighborhood school was a community center, with a PTA [Parents Teachers Association] and a Block Club for adults. We would walk to school together, 5 minutes away. Everyone was 'our mother,' and we couldn't get away with anything! Then the schools were taken away with no explanation. We lost our community." Youths were still bused to another township in 1995.

The 1990 U.S. census reports indicate that of the 1,445 residents 25 years of age and older, 12% had less than a ninth-grade education; 32% completed between 9th and 11th grades and had no diploma. Therefore, 45% of the residents have less than a high school diploma. Five percent of the residents have an advanced degree.

TRANSPORTATION

Of the 819 occupied housing units cited in the 1990 census, 33% of the households had no available vehicle and 31% of the households reported having two or more cars. Public transportation was used by 23% of the workers in the community. Bus service runs on a major north-south avenue adjacent to the community.

RECREATION

There are limited recreational facilities for youths in the community. The older youths play along a grassy area by a riverbed, but they cross five lanes of traffic on a major parkway do so. There is a very small area near the church that has been designated as a city park. However, the children play on the church's blacktopped parking lot, which is equipped with a basketball hoop.

A neighboring church, one of many religious institutions in the community, has a large sports program serving the community at large. According to the church's social worker, the recreation program is held 12 months a year and includes soccer, football, softball, cheerleading, and two basketball sessions with 500 participants in each session. To play basketball, youths must attend tutoring sessions. The tutoring-basketball program teaches life skills and decision making for youths 12 to 18 years of age. There are usually 5 to 35 youths in attendance at each session.

POLITICAL FORCES

The 1994 political election suggests that the residents are not involved in the political process. Of the 750 registered voters in the church precinct, only 125 voted. Only one campaign poster was visible in a yard during a windshield community survey. One key informant stated, "Nothing has happened to make people feel they have a say." Another resident said, "We would like to be empowered to face the city, to get needed repairs for sidewalks and streets, . . . [but] we are not invited to meetings where decisions about the neighborhood are made." Residents indicated that they felt powerless against absentee landlords who own houses that have been abandoned or condemned by the city.

COMMUNITY SOCIAL SERVICES RESOURCES AND AGENCIES

The community's strength lies in the presence of its many social service, governmental,

and nonprofit agencies. These agencies were designed to strengthen the community and to assist the residents with housing, social, cultural, and economic needs. Some of the resources include a multichurch council, a housing development corporation, a neighborhood housing program, the township trustee, and the community church and its sponsored Summer Youth Program (SYP).

The multichurch council is an organization composed of five churches in the community. The council formed to provide support for community initiatives sponsored by neighborhood residents and social service agencies. This council formed the first food bank in the community.

The *housing development corporation* offers eligible residents low-interest loans and grants for home purchases and home repairs. It is considered a banking agency that grants a 20% loan on the full purchase price of a house at a 6% interest rate. It provides the rest of the mortgage at fair interest rate. The corporation also offers education and counseling on money management, weatherization of homes, reclamation of duplexes for affordable rentals, and job training for development in construction skills. Approximately, 200 to 300 people were served by the agency according to 1994 documents.

A *neighboring church* provides outreach services for the community as well as the recreation program previously described. A staff social worker located at the church provides counseling to community residents 2 days a week. The church also purchases school clothes, including winter coats, and supplies for more than 100 children each fall. The church owns a building in the community that houses the Neighborhood Association, the Community Christian Legal Service Center, and a food bank. The Neighborhood Association organizes to provide support services for the community. The Legal Service Center provides affordable legal services by volunteer lawyers to residents who meet the income guidelines. The food bank provides food for community residents in need.

The *township trustee* is another resource available to the community residents. Each of the county's nine townships elects a trustee who is mandated by law to be an overseer of the poor. The township trustee in this community provides emergency assistance for food, housing, and utilities for township residents who meet income eligibility guidelines. For a family of four living in the township, the maximum income for the preceding month in 1994 was set at $678.33. The township office also houses other services, such as the state's child welfare and food stamp programs. According to a key informant in the trustee's office, plans are underway to make the township building a "holistic center housing 14 governmental and social services providers."

Health Services. There are multiple health services available in the township for the community residents. The county hospital provides outpatient, inpatient, and emergency services at its main site. To get to the main hospital facility, residents without transportation must take a lengthy bus ride, seek transportation through a friend or neighbor, or take a taxi.

The hospital's outreach community health centers consist of multidisciplinary teams that provide primary health services for adults, children, and adolescents. The hospital's satellite outreach health centers are geographically closer to the community but do not seem to be used as much as the main hospital facility. Services are free to adolescents if the visit is not authorized by a parent.

Other hospitals and agencies within the township include a large private nonprofit hospital and the county's public health department. The latter also has satellite clinics in the county and township. Within the community is a nurse practitioner-managed wellness center, located in the church. It will be discussed in the next section.

THE COMMUNITY CHURCH

The church, the source of this study, stands majestically at the perimeter of the community, one of many churches in the community. During the transition of the community from a predominantly white to black area, many of its members moved out of the community. Currently, the church is attended largely by white parishioners, yet it is surrounded by a community that has a 95.5% black population. During the community's transition in the 1950s and 1960s, the church was challenged to rethink its outreach mission.

In 1957, a magnetic and visionary minister was appointed to the church. He personally reached out to the community, offering residents support. He proposed to the members of the congregation that they too should reach out to the community. Not all the church members agreed

with his direction, and some left the congregation. Other members agreed with the mission, and many more came to the congregation, including members from diverse ethnic groups. The outreach mission to the local community continues to this day.

One of the church's outreach missions was to provide a safe haven for community residents, through programming to meet some of the community's needs. Through its outreach to children, the church has developed a bridge to the community through its educationally based afterschool programs, tutoring programs, and its SYP. More recently, a church-based wellness center has been opened to serve families in the community.

The tutoring program began in the early 1980s and is jointly sponsored with another church located in a suburban area within the city. A volunteer coordinator from each church recruits the children and the tutors. Tutoring is held three afternoons a week. An afterschool program was also implemented to provide a safe haven for neighborhood children to do homework, work on crafts, or engage in reading for leisure. In addition to tutoring and afterschool programs, volunteers offer a violin and piano program for children interested in learning to play these instruments.

The *wellness center* opened in 1994 within the church. It was conceptualized and designed by two professors at a midwestern university school of nursing and was funded by grants from a state agency and private foundations. It uses a rural health clinic model and parish nursing model to provide care to community residents. It is staffed by nurses, an outreach worker, and a secretary who are from the community. The clinic provides health screenings, symptom management, and referrals and is designed to be a partnership with the community. The foci of the clinic are wellness, prevention, and health promotion. The clinic staff offers a variety of classes, including, for example, classes on nutrition, stress management, exercise, and smoking cessation.

The Summer Youth Program (SYP). In 1972, the church began a recreational program for youths. This program grew in size each year and provided the foundation of service to youths in the community. In 1988, educational activities, field trips, and invited guest speakers were added to the summer program to expand the participants' experience beyond their neighborhood. The summer program's advisory board addresses the overall management needs of the program and works all year in planning future programs.

In 1995, the SYP consisted of a 9-week, full-day Afrocentric summer program that included education, recreation, fine arts, community service, and social skills training to 100 participants ages 4 to 13 years of age. According to a published bulletin from the church, the purpose of the church-based SYP is to "provide school-age youths [living in the community] with a summer experience that promotes self-respect and achievement, builds an understanding of community, broadens cultural understanding and enriches spiritual life." An enrollment fee of $15 per family was implemented, based on an ability to pay. Adult volunteers from varied ethnic, social, economic, and religious backgrounds are a key to the yearly success of the SYP, with more than 140 adults participating in the summer of 1994 and 1995.

The youths attend an all-day academically based program from Monday through Friday, participating in enrichment field trips on Fridays. The program incorporates teenagers from the community who serve as peer counselors and role models for the younger children. Approximately 20 teenagers volunteered as teen counselors in 1994 and 1995. According to the church's volunteer director who coordinates the SYP, teenagers are selected from those who were previous participants in the program. The church is committed to developing leadership skills, improving self-worth, and promoting decision making and empowerment in the youths.

Children and youths are grouped according to age into a family unit, supervised by teen counselors. They participate in a variety of educational, social, and recreational programs. Examples of activities that 4- to 5-year-old SYP participants engage in are daily story time, health education programs, recreation programs, and field trips.

Youths 6 to 13 years old are engaged in activities such as math, reading, and writing enrichment classes with an Afrocentric focus; weekly access to bookmobiles and the SYP library; weekly health education classes; art, culture, or music sessions that may include things such as singing in a gospel choir, violin or piano lessons, or art classes. Violin lessons are available for beginning, intermediate, and advanced students and are given at no charge to SYP participants. Twelve to 30 children participate in lessons throughout the year, and students perform at nursing homes and functions such as the SYP closing ceremony.

COALITION BUILDING BETWEEN COMMUNITY HEALTH NURSES AND THE SYP

The SYP provides a bridge for two community health nurses to work toward fulfilling their respective goals within the framework of the church's common goals in the SYP program. The community health nurses, from European American and African American backgrounds, had common goals related to youths and formed a coalition with the church to meet their respective goals. Both community health nurses were affiliated with a large midwestern university in the city where the community is located when the coalition was formed. One community health nurse, "Lou," was a master's student at a large midwestern university with 20 years of varied community health nursing experiences. She had also served as a volunteer in a number of the church's outreach programs during 1993 and 1994. Her commitment to the church's programs fostered trust and promoted the development of coalition building among the church, community health nurses, and the community's youths. Through Lou's connection with the church and the SYP, the second community health nurse, "Lee" became involved with the SYP in the summer of 1995.

Lee has a doctorate in nursing and more than 15 years experience working as a public health nurse and community health nursing educator and researcher of adolescents' health needs. Lou introduced Lee to the SYP coordinators and executive director who felt that her specialized skills could enhance the SYP, especially in meeting one SYP objective, "to understand communities." Because Lee had conducted research related to "caring" in urban adolescent samples, caring was also added to the theme of the SYP.

Two particular programs will be discussed that were initiated by Lou and Lee within SYP's program purposes. Lou's project demonstrated partnership and coalition building during the assessment and data collection, planning, and implementation of a conflict resolution project. Lee used the SYP theme of caring and one SYP programmatic goal, "to understand the community" to develop a program titled, Creating a Caring Community, or the 3-Cs Project. Coalition building was an integral aspect of both programs because people from various groups came together for the common goal of enhancing the health, education, social skills, recreation, and well-being of an urban, inner-city group of children and youths in the community.

COALITION BUILDING

Coalition building was an integral aspect of all phases of the community health nurses' interactions with the SYP, including meetings with the church leaders, other community organizations directly involved in the SYP, teens, parents, and counselors from the community and, finally, with the youth participants in the SYP.

Problem Identification. Identification of a single health issue for programming was difficult in a community with multiple problems caused by poverty and other socioeconomic and political issues. A bridge to the community was needed to nurture partnerships and form coalitions between the community health nurses and the church-based SYP. The church leaders and youths in the SYP provided the bridge. In coalition with church leaders and adolescents in the community, the nurses were assisted in identifying problems and programs to be addressed in the SYP during 1995.

Adolescents assisted in this process because they were able to think more abstractly than their younger peers and because they served as teen counselors and role models for the younger children. They also offered a link to the adult community, which was difficult to access. This collaborative, coalition-building process of problem identification assisted Lou to bridge the gap between her ethnicity and social class, which was European American, suburban, and an outsider, and those of the participants—African American, urban, and insiders. Lee attended some of the SYP planning meetings to enhance the African American nursing perspective to a group of African American youths. The diverse, collaborative team of Lou and Lee was beneficial in the

coalition-building process. Lou's background was similar to that of the church members, and Lee's background was similar to that of the participants in the SYP.

Eliciting the assistance of the SYP executive director, a lifetime community resident and an SYP graduate, was crucial to the success of any community health nursing programs geared to the SYP youths. The SYP executive director arranged the initial meeting between Lou and the SYP teens to discuss their health needs and those of younger children. The executive director's willingness to convene the meetings and participate in the problem identification process gave credibility to the community health nurses' efforts. The teenagers attending the meetings ranged in age from 13 to 17 years. The teens were told that their ideas would be used to direct the activities of the SYP for 1995. They were also informed that their input promoted their ownership, involvement, self-responsibility, and problem-solving skill building for the SYP. A brainstorming process was initiated to produce a list of health problems or needs that youths thought they wanted addressed by the SYP. They were told that there were no wrong answers. Following the identification of issues, the areas focusing on health were reviewed. The teens then prioritized the list and considered possible programming needs for children 12 years and under and for teens 13 years and older.

The prioritized list identified by the teens for the 12-years-and-under group included the following needs:

- For personal hygiene education
- To control behavior
- For parent participation in the SYP
- For nutrition education
- For clinic services
- For physical fitness

Prioritized needs identified for the 13- to 18-year-old group were these:

- To get along—for example, how to control one's temper
- For teens to socialize together
- For educational and job counseling
- For help with issues such as self-esteem, decision making, and birth control

Common to both groups was a need for conflict resolution strategies (i.e., a need to control behavior, a need to get along with others, a need to control one's temper). Conflict resolution strategies were within the community health nurses' arena of preventive health interventions.

The teenagers' ability to assess their needs and environment was noteworthy. Police reports supplied data supporting the need to "get along" and to "control behavior." The number of arrests for aggravated assaults in the community was the highest for any district in the city during 1990 through 1992. A community mural outside the church memorializes the people within the community who had been murdered. The mural, funded by the church, contains the names of 23 persons who were killed between September 13, 1991, and May 8, 1994.

The fact that the teenagers wanted to learn how to resolve conflicts was perhaps testimony to the positive impact that the SYP program had on the youths. One key informant said, "The law of the streets in the community was resolution by force, and disgrace was bestowed on those who refused to fight for their rights." The acknowledgment that there are alternative ways to resolve conflict was part of the SYP philosophy of noncombative resolution of differences.

Meetings were held to discuss and clarify the prioritized needs, establish some content for programs, meet the identified needs on the list, and set objectives for each age group. Throughout the problem identification process, Lou was impressed with the ability of the teenagers to identify issues, stay on task, work together, and set priorities. The teens took their roles very seriously and were committed to the process.

Planning and Implementing the Conflict Resolution Program. Planning for the conflict resolution program involved setting goals and objectives, planning activities and strategies, and gaining the necessary funds to implement the program. The goals and objectives for the conflict resolution program in the SYP were mutually established by the community health nurse, the teens, the executive director of the SYP, church administrators, some parents, and adult volunteers. The major goals of the SYP program were (a) to develop and implement techniques for resolving interpersonal conflict, managing anger, and using conflict mediation skills and (b) to increase competence in managing conflict-provoking situations and empower youths to use conflict resolution techniques in a safe environment. Major objectives were established to meet the identified goals, and activities were written to support program objectives.

Some of the objectives and activities identified were these:

- Identify the content of the conflict resolution program

- Identify, evaluate, select, and purchase relevant conflict resolution and educational materials

- Identify resources that will assist in funding the conflict resolution program

- Develop teaching strategies to be used by teens and/or other staff in the conflict resolution program

- Plan and implement a 1-day training session for church staff, teen counselors, and adult volunteers—conducted by a person trained in conflict management techniques

- Plan activities to promote conflict resolution principles, including skits, role plays, small-group work, and so on

- Implement and evaluate the program

On the basis of goals, objectives, and activities planned for the conflict resolution program, the coalition-partner group identified funding as a major need for implementing the program. Lou spearheaded writing a grant proposal to a local foundation to acquire funds for the church-based conflict resolution project. As a result of her efforts, the church was awarded the grant for the program.

The church administrators and executive director in coordination with the community health nurse and teen counselors decided to hire a specialist in conflict resolution training for 8 weeks during the SYP. Lou remained the overall program coordinator for the 10- to 12-year-old age group. As such, she was responsible for ensuring that programs in the SYP were implemented as planned (described in another section).

The conflict resolution program was effective in improving knowledge, skills in decision making, and choices in solving conflicts. This evaluation was based in part on staff members', volunteers', and teen counselors' observations of the youths' verbal and physical behaviors.

PLANNING AND IMPLEMENTING THE CREATING A CARING COMMUNITY PROJECT

On the basis of youths' identified need to "get along," the SYP's theme of caring, and the church leaders need to assist youths in understanding their community, the Creating a Caring Community Project (3-Cs Project) was developed and implemented by Lee, with Lou's assistance in coordinating the youths involved. Lee volunteered 2 hours weekly to lead this 8-week program at the church's SYP.

Goals. The identified goals of the 3-Cs program were to (a) develop SYP youths' understanding of communities and caring communities, (b) help SYP youths discover their special talents that help to create caring communities, and (c) assist SYP youths to identify and develop projects that help create caring communities. During each of the eight sessions, objectives and activities were planned for the youths.

During Weeks 1 through 3, the major objectives centered around a discussion of the meanings of community, caring, caring community, and creativity. These discussions, based on a focus group format, established the base for the next 4 weeks' objectives. The fourth week of the project involved youths in identifying their creative skills. Games were used to assist in this process and to assist youths in overcoming their reluctance to relate their special talents and skills. Some youths found it difficult to find any creative talents or skills.

During the fifth week, the youths were divided into three teams, with four persons to a team. Each team was given 10 minutes to write down as many community problems as they could. In all, 38 separate community problems were identified by the teams. The teams were asked next to identify two problems that they thought were the most significant to resolve in their community. The six most significant problems identified were violence, rape, drug dealing and using, too many liquor stores, teenage pregnancy, and blacks being pushed out of their community by whites (urban renewal). Last, each team was asked to identify what they thought was the Number 1 problem in their community from the six listed. All but one youth identified violence as the Number 1 problem in their community. The one dissenting youth identified "too many liquor stores" as the major

problem. After this problem-assessing session, youths were asked to identify one problem they would personally like to become involved in solving.

During the sixth session, youths were given a typed list of all the problems they had identified and the six most significant problems. They were asked to write down and discuss a problem from the list, and what they thought could be done to resolve the problem. Again, they were asked to work in groups and discuss their responses.

From the end of Week 6 through the beginning of Week 8, youths were encouraged to use their creativity to identify possible solutions to a problem of concern to them. They were also invited to complete some project related to the problem during a 2-week period of time between Weeks 6 and 8, when the project ended.

Youths were active participants in this process and formulated several personal, workable solutions. Some of the ideas formulated and projects completed included the following:

- Starting a petition signed by community youths and adults to voice concerns about the number of liquor stores in the community, especially near schools

- Recycling cans and other products to reduce the waste on the streets

- Volunteering to help the elderly in their community with their chores

- Advising friends not to "hang out on corners" and to "avoid getting into drugs"

- Keeping the streets clean

- Telling girls to walk with someone to prevent being raped

- Joining a group that helps the earth, "clean up my own yard," and recycle

During the final session, youths were encouraged to continue their involvement in community projects. In many instances, youths in inner cities may feel powerless in the face of seemingly unsurmountable problems. The 3-Cs project highlighted the benefit of youths' training to create caring communities. The project also helped youths to realize that there were small workable solutions to many problems, within their power to perform. Adult sponsorship through coalition building will do much to strengthen such programs in the future. Participants were awarded certificates for their involvement in the 3-Cs Project.

DISCUSSION

This case study describes community health nurses' role in building coalitions with a local church and community teens to develop and implement specific programs for youths in an inner-city community. The case study points to the possibilities inherent in building coalitions among (a) community health nurses from diverse ethnic backgrounds, educational levels, and practice settings; (b) churches and community health nurses; and (c) community health nurses and inner-city youths who are not usually accessible through community agencies.

The case study also points to the influential role of the church in local communities. As the focal point and center of many urban communities, the church can serve as the bridge for the assessment, problem identification, planning, and implementation of many health promotion programs. It means that community health nurses must consider nontraditional settings to meet the diverse health, educational, and social needs of youths in the 21st century, such as the church in urban settings. This case study exemplifies the need for community health nurses to be partners with local churches and community residents in designing and implementing these needed programs.

REFERENCES

American Association of University Women. (1981). *Community action tool catalog: Techniques and strategies for successful community action programs*. Washington, DC: Author.

Bracht, N. (1990). *Health promotion at the community level*. Newbury Park, CA: Sage.

Chavis, D. (1995). Building community capacity to prevent violence through coalitions and partnerships. *Journal of Health Care for the Poor and Underserved, 6,* 234-245.

Cohen, L., Baer, N., & O'Keefe, K. (1991). *Developing effective coalitions: An eight step guide*. Contra Costa, CA: Contra Costa County Health Services Department.

Cooley, C. H. (1902). *Human nature and social orders*. New York: Scribner's.

Cottrell, L. S. (1976). The competent community. In B. H. Kaplan, R. Wilson, & A. H. Leighton (Eds.), *Further explorations in social psychiatry*. New York: Basic Books.

Dahl, S., Gustafson, C., & McCullagh, M. (1993). Collaborating to develop a community-based health service for rural homeless persons. *Journal of Nursing Administration, 23*(4), 41-45.

Davidson, L., Durkin, M., Kuhn, L., O'Connor, P., Barlow, B., & Heagarty, M. (1994). The impact of the Safe Kid/Healthy Neighborhoods Injury Prevention Program in Harlem, 1988 through 1991. *American Journal of Public Health, 84,* 580-586.

Dluhy, M. J. (1990). *Building coalitions in the human services*. Newbury Park, CA: Sage.

Elder, J., Sallis, J., Mayer, J., Hammond, N., & Peplinski, S. (1989). Community-based health promotion: A survey of churches, labor unions, supermarkets, and restaurants. *Journal of Community Health, 14,* 159-168.

Eng, E., & Parker, E. (1994). Measuring community competence in the Mississippi Delta: The interface between program evaluation and empowerment. *Health Education Quarterly, 21,* 199-220.

Eng, E., Salmon, M., & Mullan, F. (1992). Community empowerment: The critical base for primary health care. *Community Health, 15*(1), 1-12.

Florin, P., & Wandersman, A. (1990). An introduction to citizen participation, voluntary organizations, and community development: Insights for empowerment through research. *American Journal of Community Psychology, 18*(1), 41-54.

Flynn, B., & Rains, J. W. (1990). Establishing community coalitions for prevention: Healthy cities Indiana. In R. Knollmueller (Ed.), *Prevention across the life span: Healthy people for the twenty first century.* New York: American Nurses Association.

Flynn, B., Ray, D. W., & Rider, M. S. (1994). Empowering communities: Action research through healthy cities. *Health Education Quarterly, 21,* 395-405.

Freire, P. (1973). *Education for critical consciousness.* New York: Seabury.

Gerschick, T. J., Israel, B. A., & Checkoway, B. N. (1990). *Means of empowerment in individuals, organizations, and communities: Report on a retrieval conference.* Ann Arbor: University of Michigan, Program on Conflict Management Alternatives.

Israel, B. A., Checkoway, B., Schulz, A., & Zimmerman, M. (1994). Health education and community empowerment: Conceptualizing and measuring perceptions of individuals, organizations, and community control. *Health Education Quarterly, 21,* 149-170.

Kent, J. (1970). *A descriptive approach to a community clinic.* Unpublished report, Denver, CO.

Kreisberg, S. (1992). *Transforming power: Domination, empowerment and education.* New York: State University of New York Press.

Lacey, L., Turkes, S., Manfredi, C., & Warnecke, R. (1991). Use of lay health educators for smoking cessation in a hard-to-reach urban community. *Journal of Community Health, 16,* 269-282.

Leavitt, J., & Herbert-Davis, M. (1993). Collective strategies for action. In D. Mason, S. Talbott, & J. Leavitt (Eds.), *Policy and politics for nurses* (pp. 166-183). Philadelphia: W. B. Saunders.

Mayster, V., Waitzkin, H., Hubbell, F. A., & Rucker, L. (1993). Local advocacy for the medically indigent. *Journal for Health Care for the Poor and Underserved, 4,* 254-267.

Michielutte, R., & Beal, P. (1990). Identification of community leadership in the development of public health education programs. *Journal of Community Health, 15*(1), 59-68.

Meister, J., Warrick, L., deZapien, J., & Wood, A. (1992). Using lay health workers: Case study of a community-based prenatal intervention. *Journal of Community Health, 17*(1), 37-51.

Millar, J. D. (1988). Summary of proposed national strategies for the prevention of leading work-related diseases and injuries, Part 1. *American Journal of Industrial Medicine, 13,* 223-240.

National Institute of Occupational Safety and Health. (1989). *National preventive strategies for the ten leading work-related diseases and injuries.* Atlanta, GA: Centers for Disease Control.

Nelson, G. (1994). The development of a mental health coalition: A case study. *American Journal of Community Psychology, 22,* 229-255.

Poland, M., Giblin, P., Waller, J., & Hankin, J. (1992). Effect of a home visiting program on prenatal care and birthweight: A case comparison study. *Journal of Community Health, 17,* 221-229.

Rappaport, J. (1984). Studies in empowerment: Introduction to the issue. *Prevention in Human Services, 3,* 1-7.

Rappaport, J. (1987). Terms of empowerment/exemplars of prevention: Toward a theory for community psychology. *American Journal of Community Psychology, 15,* 121-148.

Rogers, E., & Shoemaker, F. (1971). *Communication of innovations: A cross-cultural approach.* New York: Free Press.

Rosenthal, G., & Harper, D. (1994). Cleveland health quality choice: A model for collaborative community-based outcome assessment. *Journal of Quality Improvement, 20,* 425-442.

Ross, S., Loening, W., & Mbele, B. (1987). Breast-feeding support. *South African Medical Journal, 72,* 357-358.

Rothman, J. (1970). Three models of community organization practice. In F. M. Cox & J. E. Trotman (Eds.), *Strategies of community organization* (pp. 20-36). Itasca, IL: F. E. Peacock.

Shipley, R., Orleans, C., Wilbur, C., Piserchia, P., & McFadden, D. (1988). Effects of the Johnson & Johnson Live for Life program on employee smoking. *Preventive Medicine, 17,* 25-34.

Simons-Morten, D., Simons-Morten, B., Parcel, G., & Bunker, J. (1988). Influencing personal and environmental conditions for community health: A multilevel intervention model. *Family and Community Health, 11*(2), 25-35.

Smith, E. (1989). The role of black churches in supporting compliance with antihypertensive regimens. *Public Health Nursing, 6,* 212-217.

Stunkard, A., Cohen, R., & Felix, M. (1989). Weight loss competitions at the worksite: How they work and how well. *Preventive Medicine, 18,* 460-474.

Statistical Abstracts of the U.S. (114th ed.). (1994). Washington, DC: Government Printing Office.

Sung, J., Coates, R., Williams, J., Liff, J., Greenberg, R., McGrady, G., Avery, B., & Blumenthal, D. (1992). Cancer screening intervention among black women in inner-city Atlanta: Design of a study. *Public Health Reports, 107,* 381-388.

Swift, C., & Levin, G. (1987). Empowerment: An emerging mental health technology. *Journal of Primary Prevention, 8,* 71-94.

Wallerstein, N. (1992). Powerlessness, empowerment, and health: Implications for health promotion programs. *Health Promotion, 6,* 197-205.

World Health Organization. (1978). *Alma-Alta 1978 primary health care.* Geneva: Author.

Zerwekh, J. V. (1992). The practice of empowerment and coercion by expert public health nurses. *Image: Journal of Nursing Scholarship, 24,* 101-105.

Zimmerman, M. (1990, Autumn). Citizen participation in rural health: A promised resource. *Journal of Public Health Policy,* pp. 323-340.

Zimmerman, M., & Rappaport, J. (1988). Citizen participation, perceived control, and psychological empowerment. *American Journal of Community Psychology, 16,* 725-749.

CHAPTER 12

COMMUNITY INTERVENTIONS
Nursing Centers, Mass Clinics, Partnerships, and School Services

OBJECTIVES

1. Define nursing centers.

2. Discuss the types of nursing centers and services offered.

3. Discuss the establishment and marketing of a nursing center.

4. Evaluate mass clinics as a community aggregate intervention.

5. Evaluate partnerships as an aggregate intervention.

6. Discuss sources and focuses of partnerships.

7. Discuss school nursing as an aggregate-focused intervention.

8. Discuss health problems of the school population.

9. Discuss models for school nursing practice.

In previous chapters, the interventions discussed are appropriate for either the total community or aggregates. Interventions in this chapter are useful with aggregates. These include nursing centers, either stationary or mobile, used with the elderly, the homeless, low-income groups, and other aggregates. A second implementation discussed in the chapter is mass episodic immunization clinics, used with the elderly during the flu season or with school-age children just prior to school enrollment.

A third aggregate intervention is partnerships. These have been established to provide immunizations to preschool-age children, to provide prenatal

AUTHOR'S NOTE: I wish to acknowledge Susan R. Opas, PhD, RN, CPNP, Assistant Professor, School of Nursing, University of California—Los Angeles, for assistance with parts of the school nursing literature review.

care for childbearing women, safety education for school-age children, and for other purposes. The last intervention to be discussed is school nursing services. Interventions with other aggregates may be found in Chapter 4 (on occupational nursing) and in Chapter 5 (on health care for migrants and the homeless).

NURSING CENTERS

Nursing centers can be traced to the Henry Street Settlement founded by Lillian Wald in 1893. However, nursing centers as operated today extend back to the establishment of the nurse practitioner role in 1965. This role allowed nurses to provide primary care to clients and to manage and monitor their health needs in addition to the more traditional roles of health promotion and disease prevention. Nursing centers offer care for aggregates in the community who might not otherwise receive care, such as the homeless and low-income populations. Although providing individual care for these aggregates may not be within the sphere of advanced practice nurses, they may have responsibility for assessing, planning, and evaluating care for these populations.

DEFINITIONS

Various names have been used interchangeably to identify nursing centers, including *nursing center, nurse-managed center, community nursing center, nurse-run clinic,* and *community nursing organization* (Aydelotte et al., 1987; Riesch, 1992). Kos and Rothberg (1981) define nursing centers as "nurse-anchored systems of primary care delivery or neighborhood health centers" (p. 53). According to Lang (1983), nursing clinics are "places where clients/patients receive care that is completely managed by nurses and where education and research components are built in" (p. 1291). Lockhart (1995) says that nursing centers are those with nurses in chief management positions, with nursing staff responsible for client care and nurses as the primary providers of care.

TYPES OF CENTERS AND SERVICES

Riesch (1992) identifies the following types of centers: (a) community outreach centers, which are similar to traditional public health clinics; (b) institutional-based centers following the mission of a large institution, such as a hospital or university; (c) wellness/health promotion centers, which offer screening, education, counseling, triage, and health maintenance services; and (d) independent practice (Aydelotte, Hardy, & Hope, 1988). Some nursing centers are stationary sites in buildings, whereas others are mobile and travel to various locations within a community. Nursing centers are more than a setting; they are a concept of services provided by nurses in practice arrangements in a community (Aydelotte et al., 1987; Riesch, 1992; Sharp, 1992).

Nursing centers offer a variety of services, ranging from primary care provided by advanced practice nurses with distant medical backup to the more traditional education, health promotion, screening, wellness, and coordination services. Some services, such as the care provided by advanced practice nurses, may be reimbursed under various insurance plans in some instances and states, whereas others, such as preventive and educational services, are not. Thus, lack of reimbursement has threatened the survival of some centers. The *American Journal of Nursing* ("Community Nursing Centers," 1992) says,

> Slightly more than a quarter of their [community nursing centers] services were paid for out of pocket while 19% were covered by private insurance and 24% by Medicare or Medicaid. The centers reported that 13% of care provided was uncompensated and that 17% was reimbursed by other methods. (p. 70)

In addition, some practice nurses in the centers, such as nurse midwives and nurse anesthetists, may have difficulty accessing hospital privileges due to state laws or physician pressures.

THE CENTER'S PLACE IN THE COMMUNITY

Initially, staff should determine the nursing center's role in the community. Because the local health department has traditionally been considered the lead agency in relation to community assessment and planning for unmet needs, it is important to work closely with this agency to determine gaps that might be filled by the center.

Community involvement in planning for the center should be solicited early. An assessment of community needs using community agencies and individuals should be completed to determine appropriate services for the population. A community advisory board for the center should be established early. Potential consumers, influential community leaders, and health care professionals should be included on the board. This group is useful for reviewing assessment data and for assisting in planning. They are also helpful in marketing the nursing center and providing community feedback about the services.

Cooperative relationships with other community agencies are important to ensure referrals of clients to and from the center. For example, social services may refer low-income clients in need of care if this is the focus of the center. In addition, referrals may be made from the center to health departments for child care, immunizations, and testing for sexually transmitted diseases (STDs).

LOGISTICS OF CENTER START-UP

A variety of preparations must be made before the center is ready to open. After the location of the center is determined, a needs assessment completed, a community board appointed, and other activities identified above are carried out, staff members must be interviewed and appointed; supplies, equipment, and medications ordered and put into place; X-ray and medical backup arranged; and a laboratory established or arranged through other facilities. In addition, clinic hours should be established.

Often, nursing centers serve as learning sites for a variety of students, from both nursing and nonnursing disciplines. Nursing students may include graduate students in family nurse practitioner roles, community health nursing, and nursing administration. Undergraduate nursing students in community health nursing may also be involved. Nonnursing students may include those from areas such as medical laboratory sciences, dental hygiene, dentistry, business administration, and health education. Coordination, supervision, and evaluation of students is an important aspect of student involvement in clinics.

Research and patient evaluation is also an important aspect of nursing centers and should be planned early in the endeavor. Some of the tools useful in assessing patient outcomes[1] include the "Assessment of Quality of Life in Rheumatoid Arthritis" (Bendtsen, 1994); "Reliability and Validity of a Diabetic Quality-of-Life Measure for the Diabetes Control and Complications Trial (Ware, 1988); "Quality of Life Measures in Cancer Chemotherapy" (Ganz, 1994); and "Quality-of-Life Instruments for Severe Chronic Mental Illnesses" (Becker, 1995). *The SF-36* (Ware, Snow, & Kosinski, (993) is a good general tool to measure the following dimensions: physical functioning, physical role, bodily pain, general health and vitality, social functioning, role of emotional and mental health.

MARKETING

Marketing is another important aspect of a nursing center and should be planned after services have been determined. Marketing is an ongoing process of promoting the center; it assists in making clients aware of and committed to the services of the center. Strategies for marketing may include brochures, television and radio announcements, and newspaper announcements or human interest stories. Presentations may also be made to various local organizations. The most important strategy is word of mouth. Barger and Rosenfeld (1993), for example, found that more than half of the clients recruited in a nursing center were from the recommendations of others.

Interventions by the advanced practice nurse may include primary care with screening, health promotion, and wellness activities for an aggregate (the homeless, the elderly). These nurses are also involved in the assessment of needs for the population, planning of appropriate sites for nursing care when units are mobile, marketing and coordinating plans, and many of the activities discussed earlier.

NURSING CENTER CASE STUDY

A nursing center case study in a southeastern community is presented at the end of this chapter. The nursing leader obtained funding for this project from the Division of Nursing, U.S. Department of Health and Human Services (U.S. DHHS). A fair number of competitive grants for nursing centers have been funded by this agency.

MASS IMMUNIZATION CLINICS

Mass immunization of aggregates may be required annually prior to influenza season, when there is an outbreak of diseases such as hepatitis A, or prior to school enrollment if many children are unimmunized. The advanced practice nurse may or may not be involved in implementing the immunization programs but will assess, plan, and evaluate them.

During a flu season, primary preventive measures may require immunization programs and education about protecting oneself from exposure. Education may be presented by the advanced practice nurse on a variety of topics and sources (see Chapter 9). New strains of the influenza virus are usually present each year, and consequently, new vaccines are developed to protect from these. Those at greatest risk include the elderly, infants, and those with chronic or disabling diseases; these populations should be immunized. The Advisory Committee on Immunization Practices (1993) recommends yearly influenza immunization for health care workers, the elderly, and persons with chronic illnesses, such as chronic pulmonary or cardiovascular diseases; asthma; chronic metabolic diseases, such as diabetes; renal dysfunction; hemoglobinopathies; and immunosuppressive diseases.

Those in contact with high-risk individuals (e.g., household members) should also receive immunizations to reduce exposure. In addition, individuals with HIV infections and those traveling to high-incidence areas should be vaccinated.

Following an outbreak of hepatitis, it is usually necessary to provide immune globulin within 2 weeks to those exposed. This will reduce further diseases. For example, following an outbreak of hepatitis traced to a local restaurant in an eastern city, community health nurses assessed the population and provided immune globulin to those who had eaten in the restaurant during the critical period. The media were used for case-finding purposes and to notify the potentially infected about the preventive mass immunization program. Eventually, the epidemic subsided.

Immunizations prior to school enrollment may also be necessary for unimmunized children. In such instances, if large numbers of preschoolers are unimmunized, mass clinics may be established on a temporary basis.

PARTNERSHIPS AS COMMUNITY INTERVENTIONS

Community partnerships are currently being developed as a way to improve community health care at a time when health care funds are decreasing. Baker et al. (1994) say financial and program constraints at all levels of government during the 1990s have forced health departments to "aggressively seek partnerships, coalitions, and shared resources wherever possible to achieve objectives" (p. 1276). Economic forces are moving health departments away from the provision of individual clinical services for segments of the population, such as the economically and medically indigent populations, while retaining basic population-focused services, such as finding cases of disease in the community, environmental assessment, and interventions (see case study in Chapter 3). Partnerships are a part of this rethinking and restructuring of services. These partnerships are proving successful because the community members and professionals who form the partnerships and make decisions jointly have a vested interest in the success of the efforts to provide care (Rienzo & Button, 1993).

PARTNERSHIP DEFINED

Schuster and Goeppinger (1995) define partnership for community health as "the informed, flexible, and negotiated distribution (and redistribution) of power among all participants in the processes of change for improved community health" (p. 295). They highlight the concepts of *informed, flexible,* and *negotiated* and say the partnership is informed because all participants must be aware of their perceptions, rights, and responsibilities and those of others in the partnership. It is flexible because partners recognize the unique and similar contributions made by each other. It is negotiated because the contributions vary and situations differ, and therefore, power must be negotiated at each stage of change.

Courtney, Ballard, Fauver, Gariota, and Holland (1996) enlarge on this concept of partnership; they say it is "the negotiated sharing of power between health professionals and individual, family, and/or community partners . . . mutually determining goals . . . to enhance the capacity of individuals, family, and community partners to act more effectively on their own behalf" (p. 177).

PARTNERSHIP MODEL AND PROCESS

Courtney et al. (1996) compare the professional model with the partnership model. In the partnership role, the *practitioner* focuses on strengthening the skills and capacity of the partner rather than focusing on the problem; the professional's role is to work with, facilitate, or enable rather than be an expert who does "to" or "for" or serves as a decision maker. The *partner's* role is active rather than passive. Goal setting, assessment, and planning are mutual rather than done by the professional. The outcome is an increase in the partner's effectiveness rather than the professional's solving the problem. The reader will recognize these two models (professional and partnership) as two of the community development models discussed in Chapter 8.

The authors also discuss the partnership process. Steps identified in this process include (a) exploring potential partners, which involves becoming familiar with the community and facilitating dialogue with potential partners; (b) inviting partnerships, which includes risk taking and making a commitment to changing roles; and (c) partnership action, which involves initiating partner actions, working with partners, and evaluating accomplishments.

SOURCES OF PARTNERSHIPS

A wide range of organizations and agencies form partnerships with local health departments, and the advanced practice nurse is an important participant in this process. Some potential partners include public schools; nonhealth governmental agencies, such as for welfare and housing; churches; hospitals; universities; and community-based nonprofit organizations. Partnerships in eastern Virginia have been established between hospitals, private doctors, and the health department to provide immunizations to children, and in Chicago, a partnership was established between four hospitals, 150 physicians, a freestanding community health center, community-based organizations and the local and state health departments for prenatal care and immunizations (Greenspan, 1994). Another partnership was established in New York City between the pediatric trauma division at Harlem Hospital, the New York City Board of Education, and the New York State Department of Parks to deal with safety instructions in schools and on the streets and to teach stress management to school and hospital personnel. This resulted in a decrease in pedestrian injuries and gunshot wounds (Shoemaker, James, King, Hardin, & Ordog, 1993).

PARTNERSHIP FOCUSES

Three focus areas for partnerships of essential public health services have been proposed by Baker et al. (1994). First, providing the community with information from an assessment of the health needs and resources based on a disease and injury surveillance, the identified behavioral risks, environmental hazards, and health determinants. The second area is to lead others in the community in planning and mobilizing appropriate resources. The third area is to ensure that individuals, families, and the community receive quality public health services. Each of these areas is elaborated on in the article. Partnerships are basically a way of financing and providing more services to the community population than would be possible without the partnership. For this reason, it is included as an intervention in this book, but the reader should realize that some liberties have been taken with the concept of partnership as an intervention. The effectiveness of the services are based on the approach used by the partnerships. Many of the partnerships discussed in the literature use a community development (locality development model) to carry out the programs. This concept was discussed in Chapter 8 and is effective in bringing about change.

The role of the advanced practice nurse in community development was discussed in Chapter 8. The role of the nurse in forming partnerships has been discussed by Mahon, McFarlane, and Golden (1991), Wainwright (1996), and others.

INTERVENTIONS WITH THE SCHOOL-AGE POPULATION

From a systems point of view (see energy theory in Chapter 2), a school or an industrial setting is a community subsystem (aggregate of the population), and all of the concepts presented in the theory will apply to these populations. A brief review of school nursing is presented next. Occupational health nursing was presented in Chapter 4. As with other interventions in this chapter, the advanced practice nurse may not carry out the day-to-day assessment of and interventions with individual students but will be involved in the overall assessing, planning, and evaluating of nursing care for the aggregate.

SCHOOL POPULATION AND HEALTH PROBLEMS

As of 1989, there were more than 46,000,000 children and adolescents attending 110,000 public and private school in the United States (U.S. Department of Education, 1989). This is a large population that can be reached at an early age to prevent health problems through health promotion and wellness activities and to detect and correct health problems through case-finding activities.

HEALTH PROBLEMS: MORTALITY

Health problems for this aggregate vary by the age of the student. In 1990, the leading causes of death per 100,000 population for 5- to 9-year-olds included injuries (9.8), malignant neoplasms (3.2), congenital anomalies (1.6), homicide (0.9), and diseases of the heart (0.7); for 10- to 14-year-olds: injuries (11.0), malignant neoplasms (3.1), homicide (2.1), suicide (1.5), and congenital anomalies (1.1); for 15- to 19-year-olds: injuries (42.3), homicide (17.0), suicide (11.1), malignant neoplasms (4.2), and diseases of the heart (1.3) (U.S. DHHS, 1993a).

Deaths from unintentional injuries are decreasing but remain the leading cause of death for all school-age children. The single largest contributor to this category for all ages is automobile accidents (U.S. DHHS, 1993a), and this increases by five times for adolescents. Risk-taking behaviors may be involved. For example, data from the national school-based Youth Risk Behavior Survey in 1990 showed that less than one fourth (24.3%) of all students "always" use seat belts when in an automobile (Centers for Disease Control [CDC], 1992b, p. 111). Alcohol use among adolescents is prevalent and may also be related. Alcohol-related accidents have decreased, but alcohol use remains a problem. For example, the national survey on drug use in 1992 found that 88% of students had tried alcohol by the 12th grade and more than one half (51%) of the seniors reported using alcohol during the past month (Johnston, O'Malley, & Bachman, 1993, p. 45). In addition, 30% of the seniors reported being drunk in the past month. Fires and related burns and drowning are a second source of deaths, but these affect mainly the younger age groups.

Homicide is a major cause of death of all school-age children and has nearly tripled since 1960. Factors related to this cause of death include (a) poverty (high incidence of homicide among low-income cultural groups); (b) the use of or dealing in drugs (U.S. DHHS, 1991, p. 239); and (c) others, such as family breakdown, handgun availability, societal attitudes of violence as an acceptable way to solve conflict, teenage proneness to violence, the number of juvenile offenders, fighting and victimizing behaviors, gang membership, dropping out of school, homelessness and unemployment among youths, and abuse and neglect of youths (CDC, 1992a; U.S. DHHS, 1991).

Suicide has increased in the school-age population since 1960, and in 1990, it was the third leading cause of death for those aged 15 to 19 and the fourth leading cause of death for those aged 10 to 14 (U.S. DHHS, 1993a). Suicide attempts are also high. The CDC Youth Risk Behavior Survey in 1991 reported the following: Of 12,272 students surveyed in Grades 9 to 12, 29% had seriously considered suicide; 19% had made a specific suicide plan; and 2% had made an attempt resulting in the need for medical attention (CDC, 1992c, p. 771).

Children in this age group also die from cancer. It is the leading cause of death from diseases for those under the age of 14. Leukemia is the most common type of cancer among children under the age of 9, and lymphoma is the most common type for those between ages 10 and 14. One third of all deaths from cancer in children are from leukemia (American Cancer Society, 1994).

HEALTH PROBLEMS: MORBIDITY

Mortality is only part of the problem affecting the health of children. Morbidity affects health and causes a loss of school days. The major types of acute illnesses for school-age children under the age of 16 include respiratory conditions, infectious and parasitic diseases, injuries, and conditions of the digestive system. Schoolchildren average 3.8 days of absences per year from these conditions. The number of days lost per year by students for these conditions has not changed significantly for 20 years (U.S. Bureau of the Census, 1992). For all types of conditions, the national health survey reported that school days lost may rise to 5 days per student (Klerman, 1988).

Since 1977, acute respiratory conditions have consistently been the main reason for school absences and account for more than 50% of all reported illnesses. In 1989, 182 school days per 100 children were lost due to respiratory infections. Although the common cold is frequently ignored, it can lead to chronic conditions. For example, Heazlett and Whaley (1976) report that the common cold adversely affects the perceptions and learning of junior high students, and Hendershot (1989) reports that 25% of all children on the National Health Interview Survey stated they had repeated ear infections. Untreated otitis media can progress to hearing loss and chronic ear infections. The U.S. DHHS (1993a, p. 24) found that respiratory problems were the leading caused of hospitalization for those under the age of 9 in 1990.

Because they are contagious, infective and parasitic diseases such as scabies, impetigo, ringworm, and head lice are of concern to the school nurse. Treatment includes finding the source of a particular case to prevent further incidence of the disease.

Injuries are also of concern, and according to the U.S. DHHS (1991), they are the leading cause of death and a major cause of morbidity among the school-age population. Although the most common site for injuries is the home, about 21% of all injuries of children aged 10 through 14 occur at school (U.S. DHHS, 1989, pp. 23, 27). One in nine children is hospitalized for accidental or other injuries before the age of 15 (U.S. Congress, 1988) and sports cause more injuries in boys and girls (Ostrum, 1993, p. 335); combined with recreation, sports participation is responsible for more emergency room treatment than any other type of injuries (Verhalen, 1987, pp. 673-674).

In 1990, stomachache, vomiting, diarrhea, celiac disease, appendicitis, and other diseases of the digestive tract were the third leading cause of hospitalization of schoolchildren under the age of 14 (U.S. DHHS, 1993a, p. 24). Some of these were related to psychosocial factors such as family conflict; separation due to death, divorce, or illness; child abuse; poor academic achievement; unfavorable emotional environment in the classroom; and lack of peer support.

Morbidity may also be related to chronic illnesses. Chronic conditions affect 10% to 15% of all children according to estimates, and in 1991, more than 4.1 million (6%) of all children under the age of 19 had activity limitations due to these conditions (U.S. DHHS, 1993a, p. 26). Hobbs, Perrin, and Ireys (1985) and Johnson, Lubker, and Fowler (1988) report that approximately 7.5 million children under the age of 18 have chronic health problems, including diabetes, cystic fibrosis, muscular dystrophy, seizure disorders, hemophilia, asthma, and spina bifida; 10% to 15% of these are classified as severe. The number of disabled children has almost tripled since 1960 (Yates, 1994). The leading causes of chronic illnesses among children under the age of 18 were hay fever or allergies without asthma, chronic sinusitis, chronic bronchitis, asthma, dermatitis, and orthopedic impairments (Collins, 1993).

OTHER HEALTH CONCERNS

Other health concerns have to do with inadequate nutrition, visual and hearing problems, drug use, and teenage pregnancy. Although there is less undernutrition in schoolchildren than in the past, there is more overnutrition and food imbalances due to foods consumed with high sugar, fat, and salt content. Obesity is a major problem.

Visual and hearing problems are common. One in 500 children is partially sighted (Lovato, 1990), and up to 20% have myopia (Committee on Vision, 1989). Of schoolchildren, 6% have hearing losses, and close to 1% are diagnosed as legally deaf (Northern & Downs, 1989).

Alcohol is the prime drug used by adolescents, but alcohol and other drug use have both declined. For example, among high school seniors in 1993, 51% reported drinking alcohol during the past month compared with 63.9% who reported daily drinking in 1988. In 1993, 21.5% reported five or more drinks at one time during the previous 2 weeks compared with 24.7% in 1988 (U.S. DHHS, 1993b, 1994). Marijuana and cocaine use also decreased during this time. Marijuana use dropped from 18% in 1977 to 15.5% in 1993, and cocaine use dropped from 3.4% in 1988 to 1.3% in 1993 (U.S. DHHS, 1993b, 1994). Despite this decrease in drug use among high school students, there is increased drug use among younger students. For example, daily drinking among eighth graders showed an increase from 25.1% in 1988 to 26.2% in 1993; marijuana use was at 5.1%, and cocaine use was at 0.7% in 1993 (U.S. DHHS, 1993b, 1994).

Teenage pregnancy and STDs are other important health concerns among school-age students. Recurrent sexual activity among teenagers increased rapidly during the 1970s and has remained around 46% since 1980 (Forrest & Fordyce, 1988). Sexual activity increases with age in the school-age population, and between the ages of 15 and 17, 50% of all males and 33% of females are active; by age 19, 80% of the males and 70% of the females are active ("Health Objectives," 1992; Zelnik & Kantner, 1978). In America, 1 in 10 of 15- to 19-year-old female students becomes pregnant each year compared to 1 in 20 in Canada, England, and France (U.S. DHHS, 1989). Between 1973 and 1984, the pregnancy rate for adolescents increased by 20% from 82.1 to 109 per 1,000 population (Alan Guttmacher Institute, 1986; Hayes, 1987). In addition, STDs affect 2.5 million teenagers in the United States each year, and 75% of all STDs are reported among 15- to 24-year-old Americans. By 1993, there were 456 cases of AIDS in adolescents between 13 and 19 years of age, and the prevalence of HIV infections was rising (Coupey & Klerman, 1992).

HEALTHY PEOPLE 2000 OBJECTIVES

Recognizing the extent of health problems in the school-age population, *Healthy People 2000* (U.S. DHHS, 1991) addresses some of these. This document advocates (a) education to prevent HIV infections and STDs; prevent the use of alcohol, drugs, and tobacco; and prevent injuries; (b) increased nutritional education; and (c) education about human sexuality and nonviolent ways to resolve conflict. The document also includes objectives for expanding immunization laws, reducing the risk of multiproblem behavior and poor mental health and physical health, and providing for dental screening and follow-up. Objectives for each area are included.

SCHOOL NURSING PROGRAM

DEFINITION

The school nurse is defined by the National Association of School Nurses (NASN, 1994) as one who "provides physical care for acute and chronically ill students; assesses for potential or actual health impairments; manages student medications; counsels students, families, and staff; and serves as liaison with community health resources, among numerous other responsibilities" (p. 1).

CONCEPTUAL FRAMEWORKS

Four major conceptual frameworks for school health nursing will be discussed briefly here. These were developed by Wold (1981), the NASN (Proctor, Lordi, & Zaiger, 1993), Nader (1990), and Rustia (1982). The Wold (1981) framework is the oldest school nursing model and was developed to assist nurses in the organization of their work. Five interacting concepts supporting school nursing activities were developed: public health, adaptation, helping relationships, tools, and systematic process. The central concept, school nursing, says school nurses are public health nurses who provide primary, secondary, and tertiary care to an inclusive community. The school is seen as a subsystem of the total community in which the nurse provides distributive rather than episodic care. Wold assumes that the care is effective and says outcomes for the nurse and client are positive when nurses use a helping relationship and systematically apply nursing tools such as nursing process and health assessment to assist adaptive clients over long-term situations.

The NASN model (Proctor et al., 1993) is the current practice model for school nursing. In this model, school nursing roles are conceptualized as an umbrella over 10 school nurse practice standards that fall under six role concepts:

1. Provider of student health care with standards for clinical knowledge, special health needs of students, and nursing process
2. Communicator with standards for communication
3. Planner and coordinator of student health care with standards for collaboration with community health systems, collaboration within the school health system, and program management
4. Investigator with standards for research
5. Teacher with standards for health education
6. Having a role within the discipline of nursing with standards for professional development

Guidelines for the implementation of the six roles to achieve the standards of care were included. This model was developed using literature written by nurses and those from other disciplines.

The Nader (1990) model uses the three constructs of school nursing—service, education, and environment. This problem-solving model has a triangle with the student's health status and educational achievement at the apex. Other aspects of the model are factors that influence the student's health and learning: (a) family and friends, (b) agencies and programs in the school and community, and (c) media influences about health and education that may be positive or negative. Five steps of the model's intervention plan relate to the service, education, and environment constructs.

The basic message of the model is that resources are limited and the best health and educational outcomes are achieved when families, the school, and the community cooperate in planning programs and providing services.

Rustia's (1982) model is a health promotion model that proposes a comprehensive program to promote optimal health, which influences the learning process. At the center of the model is the school health triad of service, education, and environment. The model provides a framework for a team approach by organizing a link between health services and school personnel and between administrators, teachers, and maintenance staff, with the nurse serving as the school health services administrator. The model also links the school with families and the community through services that meet student's health-related needs.

SCHOOL HEALTH NURSING SERVICES

Three basic components to a school nursing program are identified in the models above: (a) health services, (b) health education, and (c) a healthy environment.

Health Services. Health services provided by nurses in schools usually include screening, treatment of minor problems, medication administration, case finding and case management, immunization level surveillance, and primary health care, if appropriate staff members are available. Medical and psychological consultation may also be available.

Screening may have to do with height and weight, vision, hearing, scoliosis, dental problems, cardiovascular risk, tuberculosis, and other specific testing, such as wellness behaviors (nonsmoking, nonuse of drugs, diet, exercise). The nurse's role in screening includes (a) determining parameters of screening, (b) establishing a plan for screening and management of the data, (c) teaching and assisting others to carry out screening, (d) referring identified students for follow-up diagnostic testing or treatment through parents, and (e) evaluating treatment provided and making necessary arrangements, when required, for altered school activities. The advanced practice nurse may be involved in some of these responsibilities.

In some schools, nurses are present on a limited basis, and teachers carry out most of the management of minor complaints. Nurses may teach them first aid skills or refer them to classes at organizations such as the American Red Cross. First aid kits should be available in all classrooms or in a central location accessible to teachers. When nurses are in schools for longer periods of time, physical assessment skills are helpful. A system should also be established for parental notification. In a study by Bowen (1996) involving teachers concerns about emergency situations with children who have epilepsy, asthma, and diabetes, researchers found that neither basic teacher education nor in-service prepared teachers to deal with the care of these children and that they wanted current knowledge and regular updates. The author presented training sessions to fill this need. Thus, teachers may be deficient in the area of health assessment and care that may be expected of them.

In another study that looked at teacher competence in carrying out health promotion in schools in Australia, Thyer (1996) found that teachers lack an understanding of child health issues and health promotion strategies. Teachers also wanted assistance from nurses to carry out this role.

Medication administration may be carried out by nurses or other school personnel if allowed by state laws. It has been reported by the National Council on Patient Information and Education (1989) that during a 2-week period, about 13 million Americans under the age of 18 are on medications prescribed by a physician and 46% have problems with correct administration. Many of these medications are needed during the school day. For legal purposes, medication policies should be identified. Requirements for policies include the following: (a) Medications should be given only with written permission of a parent and physician authorization, if prescribed; (b) meds prescribed must be individually bottled in a pharmacy-labeled bottle; (c) meds must be stored in a locked cabinet, and (d) meds given must be recorded on a record including student's name, medication, dosage, time given, and person giving the medication.

Nurses also find cases of need and manage cases in the school. In case finding, they often concentrate on students with the following potential risks: (a) excessive absenteeism (over 10% of the time); (b) frequent illness or acting-out behavior identified in the classroom; (c) emotional problems or chronic illnesses assessed by teachers; (d) seriously injured or injury-prone students; (e) predispositions to selected genetic diseases, such as sickle-cell anemia; and (f) students with nonspecific complaints frequently attended to by the nurse. Data may be collected from teachers, principals, or from observations by the nurse.

Case management involves communicating with parents, teachers, physicians, and others on behalf of the student's health. Parents are contacted to obtain permission to discuss the student's health with the physician or to report potential problems identified or occurring at school that may need medical follow-up. Teachers are contacted about health problems or conditions of students that require special consideration during the school day.

Immunization surveillance is an important aspect of school nursing. Most students are required to complete an immunization series prior to school enrollment, and in some instances a booster during adolescence may be required. Frequently, immunizations are required for diphtheria/tetanus, measles, mumps, polio, pertussis, and rubella. A procedure is needed to evaluate the immunization status of students; to exclude those who are unimmunized, if appropriate; and to provide truancy notification if immunizations are not obtained and the child is not returned to school within a reasonable time. As with other school nursing tasks, the advanced practice nurse will not be involved in the day-to-day operation of the program but may assist the school nurse in (a) establishing a plan for immunization surveillance and procedures, (b) evaluating changes in immunization levels as they potentially influence the health of the population, (c) finding ways to best meet the needs of large groups of unimmunized students (special clinic vs. referral), and (d) other aspects of the role involving assessment, plans, or evaluation of this population.

In some schools, primary health care services may be provided. This involves obtaining health histories, providing physical examinations and necessary laboratory tests, and diagnosing and treating health problems. A referral system for problems beyond the scope of the primary care practice in the school should be established. In a study by Chen, Fitzgerald, DeStefano, and Chen (1991), it was found that a school-based, nurse-run prenatal counseling program was effective in ensuring that students obtained adequate prenatal care. For additional information, see discussion below on school-based clinics.

Research Related to Service. Some research has shown that most of the school nurse's time is spent providing service. White (1985) surveyed 403 school nurses in New York and found they provided five categories of services, presented here in rank order: (a) providing physical care, (b) facilitating optimal health, (c) instructing students and staff, (d) giving administrative input to school health services, and (e) keeping records. Statistics showed that 62.3% of the nurses spent most of their time assessing the health complaints of students, and 51.9% of their time was spent providing first aid. Although 57.6% said they were prepared to teach students and teachers, 45.4% said they spent little or no time with this activity. The author concluded that school nurses were not viewed as having teaching or administrative abilities.

Wiley, James, Jonas, and Crosman (1991) surveyed 7 of the 1,056 school districts in Texas and found that all districts reported the following primary responsibilities for the nurse: conducting screening among students, record keeping, and illness and accident treatment for students and school personnel.

Miller and Hopp (1988) developed a questionnaire using California's school nurse standards and surveyed parents and employees in multiple positions in six California school districts. Participants prioritized services that they wanted provided in schools and their perceived availability from a certified school nurse. Screening was ranked highest by principals, whereas, teachers, parents, staff members, and others ranked emergency care as their first priority. The priority for nurses was prevention and control of communicable diseases. All nurses believed emotional health counseling was important, but none of the others agreed. The researchers concluded that nurses need to better articulate their skills and competencies to the public.

Health Education. Health education takes place in a variety of settings and situations in school. One situation involves the informal teaching that takes place when interacting with students, staff members, and parents. For example, children with colds should be identified and kept out of school to prevent the spread of disease to other children. The child and parents may be taught about ways to prevent colds and about treatment of sick children. Teachers may be taught about signs and symptoms of colds that should be identified in students who should then be referred to the nurse or kept out of school.

There is also formal health teaching in schools. For example, a group of obese students might be organized and taught aspects of a proper diet, the role of exercise in weight loss, how to deal with peer pressure and stress that influence eating patterns, how to select foods when eating at or away from home, how to write a self-contract, and other methods to motivate weight loss. This could be taught by the nurse or team taught with the home economics or physical education teacher. Teaching to the appropriate stage of behavior change is important (see Chapter 9). Also, multiple interventions (written and visual materials, lectures, support groups, and incentives) are more effective than single interventions (see Chapter 9).

Health teaching may also supplement classroom teaching. For example, the nurse may provide written and audiovisual materials on growth and development of the fetus to the biology teacher who is presenting classes on growth and development throughout the life span. The nurse may also offer to assist with the class.

School nurses may also provide assistance in integrating health education throughout the curriculum. Nurses may teach health aspects or work with teachers to integrate this material throughout the school years. Wold's (1981) goals may guide this integration. She says goals of health education in school health include teaching students about their bodies and how to keep them well, helping them develop lifelong healthful habits, and giving them the knowledge that will help them make responsible decisions regarding their health.

Research on Education Role of the School Nurse. Hacker, Fried, Bablouzian, and Roeber (1994) report on a telephone survey on school health. This is the only data-based article that identifies a major nursing role beyond the traditional tasks of record keeping, screening, and first aid. In their survey of 33 major metropolitan cities, the services of school nurses most commonly reported were education and counseling, followed by screening services, direct services, and prevention in that order. These results were contrary to all other documented reports.

Healthy Environment. The environment in the school has physical, mental, and psychosocial components (see theory in Chapter 2). Concerns about the physical environment include areas such as sanitation, heat and light, and safety. Some of the factors discussed in Chapter 4 on the internal environment, such as the presence of lead and asbestos, may also be a threat to the health and safety of the students. Other safety factors for schools that must be considered include (a) having off-street parking and areas to release children from buses or cars to reduce traffic accidents, (b) having fenced play areas, (c) being located away from industrial waste and noise, and (d) having ramps and ground floor entrances and elevators to accommodate handicapped students. Other safety considerations in school activities include (a) protection from falls and injuries in sports activities, (b) protection from contaminated water in swimming pools, (c) supervision on the playground to avoid injury, (d) protection from hazards in metal and woodworking shop activities, and (e) protection from chemicals or dust in print shops or other school areas.

Heating and ventilation in a school should allow for a temperature of 68 to 70 degrees with 50% humidity. Because radiant heat from bodies raises the temperature of the room, the thermostat should be adjusted accordingly. Fresh air usually requires an air change of 15 cubic feet per person per minute. Nervous tension and fatigue may result from inadequate lighting conditions, and standards have been established for classrooms, lecture halls, and shops, as well as for doing fine work and for partially sighted children.

Students should also be protected from communicable diseases, overcrowding, and unhealthy foods. Identified problems should be discussed with the appropriate school personnel. In addition, unfavorable influences such as cigarette machines and smoking areas should be discontinued.

The psychosocial environment is also important. For example, stress may be produced by a curriculum that is too crowded or difficult or a curriculum that does not allow adequate time to get from class to class or for adequate breaks between classes. A limited curriculum may also lead to boredom.

ASSESSMENT

The assessment process in the school is the same as in the community, although assessment data may vary. See Chapter 6 for community assessment. The advanced practice nurse will determine the leading causes of morbidity and the major health problems and wellness behaviors practiced by students as a basis for planning. These data are compared with state and national data to determine how well the school population is doing, what plans should be made, and what services should be provided. Periodic reassessment should be carried out to evaluate changes.

PLANNING AND IMPLEMENTING THE SCHOOL HEALTH PROGRAM

An important aspect of school nursing is planning and implementation. Data is collected on the health and immunization status of students entering school and periodically thereafter. Data forms for health and immunization histories are sent to parents and when returned, records are opened or updated. If data are not returned, parents may be invited to school and physical exams may be scheduled. In addition, screening activities must be scheduled and the volunteers and others used in the screening process must be trained.

Defect follow-up of students is another important part of the program. Often, it is necessary to contact parents about follow-up care for defects, such as vision, hearing, and heart problems, identified during school physicals or on exams by family physicians. Information is then solicited from parents on the care provided and recommendations so that school records on the child can be updated and the appropriate school personnel notified. Following this process, records are tagged so that nurses will know when additional follow-up care or recommendations are needed and a reminder can be sent to parents.

Nurses should also be available at selected times to evaluate children referred by teachers or to be available for consultation with teachers. Depending on their assessment, nurses may send referred children back to class, allow them to remain in the nurse's office for a while, or send them home.

Planning also involves the health education activities discussed above. Nurses must arrange with teachers for teaching formal classes, integrating information into the curriculum, and so forth. In addition, nurses may meet with teachers to discuss each student's health during a teacher-nurse conference and may teach about assessing illness and wellness activities and any diseases that are reported to have an increased incidence in the community. At this time, nurses also reinforce special health recommendations for selected students in the classroom.

Emergency care for students should also be planned. A system should be established for obtaining care for students following an emergency. For example, the parent may be notified to pick up the child and take him or her for care; parents may leave directions for obtaining care from their family physician or from some other source.

EVALUATION IN SCHOOLS

Evaluation of the total school health program may be difficult because of the numbers of people involved. Teachers integrate health into the curriculum and supervise students on the playground and in a variety of school settings. They may also be responsible for assessing and referring sick students. Some aspects of the program may be evaluated, however. Health information taught in classes can be assessed on examinations. In addition, following identification of illnesses and defects the care received and the results of the care implemented can be evaluated. Statistical data on numbers of illnesses and defects can be enumerated and viewed for trends. In addition, environmental problems identified and discussed with appropriate personnel and thereafter corrected can be enumerated.

SCHOOL-BASED CLINICS

It is estimated that 20% of the 31 million adolescents in America have at least one serious health problem, such as asthma, heart disease, hearing or vision impairment, depression, or other psychological problems (American Association of Colleges of Nursing [AACN], 1994). In addition, they use health services less frequently than any other age group, and 25% are poor or near-poor and thought to be at risk of teen pregnancy, drug or alcohol abuse, and sexually transmitted diseases such as AIDS (AACN, 1994). Other problems of this age group include motor vehicle accidents, cigarette smoking, and suicide attempts. McClowry et al. (1996) say children from inner cities are particularly disadvantaged by limited access to and availability of health care.

In addition to those who do not use health services, many use the school nurse as their primary or only contact with health care professionals (Feeg, 1991). A relatively recent innovation to meet the health needs of the school-age population is the school-based clinic.

These clinics started in the 1960s, and today there are more than 600 clinics in elementary, middle, and high schools (Robert Wood Johnson Foundation, 1994). These clinics offer a wide range of diagnostic and treatment services for conditions such as respiratory infections, ear and stomach problems, asthma, menstrual cramps, cuts and bruises, and injuries. Clinics are staffed by nurse practitioners, physicians, nurses, social workers, and health educators and may provide counseling to students and their parents. Not every student will be seen in these clinics. Those seen have been enrolled by their parents, who give written consent for care.

The effectiveness of nurses to resolve problems in the schools was found in a study carried out from 1980 to 1985 (AACN, 1994). In this study, it was found that school nurse practitioners could manage 87% of the student health problems independently and resolve 96% of those cases. Most of the needed interventions were within the scope and competence of the nurse practitioner. Cases were referred to physicians when needed.

Clinics may be operated by school districts, primary care centers of local hospitals, health departments, academic health centers, or community health centers. These centers are similar to the nursing centers discussed previously.

SCHOOL-BASED CLINIC IN PARTNERSHIP

McClowry et al. (1996) report on a school-based clinic that was supported by a partnership between New York University, Brooklyn Community School District, and the Brooklyn Hospital Center. Expert nurses from the faculty and student body were provided by New York University to provide care and research capability; the school district offered space and access to students. It also made a commitment to active participation in obtaining parental, community, and teacher support for planning and maintaining the clinic. The hospital provided physician collaboration, referral sources, a 24-hour backup service, its experience in administering-based clinics, and licensure. Overall goals were similar to those discussed above for nursing centers—that is, the provision of service, education of nursing students, and conducting of research.

The authors discuss the patient population, services offered, education offered to nursing students, research studies, current status and future goals, and the practical implications of the project.

Case Study 10

Primary Care Nursing Center

DORIS GLICK
BARRIE CARVETH
SHERRY WEINSTEIN
CYNTHIA WESTLEY

The University of Virginia (UVA) School of Nursing has established the Primary Care Nursing Center, which includes three nursing clinics. The clinics provide direct access to nursing services for populations that otherwise lack access to adequate health care services, provide opportunities for nursing students to gain experience in the delivery of care for vulnerable groups in the community, and establish a setting for nursing research and practice.

The overall objectives of the Primary Care Nursing Center are as follows:

1. *Service:* To provide high-quality, cost-effective primary care services for vulnerable populations in the community.

2. *Research:* To develop, test, and evaluate a model for the planning and delivery of primary care in community health settings.

3. *Education:* To provide educational opportunities for nursing students to practice in partnership with faculty in providing primary care to underserved and disadvantaged populations in the community.

4. *Practice:* To provide opportunities for faculty practice in primary care settings in the community.

The project began with two clinics for residents of public housing in Charlottesville through a collaborative effort between the UVA School of Nursing and the Charlottesville Redevelopment and Housing Authority. The third clinic, a school health cottage, was developed in a rural county based on a collaborative effort between the Greene County Public Schools and the UVA Primary Care Nursing Center. The clinics are organized around a case management model that emphasizes appropriate use of existing health and social services to best meet the needs of residents. The clinics operate collaboratively with physicians, with the District Health Department, mental health services, the local Area Agency on Aging, and with other health providers and social agencies in the region.

Initial support for the development of the Primary Care Nursing Center was provided by combined support from five private foundations. These gifts documented community support for the project, and in 1993 grant funding was obtained from the Division of Nursing, U.S. Public Health Service, Department of Health and Human Services for 5 years for the two clinics in public housing. Space for these clinics has been provided by the Charlottesville Redevelopment and Housing Authority. The third clinic was begun in July 1994 by the UVA School of Nursing Primary Care Nursing Center in collaboration with the Greene County School System. Initial funding was provided through a grant from the Virginia Health Care Foundation, and subsequent funding was obtained from the Virginia Department of Education, Department of Medical Assistance Services. Funding was provided to plan and implement the primary health care model in the rural Greene County Schools.

Each of the three clinics is staffed by a secretary and an advanced practice nurse who is a member of the faculty of the UVA School of Nursing. The clinics operate through the coordinated efforts of the Primary Care Nursing Center using a case management model and provide practice opportunities for undergraduate, graduate, and nurse practitioner students. Each clinic provides services appropriate for the unique target population served. The project is developed around a community development model in which community members are included in the planning and delivery of services (Glick, Hale, Kulbok, & Shettig, 1996). Research focuses on evaluation of the costs and outcomes of these services for vulnerable populations in the community.

Healthy People 2000 health initiatives are used in the clinic to guide health promotion, health protection, and preventive services. *Healthy People 2000* identifies 22 priority areas and 300 objectives to set a prevention agenda. The goals of the initiative include (a) increasing the span of healthy life for Americans, (b) reducing health disparities among Americans, and (c) achieving access to preventive services for all Americans (Burns, 1994). The mission of nursing centers supports this initiative.

CRESCENT HALLS NURSING CLINIC

Crescent Halls Nursing Clinic, the first to be established, provides health care services for 115 low-income elderly and disabled residents of a public housing high-rise apartment building. Accessibility of health services is an important consideration for these residents, who suffer from poor mobility and lack of transportation. Many are elderly and have chronic, disabling diseases such as hypertension and diabetes. Some of the residents have seizure disorders, kidney failure, or heart disease; many people have several of these problems.

In the 1980s and early 1990s, UVA School of Nursing students and faculty visited Crescent Halls on an intermittent basis to take blood pressures and offer health assessments and education. As residents came to rely on these nursing services, it became apparent that what started as an academic site for students had identified the need for ongoing nursing services.

The Crescent Halls Nursing Clinic was opened in 1993 when federal funding was obtained to develop the Primary Care Nursing Center. Services provided include case management and referral, physical and functional assessment; health promotion classes and health screenings; nursing treatments, including foot care and medication monitoring; and individualized counseling. In addition, the nursing center has entered into an agreement with a local home health agency

for the case manager to provide reimbursable skilled nursing visits to qualified clients.

The residents of Crescent Halls value their independence and fear having to depend on others. According to Heine (1992), older adults define their health in relation to their ability to do things for themselves. Interaction of functional health, economic resources, and support systems is necessary for independent living. The nurse case manager helps to promote wellness activities and identifies when to access medical care. The goal of the services is to assist residents in attaining and maintaining their optimal level of physical, social, and psychological health.

Carey (1996) lists the roles of a case manager as these:

- *Facilitator*—supports all parties to work toward mutual goals

- *Liaison*—provides a formal communication link between all parties concerning the plan of care

- *Coordinator*—arranges, regulates, and coordinates needed health care services for clients at all necessary points of services

- *Broker*—acts as an agent for provider services that are needed by clients to stay within coverage according to budget and cost limits of health care plan

- *Educator*—educates client, family, and providers about case management process, delivery system, community health resources, and benefit coverage so that informed decisions can be made by all parties

- *Negotiator*—negotiates the plan of care, services, and payment arrangements with providers, uses effective collaboration and team strategies

- *Monitor/reporter*—provides information to parties on status of situations affecting patient safety, care quality, and patient outcome and on factors that alter costs and liability

- *Advocate*—acts as advocate, provides information, and supports benefit changes that assist member, family, primary care provider, and capitated systems (p. 359)

The case of Mrs. A. illustrates how these roles are integrated into the process of case management at the Crescent Halls Nursing Clinic. Mrs. A. is a 68-year-old, morbidly obese black woman who lives alone at Crescent Halls. She has no children and relies on a cousin who calls daily and comes once a week to help with groceries. She was originally referred to the clinic for a home visit in March 1994 by her physician and social services when she was newly diagnosed with diabetes. The nurse case manager was asked to provide diabetes education and medication monitoring.

A holistic assessment was carried out using the clinic's comprehensive assessment tool, and a home safety evaluation was carried out using a standardized tool. Mrs. A.'s one-bedroom, one-bathroom, handicapped-accessible apartment was dirty, cluttered, and bug infested. Arrangements were made for the client to receive personal care services from the local Area Agency on Aging, and slowly the environment improved (coordinator role).

The nurse taught Mrs. A. about diabetes management and self-care (educator role). Mrs. A was given a medication box that was filled weekly, and she was counseled about the reason for taking each medication. Her medication compliance was monitored and reported to the physician (monitor/reporter role). Arrangements were made for Mrs. A. to attend the local adult day health care center, which provided her social stimulation (broker role).

In April, Mrs. A. had a stroke. She was hospitalized and sent to a nursing home for physical therapy. The clinic's nurse case manager worked with hospital and nursing home social workers to assist with discharge planning (coordinator role). In July, Mrs. A. returned to her apartment with home health nursing and personal care assistance; however, she was eager to return to her usual independence as soon as possible. Mrs. A. expressed only a rudimentary understanding of her disease processes. Her fasting and random blood sugars were consistently elevated, although her hypertension was controlled by her medication regimen. She had decreased use of her left hand and needed a cane for ambulation. She expressed an understanding of an appropriate diet, but a survey of the kitchen and a 24-hour diet recall revealed that she was not consistently following a 2,000 calorie American Diabetic Association diet.

Mrs. A's apartment was thoroughly cleaned and organized to promote safe ambulation. Her

telephone was programmed for frequently used numbers, and she was able to use it independently. Her bathroom grab bars were deemed adequate, but she expressed fear of being alone. Arrangements were made for a home health aide to assist her with bathing, housekeeping, and meal preparation. With these services in place, the nurse case manager was able to support Mrs. A.'s wish to live in her apartment surrounded by her community of friends (advocate role).

Physical assessment at this time revealed that Mrs. A. was 75 pounds above the recommended weight for her height. She demonstrated decreased sensation in her lower extremities. Functional assessment was done to define her ability to perform activities of daily living and instrumental activities of daily living. A nutritional assessment was carried out using guidelines from the nutrition screening initiative, "DETERMINE" Your Nutritional Health (Cope, 1994). Based on the assessments performed, the following nursing diagnoses were determined:

- Knowledge deficit related to lack of understanding of diabetes, hypertension, and cerebrovascular accidents and treatment
- Alternation of nutrition: more than bodily requirements related to caloric intake in excess of energy requirements
- Potential for injury related to sensory-perceptual alteration: tactile, related to diabetic neuropathy
- Self-care deficit: bathing and hygiene, dressing and grooming related to sensory-perceptual and motor deficits

Based on these nursing diagnoses, the nurse case manager and client worked together to set the following goals for healthful (facilitator role):

- Mrs. A. will demonstrate a basic understanding of diabetes, its effect on body systems, and the signs and symptoms of complications and maximize glucose homeostasis and minimize long-term diabetic complications.
- Mrs. A. will verbalize the importance of and demonstrate the use of appropriate diet and the relationship between activity level and weight.

- Mrs. A. will verbalize the importance and demonstrate healthy, independent self-care and foot care and identify the signs and symptoms of peripheral neuropathies.

The nurse case manager taught Mrs. A. about insulin preparation and administration; name, purpose, dose, and frequency of each medication; signs and symptoms of disease processes; home safety; and relaxation techniques. The nurse will monitor the outcome of interventions and alter the plan accordingly. Activities for Mrs. A. to achieve included demonstrating an understanding of risk factors, diet, medication, and reportable signs and symptoms; preventing injuries to extremities; attending arm chair exercise and weight management classes at the clinic; and returning to the day program twice a week.

Currently, Mrs. A. is seen weekly by the nurse case manager to fill her medication box and monitor her condition. She independently manages her blood sugar monitoring and insulin administration. She takes NPH insulin and uses regular insulin on a sliding scale. Because her vision remains poor, the nurse case manager fills NPH syringes for daily administration and places syringes with an assortment of doses of regular insulin in separate plastic bags for Mrs. A. to use as indicated according to her sliding scale.

Mrs. A. comes to the clinic once a month for foot and nail care. Her cousin helps her with weekly grocery shopping and provides daily emotional support by telephone. When she first returned home from the hospital, Mrs. A. received a hot lunch daily from Meals on Wheels. Now she is able to use the local transportation system for the handicapped to go to the adult day care center for a daily hot meal. She is mostly independent with her activities of daily living, and three times a week she receives 2 hours of personal care assistance from the local Area Agency on Aging.

The nurse case manager sends a clinic-specific tool, the "Physician Communication Form," with Mrs. A. when she sees her physician once a month. This means of communication with her physician provides him with up-to-date information about recent blood sugar results and any changes in her health status. In addition, the tool provides a means for the physician to communicate with the nurse case manager about any changes in the plan or providers of care (liaison role).

Mrs. A.'s care is augmented each semester by fourth-year community health nursing students. In working with Mrs. A., the students apply theory learned in the classroom, develop an assessment and care plan, and have the opportunity to put creative interventions into practice.

The case of Mrs. A. illustrates the application of case management within a community nursing center. It documents how appropriate coordination and use of resources can effectively help individuals to attain their optimal level of functioning and well-being in an independent-living environment. It also demonstrates one of the biggest rewards for this challenging role: that small functional improvements can make a big difference in the life of an individual.

WESTHAVEN NURSING CLINIC

The Westhaven Nursing Clinic provides health care services for residents of a low-income, public housing neighborhood in downtown Charlottesville. Westhaven houses 450 people who are immersed in poverty and subjected to its consequences—high rates of teenage pregnancy, infant deaths, violence, preventable health risks, and chronic diseases. These travesties are compounded by ignorance of healthy lifestyles and lack of access to appropriate health care. Turning off one of the main city thoroughfares and traveling a short distance down a narrow side street lined with overgrown weeds and rubbish, one's eye is caught by a large, colorful, vibrant mural that marks the entrance to this public housing community. A single street runs the length of the community and is lined with several two-story brick buildings that house one-, two-, and three-bedroom apartments that appear from the outside to be in good repair. The neighborhood is generally quiet for much of the day. Once the children arrive home from school and the get home adults from work, however, the street livens up with residents of all ages playing, talking, walking, or just relaxing on their front porches.

The nursing clinic is housed in a small, free-standing brick building located at one end of the community. It is identified by a hand-painted sign and is surrounded by trees and shrubs that adorn it with spring and fall colors. On one side of the clinic is the neighborhood's community center, which is used by the residents on a regular basis for recreation activities and meetings. The clinic is within easy walking distance of all of the apartments.

When visiting the clinic, one first enters a small, bright waiting area. The walls are decorated with health promotion materials, and a variety of health education and community service brochures are available for clients to pick up. A VCR is situated in the corner as well, always ready for that occasional "teachable moment."

From the waiting room, clients pass through a large office area and into one of two examining rooms. Each room has an exam table, a desk, supplies for providing primary care nursing services, colorful decorations, and more health education materials. Adjacent to the exam rooms is a small space used jointly as a clinic lab and a janitor's closet. Uncomplicated tests can be performed here or specimens collected to send out to a professional laboratory.

The clinic is open Monday through Friday from 8 a.m. to 5 p.m. A receptionist is available during those hours to greet residents of the community who walk in or call for a variety of reasons: a sick child, a school physical, a blood pressure or blood sugar check, an injury, a prescription refill, or just plain curiosity about who is there and what they have to offer. A former resident of the same community herself, the receptionist serves an important role as liaison between the residents and the clinic staff, particularly during the initial trust-building stage.

A family nurse practitioner, who is also a faculty member of the UVA School of Nursing, is the primary clinician. She provides primary care services in the clinic, makes home visits to residents who are unable to get to the clinic, and serves as the clinic case manager. Fourth-year undergraduate nursing students are available in the fall and spring semesters to work with families whom the nurse practitioner has identified as needing community health nursing care and to assist with implementing community-health focused-programs. In addition, graduate nursing and nurse practitioner students spend time in the clinic, taking advantage of the opportunity to broaden their knowledge of the advanced practice nursing role while providing needed services in the community.

Establishing a successful nurse-managed clinic is a long process that requires time, attention to detail, persistence, and commitment. Once the funding has been secured and the physical space readied, all the systems that are necessary for clinic operation must be developed and put into place, including charting, tracking, developing policies and procedures, providing for quality assurance, and setting up for computerized information management. When those tasks have been accomplished, the challenging job of initiating and expanding clinic use begins.

In laying the groundwork for use of the Westhaven Nursing Clinic, much of the first year of operation, just completed, was devoted to establishing a presence in the community and earning trust from the residents. "Marketing" strategies included door-to-door flyers that list the clinic's services, open houses, mass screenings, and scattered home visits by students, all of which have been helpful in introducing the nursing clinic to the community. However, despite these efforts, a number of residents are still not aware of the clinic's availability. Just recently, a mother of several small children who lives right next door came over to see the clinic. She had "heard something about [us] but didn't really know what [we] do." Despite the flyers and the open houses, she did not notice us until a nursing student doing home visits as a part of our immunization outreach program happened to visit her when she was ill. We have found that the most effective means of establishing a presence in the community and earning trust is to be available when the need is there for a resident. When that happens for members of one family, they tell others in the neighborhood.

Another strategy that has helped our clinic to establish an identity in the community has been collaboration with other agencies and providers used by our target population. A letter of introduction to all of the relevant agencies listed in the Yellow Pages was the starting point. Later, as clients begin to come to the clinic, they are asked about other community services and providers that they use. With the client's permission, these agencies are contacted with an offer to collaborate in serving the client. This approach has resulted in referrals back to the clinic, and its credibility with residents is strengthened when people they trust recommended it.

Nursing students have been very helpful in increasing the clinic's visibility within the public housing neighborhoods and in the broader community. One of the undergraduate nursing students' assignments is to visit community service agencies that have some relevance to the families with whom they are working. Each visit that the students make reminds these agencies of the availability of the nursing clinic as an additional resource for their clients and often results in additional referrals to the clinic.

Ongoing community input is essential as the clinic staff continues to develop its nursing services. Although community advisory committee meetings have been sparsely attended, they have resulted in some helpful feedback. More informal and less conspicuous word-of-mouth communication, however, has been a more effective means of getting meaningful feedback from our target community. As trust continues to grow, community input, like use, continues to develop.

Chronic diseases are common among the residents of our target population, most notably hypertension and diabetes. Several residents come to the clinic on a regular basis for monitoring of blood pressure and blood sugar. Most of these individuals have a primary care provider whom they see for routine visits, but those visits are usually spread out over several months and usually do not allow sufficient time for the individual instruction and continuity of care that be can provided at the nursing clinic. The availability of the Westhaven Nursing Clinic in the neighborhood makes it possible for nurses to see clients more frequently to monitor their progress and help them to achieve their optimal health and potential. Nurses work closely with other providers to ensure that services are supplemented rather than duplicated.

In this community of families with school-age children, there is often a need for school-related physical exams. The many young children who are enrolled in Head Start need an annual physical exam prior to each school year, and children preparing to enter kindergarten are required to have preschool physical exams. There are also several older children living in the community who participate in school sports and who need to have an annual physical prior to their sports participation. More often than not, parents do not realize until the last minute that their child needs a particular school physical, and at these times, the availability of our nursing clinic is much appreciated.

In addition to chronic disease management visits and school physical exams, there are appointments for episodic care. Throughout the year, women with gynecological problems, particularly menstrual irregularities and sexually transmitted infections, visit the nursing clinic for treatment. In fall and winter months, the nurse practitioner spends much of her time in the clinic treating colds, ear infections, head lice, and a variety of viral syndromes. When spring and summer arrive, people begin presenting with allergy-related illnesses, minor injuries, and other problems that often occur with outdoor activities.

The nurse practitioner in the Westhaven Nursing Clinic also serves as a case manager, and one case in particular illustrates the impact of this nursing role. Mr. W., a young man in his early 30s, first became known to the nurse practitioner when he presented for the care of an alcohol-related injury. It quickly became apparent that he was an alcoholic, and the staff began to work with him and his family and several community resources to get him into a rehabilitation program. A number of obstacles were encountered, the most difficult being Mr. W.'s initial resistance to the program. Then the clinic staff had to deal with the system's refusal of services for clients who have no health insurance. After multiple attempts and telephone calls, the clinic was successful in getting him enrolled in a long-term treatment program in another city.

The nurse practitioner remained in contact with Mr. W. and his family while he was away, offered support to them, and helped with various social service issues. He did very well in this program from the beginning. Initially, expectations were low because of his history of failed attempts in a variety of treatment programs. However, as he continued to progress, Mr. W. remained sober, developed a network of social support, and eventually secured a job. He reported feeling "pretty well," and we became confident that this time he would succeed.

To the distress of the clinic's staff, several weeks into the program Mr. W. received the devastating news that he had throat cancer. As a result, he had to leave the rehabilitation program and return home to begin treatment for his cancer. The family's need for services from the nursing clinic suddenly expanded.

It has been several months since Mr. W. had surgery and chemotherapy. Through the combined effort of the nurse practitioner, the clinic receptionist, several community health nursing students, collaborating health care providers, and his family, Mr. W. has successfully coped with his treatment and its effects, and he now functions very well on his own. He remains sober and has mastered the care of his tracheostomy. He is also adjusting quite well to his changed body image and speech deficit. He and his family have expressed, on a number of occasions, how grateful they are for the support they receive from the nursing clinic. There is no way to know how circumstances may have been different for Mr. W. and his family if the services of the neighborhood nursing clinic had not been available to them.

In addition to the services described, the Westhaven Nursing Clinic has implemented several strategies for addressing prevention, targeted to the various needs that have become apparent. The most aggressive prevention project has been to ensure the immunization compliance of the pediatric population. Several graduate and undergraduate nursing students have participated in outreach efforts to educate the community about immunization schedules and to identify needs. The clinic has also established collaborative relationships with other community agencies that have allowed it access to an immunization database that helps in monitoring the compliance of our pediatric clients and in providing the required vaccines to our clients at no charge to them. As a result of these efforts, the clinic has surpassed the *Healthy People 2000* goal of 90% compliance for required immunizations for children 2 years old and younger.

The academic nursing clinic model has proven to be an ideal mechanism for implementing community health projects. Mass screenings, health fairs, and health-related classes are all very time consuming to organize and labor intensive to implement. With the help of many enthusiastic nursing students who pass through the nursing clinic, such projects are doable and frequently become very creative. Response of neighborhood residents to different health promotion events has been mixed; for every community resident who is reached, however, some good is accomplished.

During the first year that the Westhaven Nursing Clinic has been open, nearly half of the residents of the target community have registered at the clinic, many families have been assisted by the clinic staff and by nursing students, and collaborative relationships with many community agencies and providers have been developed. Clinic staff members are currently engaged in a door-to-door outreach project to re-

mind residents about their neighborhood nursing clinic. It is anticipated that these efforts will further enhance clinic exposure and use and, ultimately, the community's health.

GREENE COUNTY SCHOOL HEALTH COTTAGE

The Greene County Public Schools and the UVA School of Nursing Primary Care Nursing Center have launched a collaborative effort to develop a nursing clinic to provide comprehensive preventive and primary health care for schoolchildren in Greene County. The project was initiated by three UVA graduate students in community health nursing who were motivated by the belief that healthy bodies are a prerequisite for healthy minds. The nursing students assessed Greene County, identified and documented unmet needs for health care among school-age children, and developed a plan for addressing those needs. Working under the guidance of UVA School of Nursing faculty and taking advantage of the resources within the school, the students were able to obtain grant funding to support initial development of the project. Greene County is a rural community with a total population of 11,593. The total student population is 2,300. Among these children are many with disabilities or chronic health problems, and 529 children are included in the special education population. Greene County is characterized by poverty and low incomes with a per capita income in the lower 10% of Virginia counties. The county is designated as a medically underserved area, and many of the children come from families who lack access to adequate services and neglect health until problems escalate and urgent care is needed. Greene County Schools are unique in that all four schools in the district, including kindergarten through Grade 12, are located together on the same campus. The clinic is centrally located between the schools and is accessible to all of the schools via walkways. The clinic, in its first year of operation at this writing, is staffed by a pediatric nurse practitioner (a School of Nursing faculty member), a secretary-receptionist, and a school nurse.

A typical school day morning begins with the telephone ringing as the health cottage secretary unlocks the clinic door. A distraught parent is calling to make an appointment for her 5-year-old kindergarten son who suddenly developed a high fever and earache during the night. His mother anxiously informs the secretary that she does not have health insurance and cannot afford to pay for a doctor's visit. While the secretary is making an appointment, a health aide from the elementary school clinic walks in with a 9-year-old girl who has a sore throat, fever, and a "strange rough rash" on her arms and legs. As the young lady is escorted to an exam room, a phone call is received from the middle school secretary reporting that a 14-year-old boy is in the school office complaining of "breathing problems" after running in gym class this morning. He breathlessly explains that his "inhalers are empty, but my parents don't have any money to get me more medicine." The student is brought to the health cottage to receive emergency care for this asthmatic exacerbation, and a follow-up appointment is made for health counseling and asthma education.

As the morning progresses, several appointments are made for students who become ill at school. A 10-year-old girl reports that she was sent to the health cottage by her teacher, who thinks she may have conjunctivitis. A 4-year-old preschool student playfully waits with his mother, who has been awake most of the previous night listening to her son cough, seemingly nonstop. A tall, gaunt, 16-year-old high school junior worries that she may have an eating disorder. A high school senior is seen immediately to determine whether a tetanus booster and sutures will be needed to close a hand laceration that he received in shop class a few minutes ago. With the exception of presenting injuries, the appointment times are made around a previously scheduled physical exam for special education that must be completed before the child's "hyperactivity problems" can be evaluated by the school's special education team.

After lunch, the school nurse refers a high school boy who "twisted" his ankle while playing basketball at a friend's house over the past weekend. His ankle is badly bruised and swollen, the dirty elastic bandage wrapped tightly around his ankle offers little relief for his obvious pain. Although concerned that his ankle "might be broken," the student's family had no means of transportation to the nearest emergency room, approximately 25 miles away. As the school bell rings to signal the end of another school day, the school nurse and nurse practitioner meet with the mother of a 9-year-old student who continues to have grand mal seizures frequently at school despite several attempts to regulate her seizure medication. As ways to implement a seizure emergency plan are discussed, a phone call is received from a third-grade teacher who reports that a young student has been seriously injured on the playground while playing after school. The panicked teacher reports that the child is lying on the ground with "his leg bone sticking out of his skin." The rescue squad is called to transport the injured child. Back at the health cottage, the answering machine records a message from a parent needing to make an appointment for her daughter because . . .

The health cottage was designed to meet the health needs of students who otherwise would not have access to adequate care. Several barriers to health care exist within this rural community. A shortage of health care providers and the lack of convenient transportation often gives rise to physical barriers that are difficult to overcome for families with limited resources. Financial barriers are compounded by the fact that many students have little or no health insurance. Without adequate health insurance, families simply cannot afford the cost of a physician's visit and subsequent prescriptions written. For those students who lack both health insurance and a primary care provider, local hospital emergency rooms have been used extensively in the past to provide care for nonemergency illness and injuries.

A primary goal of this school-based clinic is to provide accessible, cost-effective, and comprehensive services to students by bringing health care directly to them. The target population includes students who do not have a primary care physician or other health care provider; however, any student with a signed parental consent form is eligible to receive services. Clinic services are available during regular school hours 5 days a week.

Necessary to the success of this program is an understanding that services provided by the health cottage should be integrated within the present school health program to provide comprehensive care without duplication of basic services. Traditional school health services are provided by a school nurse, who is responsible for maintaining the integrity of the school health program within each of the four county schools. Both the primary and elementary schools have on-site clinics staffed by paraprofessional clinic aides. The clinic aides handle minor injury and illnesses that occur during the school day. The school nurse oversees clinic operations on a daily basis and provides direct nursing care to students as needed.

Referrals to the health cottage come from the school nurse, clinic aides, teachers, and school administrators. Parents and students are encouraged to make appointments for professional care as the need arises. Because the purpose of the clinic is to provide accessible care while empowering parents and students to become responsible health care consumers, parents are strongly encouraged to be with their children during the clinic visit whenever possible. Children who become sick or injured during the school day are seen on an emergency basis, and parental involvement is still encouraged through telephone contact and written instructions sent home with the sick or injured child.

Linkages with community agencies have been established to ensure a continuum of care for those students needing services currently not provided by the health cottage staff. Limited lab services are provided on site, and students requiring more extensive lab studies or X rays are generally referred to physicians within the UVA network, with whom a collaborative practice agreement has been developed and implemented successfully.

The health cottage serves as a clinical site for several different groups of nursing students within the UVA School of Nursing. Undergraduate nursing students have helped with hearing, vision, and scoliosis screenings, and needs assessment data from the community have been collected by graduate community health students for the past 2 years. Nurse practitioner students, along with faculty preceptors, help conduct sports physicals and special education physical exams. The health cottage will also become a clinical rotation site for nurse practitioner students.

Comprehensive primary care provided by the health cottage staff goes beyond simply treating acute illness or injuries at school. Because the clinic is easily accessible to students and parents, opportunities for follow-up care and patient education may help prevent complications from illnesses that previously went untreated.

For example, Johnny T. is a 6-year-old child who has been seen repeatedly in the primary school clinic complaining of earaches and upper respiratory symptoms, indicating possible otitis media with chronic sinusitis. The clinic aide and school nurse have made numerous requests to have Johnny seen by a primary care provider but to no avail. Johnny lives in a single-parent household headed by his mother, who works in Charlottesville, approximately 25 miles away, at a minimum-wage job without fringe benefits. The family has no health insurance, and Mrs. T. cannot leave work without being docked her hourly wage. When Johnny becomes sick at school, he usually spends his day sleeping on the clinic cot and returns to school the next day without having seen a primary care provider for treatment. Johnny's teacher reports that he is becoming increasingly inattentive in class and wonders if his hearing has been affected by repeated ear infections that have gone untreated.

At the school nurse's urging, Johnny was enrolled in the health cottage program after he once again came to the school clinic complaining of an earache. Johnny was given a prescription for an inexpensive antibiotic that would treat both his ear infection and chronic sinusitis. Realizing that Johnny's health problem could be treated without an increased burden to the family, Johnny's mother followed the prescribed treatment plan faithfully and made sure that Johnny returned to the health cottage for follow-up care. With adequate treatment and care, Johnny's health problems were resolved over the next several months. An audiometric screening after treatment revealed no permanent hearing loss, and Johnny's teacher now reports that his inattentiveness during class seems much improved. Mrs. T. was referred to the county Medicaid outreach worker, who determined that Johnny was eligible for Medicaid services.

Providing health care for poor children with chronic conditions is becoming an increasingly difficult task. For families without health insurance, providing adequate health care often seems impossible. The health cottage provides care for children with special needs through a case management process that integrates care provided by medical specialists and services provided by the schools to help keep children in the classroom setting.

Common chronic illnesses such as asthma can be effectively managed through the health cottage for those children who do not have regular primary care providers. Because the cost of maintaining adequate supplies of medications for uninsured asthmatic children can be overwhelming, many children with asthma seek medical care only during exacerbations or concurrent illnesses, such as sore throats or upper-respiratory-tract infections. Often, the poorly managed asthmatic child ends up in the hospital emer-

asthmatic child ends up in the hospital emergency room in acute distress. The health cottage staff works diligently with students and their families to provide comprehensive, preventive care to children with chronic health needs. Individualized teaching and management plans are developed for children with asthma in an effort to decrease the number and frequency of acute attacks occurring at school or home. Children are encouraged to use peak flow meters as a method of monitoring their asthma and also as a way to help them assume responsibility for managing part of their health care needs. Prescriptions for medications are provided along with proper instructions on using metered dose inhalers. In the event of an exacerbation at school, emergency care can be provided quickly at the health cottage.

As we struggle to meet the health care needs of our children, it is essential that both health and educational systems find ways to work together and develop community-based, coordinated services for future generations.

EVALUATION OF THE PRIMARY CARE NURSING CENTER PROJECT

Program evaluation of the Primary Care Nursing Center focuses on studying the service outcomes of the project's three clinics. It is anticipated that availability of services and enhanced access to care will result in lower costs to families and to the health care system and in decreased use of emergency rooms for primary care services. A safe and friendly environment and trusting relationships with clinic staff will result in high clinic use, client satisfaction, and community acceptance. For school-age children, it is anticipated that preventive primary care services will result in decreased absenteeism and length of illness. And for the elderly, effective case management will result in longer length of independent living and postponed nursing home admittance.

CONTINUATION OF THE PRIMARY CARE NURSING CENTER PROJECT

It is the goal of the Primary Care Nursing Center project to continue to develop the model to pro-

vide high-quality, cost-effective community nursing services for vulnerable populations and for the clinics to become financially self-sustaining. Five sources of income for nursing centers have been identified in the literature (Elsberry & Nelson, 1993): (a) fee-for-service, (b) third-party reimbursement, (c) contracts, (d) charities, and (e) grants. Until self-sufficiency can be achieved, the project is seeking ongoing grants and gifts from local corporations and private foundations to support the services delivered by the project. We recognize that we cannot be financially strong by relying on gifts and grants, so although we continue to value these sources of funding, we are currently seeking a combination of third-party reimbursement, primarily through Medicare and Medicaid, and contracts for services. We monitor the development of managed care systems, and it is anticipated that as managed care becomes a reality, it will be possible for the clinics to contract as part of a local managed care system.

REFERENCES

Burns, C. M. (1994). Toward *Healthy People 2000:* The role of the nurse practitioner in health promotion. *Journal of the American Academy of Nurse Practitioners, 6*(1), 29-34.

Carey, A. H. (1996). Case management. In M. Stanhope & J. Lancaster (Eds.), *Community health nursing: Promoting health of aggregates, families and individuals* (pp. 357-374). St. Louis, MO: Mosby Year Book.

Cope, K. A. (1994). Nutritional status: A basic vital sign. *Home Health Nurse, 12*(2), 29-34.

Elsberry, N., & Nelson, F. (1993). How to plan financial support for nursing centers. *Nursing and Health Care, 14,* 408-413.

Glick, D. F., Hale, P. J., Kulbok, P. A., & Shettig, J. (1996). Community development theory: Planning a community nursing center. *Journal of Nursing Administration, 26*(7\8).

Heine, C. (1992). Community issues in the holistic care of the elderly. *Holistic Nursing Practice, 7*(1), 53-60.

NOTE

1. Available from Medical Outcomes Trust, 20 Park Plaza, Suite 1014, Boston, MA 02116.

REFERENCES

Advisory Committee on Immunization Practices. (1993). Prevention and control of influenza. Part 1. Vaccines. *Morbidity and Mortality Weekly Report, 42*(RR-6), 1-14.

Alan Guttmacher Institute. (1986). *Teenage pregnancy in industrialized countries: The problem that hasn't gone away.* New Haven, CT: Yale University Press.

American Association of Colleges of Nursing. (1994, June). *School nursing: Extending primary care's reach* (AACN Issues Bulletin). Washington, DC: Author.

American Cancer Society. (1994). *Cancer facts and figures—1992.* Atlanta, GA: Author.

Aydelotte, M., Barger, S., Branstetter, E., Fehring, R., Lindgren, K., Lundeen, S., & Riesch, S. (1987). *The nursing center: Concepts and design.* Kansas City, MO: American Nurses Association.

Aydelotte, M. K., & Gregory, M. S. (1989). Nursing practice: Innovative models. In *Nursing centers: Meeting the demand for quality health care* (Publication No. 21-2311). New York: National League for Nursing.

Aydelotte, M. K., Hardy, M. A., & Hope, K. P. (1988). *Nurses in private practice.* Kansas City, MO: American Nurses Association.

Baker, E. L., Melton, R., Strange, P., Fields, M., Koplan, J., Guerra, F., & Satcher, D. (1994). Health reform and the health of the public. *Journal of the American Medical Association, 272,* 1276-1282.

Barger, S. E., & Rosenfeld, P. (1993). Models in community health care: Findings from a national study of community health centers. *Nursing Health Care, 14*(8), 426-431.

Becker, J. (1995). Quality-of-life instruments for severe chronic mental illnesses. *Pharmacoeconomics, 7,* 229-237.

Bendtsen, J. (1994). Assessment of quality of life in rheumatoid arthritis. *Pharmacoeconomics, 5,* 286-298.

Bowen, C. (1996). Educating teachers in children's illnesses: A study. *Nursing Standards, 36*(10), 33-36.

Centers for Disease Control. (1992a). Behavior related to unintentional and intentional injuries among high school students—United States, 1991. *Morbidity and Mortality Weekly Report, 41,* 771-772.

Centers for Disease Control. (1992b). Safety-belt and helmet use among high school students: United States, 1990. *Morbidity and Mortality Weekly Report, 41,* 111-114.

Centers for Disease Control. (1992c). *Youth suicide prevention programs: A resource guide.* Atlanta, GA: Author.

Chen, S., Fitzgerald, M., DeStefano, L., & Chen, E. (1991). Effects of a school nurse prenatal counseling program. *Public Health Nursing, 8*(4), 212-218.

Collins, J. G. (1993). *Prevalence of selected chronic conditions, United States, 1986-88* (National Center for Health Statistics, Vital Statistics, Vol. 10., p. 182). Washington, DC: Government Printing Office.

Committee on Vision, Commission on Behavioral and Social Sciences and Education, National Research Council. (1989). *Myopia: Prevalence and progression.* Washington, DC: National Academy Press.

Community nursing centers gain ground as solution to health issues. (1992). *American Journal of Nursing, 92*(7), 70-71.

Coupey, S., & Klerman, L. (1992). Preface to adolescent sexuality: Preventing unhealthy consequences. *Adolescent Medicine, 3*(2), ix-xii.

Courtney, R., Ballard, E., Fauver, S., Gariota, M., & Holland, L. (1996). The partnership model: Working with individuals, families, and communities toward a new vision of health. *Public Health Nursing, 13*(3), 177-186.

Feeg, V. (1991). Disappearing school nurse services: Metamorphosis or endangered species? *Pediatric Nursing, 17*(6), 430-431.

Forrest, J., & Fordyce, J. (1988). U.S. women's contraceptive attitudes and practices: How have they changed in the 1980's? *Family Planning Perspectives, 20*(3), 112-118.

Ganz, B. (1994). Quality of life measures in cancer chemotherapy. *Pharmocoeconomics, 5,* 376-388.

Greenspan, B. (1994, April). *A public-private partnership.* Paper presented at the National Conference on Models for Managing Health: The Realities of Building a Healthier Community, Washington, DC.

Hacker, K., Fried, L. E., Bablouzian, L., & Roeber, J. (1994). A nationwide survey of school health services delivery in urban schools. *Journal of School Health, 64*(7), 279-283.

Hayes, C. (Ed.). (1987). *Risking the future: Adolescent sexuality, pregnancy, and childbearing* (Vol. 1). Washington, DC: National Research Council, National Academy Press.

Health objectives for the nation: Sexual behavior among high school students. (1992). *Morbidity and Mortality Weekly Report, 40,* 885-888.

Heazlett, M., & Whaley, R. (1976). The common cold: Its effect on perceptual ability and reading comprehension among pupils of a seventh-grade class. *Journal of School Health, 96,* 145-146.

Hendershot, G. E. (1989). *The 1988 National Health Interview Survey on Child Health: New opportunities for research.* Atlanta, GA: National Center for Health Statistics.

Hobbs, N., Perrin, J., & Ireys, H. (1985). *Chronically ill children and their families.* San Francisco: Jossey-Bass.

Johnson, M. P., Lubker, B. B., & Fowler, M. G. (1988). Teacher need assessment for the educational management of children with chronic illnesses. *Journal of School Health, 58*(6), 232-235.

Johnston, L., O'Malley, P., & Bachman, J. (1993). *National survey results on drug use from Monitoring the Future Study, 1975-1992* (Vol. 1; NHI Publication No. 93597). Washington, DC: Government Printing Office.

Klerman, L. (1988). School absence: A health perspective. *Pediatric Clinics of North America, 35,* 1253-1269.

Kos, B., & Rothberg, J. (1981). Evaluation of a freestanding nurse clinic. In L. Aiken (Ed.), *Health policy and nursing practice.* New York: McGraw-Hill.

Lang, N. M. (1983). Nurse-managed centers: Will they thrive? *American Journal of Nursing, 83*(9), 1290-1293.

Lockhart, C. A. (1995). Community nursing centers: An analysis of status and needs. In B. Murphy (Ed.), *Nursing centers: The time is now.* New York: National League for Nursing.

Lovato, C. (Ed.). (1990). *School health in America.* Kent, OH: American School Health Association.

Mahon, J., McFarlane, J., & Golden, K. (1991). De Madres a Madres: A community partnership for health. *Public Health Nursing, 8*(1), 15-19.

McClowry, S., Galehouse, P., Hartnagle, W., Kaufman, H., Just, B., Moed, R., & Patterson-Dehn, C. (1996). A comprehensive school-based clinic: University and community partnership. *JSPN, 1*(1), 19-26.

Miller, E., & Hopp, J. (1988). Perceptions of school nurses by school districts. *Journal of School Health, 58*(5), 197-199.

Nader, P. R. (1990). The concept of "comprehensiveness" in the design and implementation of school health programs. *Journal of School Health, 60*(4), 133-138.

National Association of School Nurses. (1994). *Membership report.* Scarborough, ME: Author.

National Council on Patient Information and Education. (1989). *Guidelines for improving prescription medicine use among children and teenagers: A report of the National Council on Patient Information and Education.* Washington, DC: Author.

Northern, J., & Downs, M. (1989). *Hearing in children.* Baltimore, MD: Williams & Wilkins.

Ostrum, G. A. (1993). Sport-related injuries in youth: Prevention is the key—and nurses can help. *Pediatric Nursing, 19,* 333-342.

Proctor, S., Lordi, S., & Zaiger, D. (1993). *School nursing practice: Roles and standards.* Scarborough, ME: National Association of School Nurses.

Rienzo, B. A., & Button, J. W. (1993). The politics of school based clinics: A community-level analysis. *Journal of School Health, 63*(6), 266-272.

Riesch, S. K. (1992). Nursing centers: An analysis of the anecdotal literature. *Journal of Professional Nursing, 8*(1), 16-25.

Robert Wood Johnson Foundation. (1994). *Access to comprehensive school-based health services for children and youth.* Washington, DC: Author.

Rustia, J. (1982). Rustia school health promotion model. *Journal of School Health, 52*(2), 109.

Schuster, G. F., & Goeppinger, J. (1995). Community as client: Using the nursing process to promote health. In M. Stanhope & J. Lancaster (Eds.), *Community health nursing* (pp. 289-314). St. Louis, MO: C. V. Mosby.

Sharp, N. (1992). Community nursing centers: Coming of age. *Nursing Management, 23*(8), 18-20.

Shoemaker, W. C., James, C., King, L., Hardin, E., & Ordog, G. (1993). Urban violence in Los Angeles in the aftermath of the riots: A perspective from health professionals, with implications for social reconstruction. *Journal of the American Medical Association, 270,* 2833-2837.

Thyer, S. (1996). The "health promoting schools" strategy: Implications for nursing and allied health professions. *Collegian: Journal of the Royal College of Nursing, 3*(2), 13-23.

U.S. Bureau of the Census. (1992). *Statistical abstracts of the U.S.* (112th ed.). Washington, DC: Government Printing Office.

U.S. Congress, Office of Technology Assessment. (1988). *Healthy children: Investing in the future* (OTA-H-345). Washington, DC: Government Printing Office.

U.S. Department of Education. (1989). *Digest of educational statistics* (NCES86-643). Washington, DC: Author.

U.S. Department of Health and Human Services. (1989). *Child health, '89* (DHHS Publication No. HRS-M-CH8915). Washington, DC: Author.

U.S. Department of Health and Human Services. (1991). *Healthy people 2000: National health promotion and disease prevention objectives, full report, with commentary.* Washington, DC: Government Printing Office.

U.S. Department of Health and Human Services. (1993a). *Child health, USA '92.* Washington, DC: Government Printing Office.

U.S. Department of Health and Human Services. (1993b). *Health United States, 1992, and Healthy People 2000 review.* Washington, DC: Government Printing Office.

U.S. Department of Health and Human Services. (1994). *Health United States, 1993* (DHHS Publication No. 73-1232). Washington, DC: Author.

Verhalen, R. D. (1987). Other intentional injuries. *Public Health Reports, 102,* 673-675.

Wainwright, M. (1996). Partnership building in a rural community: El Dorado, Arkansas. In E. Anderson & J. McFarlane (Eds.), *Community as partner: Theory and practice in nursing* (pp. 342-359). Philadelphia: J. B. Lippincott.

Ware, J. (1988). Reliability and validity of a diabetic quality-of-life measure for the Diabetes Control and Complications Trial. *Diabetes Care, 11,* 725-732.

Ware, J., Snow, K., & Kosinski, M. (1993). *SF-36 health survey manual and interpretation guide.* Boston: New England Medical Center, the Health Institute.

White, D. H. (1985). A study of current school nurse practice activities. *Journal of School Health, 55*(2), 52-56.

Wiley, D. C., James, G., Jonas, J., & Crosman, E. D. (1991). Comprehensive school health programs in Texas public schools. *Journal of School Health, 61*(10), 446-447.

Wold, S. J. (1981). *School nursing: A framework for practice.* North Branch, MN: Sunrise River.

Yates, S. R. (1994). The practice of school nursing: Integration with new models of health services delivery. *Journal of School Nursing, 10*(1), 10-19.

Zelnik, M., & Kantner, J. F. (1978). Contraceptive patterns and premarital pregnancy among women aged 15-19 in 1976. *Family Planning Perspectives, 10*(3), 135-142.

CHAPTER 13

Applying Interventions in Rural Areas

JERI W. DUNKIN

OBJECTIVES

1. Discuss the key elements of health beliefs of rural residents and how that affects health behavior.

2. Discuss the influence of culturally based mediating factors on use of health services and programming for rural residents.

3. Discuss the use of effective strategies to facilitate interventions in rural areas.

4. Analyze the role of community leadership in health-related interventions.

5. Promote understanding of the importance of natural events as they relate to health interventions.

To apply nursing interventions in the rural areas of this country, one must understand the unique culture. Rural America holds a sense of charm and nostalgia and is a place where generations of families have engaged in farming or ranching. Yet of the total U.S. residents who describe themselves as rural (45%), less than 5% of these live on farms; the remainder (40%) live in towns and villages across the nation. Approximately 25% of the population lives in communities of less than 10,000 (Human & Wasem, 1991; U.S. Bureau of the Census, 1995). A term that evolved within the past decade, *frontier,* is defined as an area having fewer than 6 people per square mile. Much of the intermountain west, several north-central states, and Alaska are designated as such (Bushy, 1994a).

Frontier regions have additional problems in delivering health care, stemming from having a few people living in large, oftentimes remote, geographical regions. Essentially, these definitions (*rural, urban,* and *frontier*) focus on population density but do not consider the cultural variations of the people who live there. These discrepancies result in a multitude of problems for those involved in rural health care delivery, including lawmakers, policy developers, program planners, researchers, demographers, and health professionals, nurses in particular (Hewitt, 1989; Lee, 1991).

Problems associated with rural health services delivery are of foremost importance given that rural residents in this country can be characterized as having relatively high rates of chronic disease and disability compared with urban residents (14% vs. 12%). However, there do not seem to be any differences between the two groups relative to acute illness (U.S. Congress, 1990). Indeed, there is a relatively low mortality rate in rural areas, with the exception of infant mortality, which is slightly higher (10.8 vs. 10.4 per 1,000 infants) and injury-related mortality, which is dramatically higher (0.6 vs. 0.4 per 1,000 residents) than for urban residents. After taking into account expected differences due to age, race, and sex distributions between urban and rural areas, mortality rates in rural areas are 4% lower than in urban areas (U.S. Congress, 1990).

There are other differences between rural and urban dwellers in this country, relative to health care services. The rural resident must overcome more physical barriers, and there are several significant economic barriers, which prevent many rural residents from receiving adequate health care and often outweigh strictly physical barriers. Rural residents are more likely than urban residents to have no health insurance coverage (18.5% vs. 16.0%). They have lower average incomes and higher poverty rates. Although some rural areas prospered in the past decade, other areas, such as those whose economies are based on farming and mining, have suffered a decrease in per capita income. Still other rural areas have been pockets of poverty for decades. These areas of persistent poverty are heavily concentrated in the South, where 88 million of the nation's 255 million residents live and where 18% of the population falls below the poverty level (National Center for Health Statistics, 1995).

RURAL CULTURE AND HEALTH

Many health care needs of rural dwellers cannot be adequately addressed by the application of nursing models developed in urban or suburban areas but require unique approaches emphasizing the special needs of this population (Long & Weinert, 1989). Thus, in the early 1980s graduate students and faculty at Montana State University began work on the development of a *rural nursing theory*. The theory development used a retroductive approach, and data were collected and refined using a combination of qualitative and quantitative methods (Long & Weinert, 1992). This led to the emergence of commonly held beliefs and practices of rural residents that affect their health behaviors and use of health care services. The key concepts identified were work beliefs and health beliefs, self-reliance, lack of anonymity, outsider/insider, old-timer/newcomer, and isolation and distance. These concepts, along with some identified by other researchers (Bushy, 1994b; Dunkin, 1991; Horner et al., 1994) are illustrated in Figure 13.1 and will be explored in some depth in the following pages.

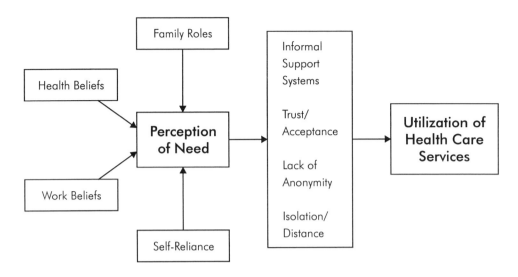

FIGURE 13.1.   Factors Affecting the Use of Health Care Services by Rural Residents

Several of the factors relate directly to the individual's "perception of need" for health care. These are health beliefs, work beliefs, self-reliance, and family roles. Others are culturally based mediating factors that influence the use of health care services: the informal support systems of the family and community and the level of trust in and acceptance of the provider—whether that person is an insider or outsider and how long that person has been known to the community (old-timer or newcomer).

DEFINITION OF HEALTH

Rules that govern one's behavior are shared within a culture, although perhaps not on a conscious level. No one is born with knowledge of these rules; rather, they are learned through verbal or nonverbal interaction within the family and community. The family unit is the first to teach the child about the culture in which he or she lives (Dunkin, Stratton, & Holzwarth, 1992). All aspects of the culture, including health beliefs, are instilled through the primary caregiver (usually the mother) as part of the socialization process of the child (Kravitz & Frey, 1989).

In general, rural residents define health as the ability to work and to do what needs to be done. One can infer that, for them, illness means not being able to do one's usual work (Bushy, 1994b; Long & Weinert, 1989; Weinert & Burman, 1994). In open-ended interviews with 80 individuals, the most frequently stated definition of health was "that you are able to get around and do your own work and enjoy life . . . Be independent" (Dunkin, 1991, p. 9). Many times, comments were made about parents working hard and caring for themselves. In addition, good health habits—"eating right," "no drinking," "get plenty of exercise" (p. 10)—were handed down from mothers and grandmothers.

WORK BELIEFS

The association of work, health, and illness reinforces the rural work ethic. This ethic can be attributed partly to rural people's being dependent on small family enterprises, another characteristic of rural environments. Small businesses, such as farming, ranching, grocery stores, and service stations, generally do not provide employee benefits, particularly health insurance. Individuals' needs may be considered secondary to the family enterprise, which is the only source of income, and lack of resources becomes a major deterrent to obtaining professional care (Bushy, 1991). Other activities often relegated to a secondary position behind work are education (Bushy, 1994b), hobbies and leisure activities (Bushy 1994a), health care (Weinert & Burman, 1994), follow-up health care appointments (Bushy, 1994a), and use of prescribed medication (Bushy, 1994b).

FAMILY ROLES

Out of necessity, self-care strategies have developed over generations of rural families, with women assuming the major responsibility for the implementation and transmission of health care and knowledge. In addition, rural women maintain links between the community and the family through involvement in community groups, including the health care system (Bigbee, 1990).

In the early 1980s, Battenfeld, Clift, and Graubarth (1981) discussed the family role of women as the carriers of the collective healing experience. The "keeper of the health" role of women was a key theme in health-related interviews reported by Dunkin (1991). Mothers and wives were viewed as the person "in charge" of the family's health. This is summed up by one man when asked from whom he sought help when he had a health-related problem. He replied, "It used to be my mother, if anything went wrong I just asked her. Now my wife takes care of all that" (p. 10). Rural women are clearly responsible for direct care of health problems as well as providing advice for self-care (Dunkin, 1991).

Making decisions about when to seek outside help is also a key role for wives and mothers. This decision-making role appears to be crucial within the rural family. Advice is sought about the problem, and the woman then decides whether a home remedy will take care of the problem. If so, she administers the remedy or guides its administration. If not, then advice is given as to where to go for help. This role was best described by one man who said "My wife . . . always seems to know what to do. She tells me what to do and when to go to the doctor. But that's only when I get real sick" (Dunkin, 1991, p. 10).

Good health practices and preventive measures are the responsibility of the women as well. Good diet is felt to be important, and it was very clear that if the food was prepared, it was good for the family or it wouldn't be prepared. Many of the informants talked at length about the need for good food, a balanced diet, and eating the right foods. In addition, the women voiced concern about family members eating away from home (Dunkin, 1991). Comments such as, "I don't like him to eat away from home. I don't know what he will eat. It might not be good for him. I know he can make choices and say no to things he shouldn't eat, but I still worry" (p. 11) were recurrent themes (Dunkin, 1991).

Another health care role rural women assume is that of advocate for the family as it interfaces with the formal health care system. Not only is it the responsibility of women to know when outside help should be sought, but they select the provider, schedule the appointment, and in many instances, arrange transportation as well (Dunkin, 1991).

SELF-RELIANCE AND INDEPENDENCE

Self-reliance and self-help have been identified as significant strategies used to cope with illness by rural persons (Bushy, 1994b; Weinert & Burman, 1994; Weinert & Long, 1991). It is a critical factor in decisions regarding health services use and may lead to failure to seek appropriate help or failure to use the health services after seeking them out, with serious health consequences. Rural dwellers often delay seeking health care until they are seriously ill or incapacitated (Bushy, 1991; Weinert & Burman, 1994). The time line for rural women may be as long as 14 days from the time of symptom recognition to professional contact. This time line is shortened for illness of a child, however. This delay in seeking health care is consistent with the rural population's function-based definition of health (Lee, 1991; Weinert & Long, 1993).

CULTURALLY BASED MEDIATING FACTORS

The rural environment is often considered to be one with strong informal support resources that enable individuals to manage health and illness. A hallmark of rural communities is the ability and willingness to enter into joint activities at times of need, such as harvesting, calving, branding, and family crises (Weinert & Long, 1991). Rural families place special importance on neighbors as sources of informal help, and neighbors are relied on for support in dealing with health problems much more often than are formal agencies or professional care providers (Bushy, 1994a; Weinert & Long, 1993). This network of support resists "outside interference." Clearly, the level of trust among the community members is high, and there is often suspicion of outsiders. Thus, the need for health care services is mediated by the availability of the strong informal support system, level of trust in the provider, sensitivity of the problem, and need for privacy.

The distance to be traveled is also a mediator. *Distance* relates not only to miles traveled but to terrain, weather, and familiarity with the city or area and is always a consideration when seeking health care (Horner et al., 1996).

INFORMAL SUPPORT SYSTEMS

Although the role of informal support systems in health has been recognized since the 1970s, the concept has long been known under the guise of friendship, community cohesion, caring, or unconditional positive regard (Weinert & Burman, 1994). Crawford and Preston (1991) found that the family was an especially important source of support for rural residents and women in maintaining selected health promotion activities. Magilvy, Congdon, and Martinez (1994) describe "circles of informal care" of both healthy and frail older rural adults that include family, friends, and neighbors who provide assistance with meals, household tasks, shopping, personal care, health-related care, errands, transportation, and companionship.

TRUST AND ACCEPTANCE

Appreciation of the strong sense of self-reliance, a consistently described characteristic of rural residents (Bushy, 1991, 1993, 1994b; Horner et al., 1996; Long & Weinert, 1989), makes it obvious that trust of outsiders to the community is always an issue. Long and Weinert (1989) identified concepts related to trust and acceptance in their early work on the development of rural nursing theory. They identified two somewhat interrelated concepts: old-timer/ newcomer and insider/outsider. These concepts are part of the rural-dwellers paradigm related to social relationships.

Old-Timer/Newcomer. This concept is related to the length of time a person has lived in a community. In Long and Weinert's (1989) initial interviews, residents who had been in a community more than 10 years but less than 20 considered themselves "newcomers" and expected others in the community to view them this way as well. Further evidence of this reluctance to accept someone new to the area is the fact that residents will preferentially seek out health care providers who have long been residents of their own community (Bushy, 1993; Horner et al., 1994; Weinert & Burman, 1994). This has serious implications for anyone planning new health-related services in a rural community.

Insider/Outsider. Rural dwellers are self-reliant and resist accepting help or services from those seen as "outsiders" or from agencies seen as national or regional "welfare" programs (Long & Weinert, 1989). Thus, help, including needed health care, is usually sought through informal rather than formal systems (Long & Weinert, 1989). If care is sought in the formal system, it will most likely be from a provider who is viewed as an "insider"—that is, one viewed as a member of the community. It is clear that there is distrust of health care providers, particularly those coming from large urban centers (Bushy, 1991, 1994a; Horner et al., 1994). The provider's attitude toward rural practice can perpetuate difficulties in relating to the rural environment as well as to the people living there. Insensitivity can exacerbate rural client's distrust of health care providers who provide outreach services (Bushy, 1994a).

LACK OF ANONYMITY

Lack of anonymity is a hallmark of small towns and sparsely populated areas. This implies a lack of privacy in the lives of these rural residents. This is of great importance for the residents as well as nurses and other health care providers. The lives of nurses and other residents are closely interwoven. Rural nurses almost always report being known to their patients as neighbors, a part of a given family, members of the community church, and so on (Long & Weinert, 1989) This is true of the residents as well. The nurses and clients know each other through several different social relationships, aside from the nurse-patient relationship. Although this familiarity accommodates rural people's preference for informal, face-to-face interactions, it infringes on the personal privacy of all involved. This lack of anonymity can be problematic for the resident who is seeking care but who knows that the vehicle parked at a clinic or physician's office will be recognized by other members of the community. The choice may be not to seek the care rather than be recognized, either by someone driving by or by the health care provider, who might be a neighbor or family member, particularly if the care needed is of a particularly sensitive nature (including mental health services) (Bushy, 1994a).

ISOLATION AND DISTANCE

Isolation can occur because of geographical remoteness, such as occurs in the upper-north-central regions of the country where there is often less than one family per square mile. This type of isolation often compels residents to be more self-reliant and use more self-care and informal systems to address their health care needs.

Horner et al. (1994), report that when rural residents exceeded their self-care abilities, they evaluate resources to decide where and to whom to go for health care. The greater the perceived seriousness of the identified health problem, the farther the individual was willing to go to obtain care. Again, distance is not limited to the miles traveled but includes the difficulties encountered due to rugged terrain, weather, and other transportation problems.

In addition, there is evidence that some rural residents, particularly the more affluent and mobile, "outmigrate" or "outshop" to larger towns or urban areas for health care services that are available locally, even though they may support local services just in case they need it. Residents who depend on the local services for health care are thus disproportionately indigent, aged, and less mobile (Shreffler, 1996). This pattern of use of local services and facilities will influence the type and numbers of health-related interventions implemented in a given rural community.

STRATEGIES TO FACILITATE INTERVENTIONS IN RURAL AREAS

There is no common culture among rural residents. Within the 50 states, every rural community is unique, with its own special groups, social structures, problems, resources, belief systems, and patterns of caring for those in need. However, one thing is clear for all people, including those from rural areas: The definition of health is a very personal thing and closely tied to family values and ethnic heritage. In addition, there is agreement among sociologists that living in small towns or sparsely populated areas as opposed to living in a more populated area creates some unique experiences for those residents, which appears to be based on similar geographical and population factors, especially in regard to health care (Bushy, 1994a).

CULTURAL COMPETENCE

To provide health care to rural residents, one must be able to work with multiple cultural groups. Multiculturalism encourages the treatment of culturally diverse group members with dignity, respect, and responsibility—the same dignity and respect that any individual receives in a particular setting. Five categories of questions are useful in examining cultural values and beliefs (Locke, 1992):

- *Time:* Is the orientation based on the past, the present, or the future?
- *Human relations:* Are individuals, collateral relationships, or lineal relationships valued most?
- *Human activity:* Is the focus on doing, being, or becoming?
- *Human nature:* At birth, are people considered basically good, bad, neutral, or mixed?
- *Spiritual:* Is the relationship with the spiritual one of control, subordination, or harmony?

Locke (1992) has provided a model from which to examine cultural differences and to enhance multicultural understanding. One can use the model by beginning with self-awareness. In helping relationships with the culturally diverse, it might be necessary and useful for those involved to share their personal experiences. Knowing one's own personal biases, values, and interests will greatly enhance one's sensitivity toward other cultures. These 10 guidelines will help:

1. Learn as much as possible about your own culture. One can appreciate another culture much more if one first has an appreciation of one's own.
2. Work at being open and honest in your relationships with culturally diverse populations. Leave yourself open to different attitudes and values and encourage those different from yourself to be open and honest with you about issues related to their cultures. Attend to the verbal and nonverbal communication patterns between yourself and your culturally diverse clients.
3. Seek to develop genuine respect and appreciation of culturally diverse attitudes and behaviors. Demonstrate that you both recognize and value the culture of those different from yourself. Respect can be demonstrated by starting with the life experiences of clients and not with the one's own.
4. Take advantage of all available opportunities to participate in activities in the communities of culturally diverse groups.
5. Keep in mind that individuals from culturally diverse groups are both members of their group and unique individuals as well. Strive to keep a

healthy balance between your view of clients as cultural beings and as unique human beings.

6. Learn to examine your own cultural biases, prejudices, and stereotypes. Eliminate all of your behaviors that suggest prejudice or racism, and do not tolerate such behaviors in your colleagues or in other members of your own cultural group. Teach your clients how to recognize bias and how to challenge stereotypes.

7. Encourage administrators and supervisors in your agency to institutionalize practices that acknowledge the diversity among your clients.

8. Hold high expectations of culturally diverse clients and encourage others who work with diverse populations to do likewise.

9. Ask questions about the cultures of ethnically diverse groups. Learn as much as possible about different cultures and share what you learn with others.

10. Develop culturally specific strategies, techniques, and programs to foster psychological development of culturally different individuals and groups.

Ethnically diverse status does not diminish or eliminate the responsibility of the person for meeting his or her own needs. These needs may be met within a different structural framework than might be used by a member of the dominant culture or by a member of another group, but the responsibility remains with the individual. Remember, however, that there is as much individualization within culturally diverse groups as within the dominant culture. What might be viewed as a particular style or pattern for the ethnically diverse group may not represent a specific style or pattern for any given individual (Locke, 1992). Indeed, these clients bring with them as many personal beliefs, values, and attitudes as any other clients. From information gained from the 10 elements of the model and using the five categories of questions, culturally sensitive strategies can be developed with which you can successfully implement interventions in these rural cultures.

RURAL-SPECIFIC STRATEGIES

Factors that will influence the effectiveness of any health-related intervention with rural residents were described earlier in this chapter (see Figure 13.1). The following sections of the chapter will explore how these factors affect the application of interventions with rural residents, both at the individual and family level and at the community level.

INDIVIDUAL-LEVEL STRATEGIES

As noted earlier, health care-seeking behaviors are influenced by values related to work, perception of healthiness, definition of illness, and preference of social support systems. It is not surprising, then, given the descriptions of the factors involved in health-seeking decisions earlier in this chapter, that rural and urban residents differ in their preventive health practices (U.S. Congress, 1990).

For example, rural residents are much less likely to use seat belts regularly, which is reflected in dramatically higher injury-related mortality rates in rural areas. In addition, rural residents are less likely than their urban counterparts to exercise consistently, and they tend to be more obese. However, rural residents smoke less than urban residents, but those who do smoke are heavier smokers. Finally, rural residents use preventive services less often than urban residents do (Dunkin, 1993; Weinert & Burman, 1994).

In planning individually focused interventions, one should ensure that the planned health service is culturally sensitive and incorporates the individual's definition of health and illness in addition to that person's informal support systems. For example, when planning a dietary intervention, it might be helpful if it is approached taking into effect things such as hot and cold properties of the food and the illness if working with a Hispanic client. In addition, because a rural dweller's health beliefs tend to revolve around work, couching the proposed change in terms of its effect on one's continued ability to function or work as "assigned" will be much more effective than a discussion of diseases or complications prevention.

The strong sense of self-reliance found in rural people implies that health promotion activities will be more readily accepted when the focus is on improving the ability to care for oneself and problem solving in regard to health issues. Exploring informal support resources with the client may help in addressing the needed care.

Because in rural areas women are the "keepers of the health," working with the wife or mother of the male client relative to dietary changes will be very important. Men consistently report that they eat what is cooked for them by their wives or mothers (Dunkin, 1991), so changes in food preparation and diet will be most effective if the changes are implemented by the "woman of the house." Also, it is important to involve the female head of the household for monitoring of health indicators, such as blood sugar, medication timing or dosage, urine checks, blood pressure, foot care, and the like. It is important to involve her in the plan of care when interface with the formal system will be needed to deliver the care, because she is often the one to schedule visits, do the transporting, and so on.

It is also important to remember that in sparsely populated areas privacy can be a real problem. There are several ways to address this issue. The first is to schedule discussion of sensitive issues, such as stress reduction and other mental health services at a regularly held meeting, so the whole group is given the information, which includes a plan for follow-up (e.g., a toll-free number) for individual contact. The lack of anonymity is an ongoing issue, but with careful thought and attention to the feelings and beliefs of the target population, it can be successfully addressed.

Timing of health promotion and preventive services is very important. Generally, attendance at prostate screening, mammography screening, and so on will be better if the program occurs during the "off" season. These activities cannot compete with planting season, harvest activities, and the like in an agrarian culture. Offer programs to groups at church, club, or community meetings rather than as freestanding meetings, particularly if the topic is sensitive in nature, such as mental health services.

When planning for an individually based intervention, one must consider the level of trust the provider has in the community. When the provider is coming from outside the community, one useful strategy is to have the endorsement and support of a recognized community leader (e.g., the public health nurse, director of nursing from the local hospital, a minister of a local church). Having an old-timer or insider to provide entrée to the clients in the community will do much to ensure participation in the intervention.

COMMUNITY-LEVEL STRATEGIES

For services to be perceived as available, accessible, and acceptable, the target population's preferences and needs must be carefully considered by program planners. To improve the outcome, comprehensive assessments should be done before planning, implementing, or modifying a program to ascertain a community's perceived problems and beliefs about how these should be resolved (Goeppinger, 1993). In planning for a new health service for a rural population, the program planners, who may also be the providers, should consider the following:

- Perceptions about space (e.g., population density of a community, being afraid to drive in a large city)
- Distances (e.g., miles to the nearest telephone, neighbor, physician, specialist, pharmacy, county nurse, hospital, and the local terrain)
- Time and season of the year (e.g., planting crops and doing farm chores; coordinating an appointment to coincide with family business or recreational activities, such as buying machinery parts, purchasing groceries, and attending community or school events, such as the annual rodeo, county fair, parent-teacher conference, or athletic tournaments)
- Potential natural events (e.g., snowstorms, tornadoes, subzero temperatures, and seasonal rain storms)

Considering these factors will go a long way toward encouraging community and client participation and enhancing the continuum of care (Bushy, 1994b).

When working with a rural community group to implement a community-based nursing or health-related intervention, it is important to involve local community leaders in the planning process. Given the lack of trust of outsiders, having local community leaders involved will increase the likelihood of a successful intervention. The health planners should work toward empowering the local community to adopt the service as their own. Community members should be involved in all aspects of the process, from assessment to evaluation. Establish partnerships with rural communities that will actively involve formal (e.g., town council, health committee, farmers unions, and schools) as well as informal community leaders and organizations (e.g., a women's missionary group from a local church) in planning and implementation of services. When possible, integrate the new service into existing and accepted models in the community, such as homemakers clubs, church circles, county fairs, church bazaars, and county extension activities (Bushy, 1993). One formal organization that carries a health-related mission and can be found in most rural communities and areas is the rural electric cooperative. Their endorsement will add acceptability to the planned health programming.

Rural political structures, too, may resist outside help. Resistance is frequently evidenced as community leaders' not providing support for a particular program. Interestingly, the political power in rural communities is often vested in an elite segment of the population that, frequently, is unaware of the needs of local underprivileged groups, such as unemployed men, homeless families, and single mothers. Powerless racial and ethnic minorities, too, may experience human service requirements to which the more affluent and powerful majority in rural communities are not sensitive or sympathetic. Their insensitivity reflects traditional rural values related to the work ethic ("If a man really wants to work, he can always find a job") and the stigma associated with a person or family seeking public assistance ("going on welfare"). Consequently, even when programs are available and accessible in the community, rural families may choose not to use those services to maintain their social reputation (Bushy, 1994a).

SUMMARY

The application of nursing interventions in a rural setting presents unique challenges. In addition to constructing the intervention in a way that addresses ethnic-based cultural beliefs and practices, one must also incorporate those rural-specific beliefs and practices that affect health practices and participation in health programming. The strong work orientation of rural health beliefs implies that successful implementation must focus the outcome of the intervention on improving the ability to work. Self-reliance meant survival in the past century as pioneers settled in remote locations. That characteristic is still very strong in rural dwellers, particularly for those who are geographically isolated. This must be addressed in planning any health-related intervention, either by demonstrating support for stronger self-reliance or as a potential delay in participation.

An individual's family role is an important consideration relative to successful application of interventions with rural clients. The role that women play in health behaviors must be incorporated into any planned intervention. For example, dietary changes need to be taught not only to the client but to his mother or wife, because she will most likely have primary responsibility for meal preparation. She is usually the one to seek care and advice from the informal system of the community and to interface with the formal health care system and can be central to the success of the intervention.

The informal support systems of the individual or group must be assessed and incorporated in a way that facilitates the trust and acceptance of the provider and program. By working through recognized long-standing community leaders (both formal and informal), the nurse can more likely ensure entrée into the community and a successful outcome of the intervention.

If the intervention deals with services of a sensitive nature, such as mental health services, the lack of anonymity becomes of critical importance. Often, presenting information about the service through a group meeting will be received better because it takes the focus off individuals and allows some measure of anonymity. The support of the community church leaders in this type of situation can be critical to success. In addition, working with a nurse from the community will enhance the trust of the community members when privacy is an issue.

Planning of health promotion activities, screenings, and the like should incorporate the seasonality of the community, relative to agricultural timing, weather, or both. In addition, distance to be traveled and the isolation of the rural dwellers should be addressed. Positive outcomes will be much more likely when the nurse works with the client, family, and community members in application of the selected intervention.

REFERENCES

Battenfeld, D. E., Clift, E. G., & Graubarth, R. P. (1981). *Patterns for change: Rural women organizing for health.* Washington, DC: National Women's Health Network.

Bigbee, J. (1990). Stressful life events and illness occurrence in rural versus urban women. *Journal of Community Health Nursing, 7,* 105-113.

Bushy, A. (Ed.). (1991). *Rural nursing* (2 vols.). Newbury Park, CA: Sage.

Bushy, A. (1993). Rural women: Lifestyle and health status. *Nursing Clinics of North America, 28*(1), 187-197.

Bushy, A. (1994a). When your client lives in a rural area. Part I: Rural health care delivery issues. *Issues in Mental Health Nursing, 15,* 253-266.

Bushy, A. (1994b). When your client lives in a rural area. Part II: Rural professional practice—Considerations for nurses providing mental health care. *Issues in Mental Health Nursing, 15,* 257-276.

Crawford, C., & Preston, D. (1991). Differences in specific sources of social support for four healthy behaviors. In A. Bushy (Ed.), *Rural nursing* (Vol. 1, pp. 215-227). Newbury Park, CA: Sage.

Dunkin, J. W. (1991, May). *Health concerns among rural families: A foundation for effective intervention.* Paper presented at the Second International Family Nursing Conference, Portland, OR.

Dunkin, J. W. (1993, February). *Relationships between family hardiness and health behaviors.* Poster presentation at the Midwest Nursing Research Society, Cleveland, OH.

Dunkin, J. W., Stratton, T. D., & Holzwarth, C. (1992). Assessment of family hardiness: A foundation for intervention. In S. B. Neister, J. M. Bell, S. L. Feetham, & C. L. Gilliss (Eds.), *Advances in the nursing of families* (pp. 247-255). Newbury Park, CA: Sage.

Goeppinger, J. (1993). Health promotion for rural populations: Partnership interventions. *Family and Community Health, 16,* 1-9.

Hewitt, M. (1989). *Defining rural areas: Impact on health care policy and research.* Washington, DC: Government Printing Office.

Horner, S. D., Ambrogne, J., Coleman, M. A., Hanson, C., Hodnicki, D., Lopez, S. A., & Talmadge, M. C. (1994). Traveling for care: Factors influencing health care access for rural dwellers. *Public Health Nursing, 11*(3), 145-149.

Human, J., & Wasem, K. (1991). Rural mental health in America. *American Psychologist, 46,* 232-239.

Kravitz, M., & Frey, M. (1989). The Allen nursing model. In J. J. Fitzpatrick & A. L. Whall (Eds.), *Conceptual models of nursing: Analysis and application* (2nd ed.). Norwalk, CT: Appleton-Lange.

Lee, H. (1991). Definitions of rural: A review of the literature. In A. Bushy (Ed.), *Rural nursing* (Vol. 1, pp. 7-20). Newbury Park, CA: Sage.

Locke, D. C. (1992). *Increasing multicultural understanding: A comprehensive model* (Multicultural Aspects of Counseling Series, Vol. 1). Newbury Park, CA: Sage.

Long, K. A., & Weinert, C. (1989). Rural nursing: Developing the theory base. *Scholarly Inquiry to Nursing Practice: An International Journal, 3*(2), 113-127.

Long, K. A., & Weinert, C. (1992). Rural nursing: Developing the theory base. In P. Winstead-Fry, J. C. Tiffany, & R. V. Shippee-Rice (Eds.), *Rural health nursing* (Publication No. 21-2408). New York: National League for Nursing Press.

Magilvy, J. K., Congdon, J. G., & Martinez, R. (1994). Circles of care: Home care and community support for rural older adults. *Advances in Nursing Science, 16*(3), 22-33.

National Center for Health Statistics. (1995). *Health, United States, 1994.* Washington, DC: Government Printing Office.

Shreffler, M. J. (1996). An ecological view of the rural environment: Levels of influence on access to health care. *Advances in Nursing Science, 18*(4), 48-59.

U.S. Congress, Office of Technology Assessment. (1990). *Health care in rural America* (OTA-H-434). Washington, DC: Government Printing Office.

U.S. Bureau of the Census. (1995). *Statistical abstract of the United States: 1995* (115th edition). Washington, DC: Government Printing Office.

Weinert, C., & Burman, M. E. (1994). Rural health and health-seeking behaviors. *Annual Review of Nursing Research, 12,* 65-92.

Weinert, C., & Long, K. A. (1990). Rural families and health care: Refining the knowledge base. *Journal of Marriage and Family Relations, 15*(1/2) 57-75.

Weinert, C., & Long, K. A. (1991). The theory and research base of rural nursing practice. In A. Bushy (Ed.), *Rural nursing* (Vol. 1, pp. 21-38). Newbury Park, CA: Sage.

Weinert, C., & Long, K. A. (1993). Support systems for spouses of the chronically ill. *Family and Community Health, 16,* 46-54.

PART V

COMMUNITY EVALUATION

CHAPTER 14

EVALUATION OF COMMUNITY INTERVENTIONS

OBJECTIVES

1. Define the concepts used in evaluation.

2. Discuss appropriate evaluation questions to ask during the planning and implementation steps of the nursing process.

3. Identify community change outcome variables.

4. Discuss the major components of evaluation.

5. Analyze methods for evaluating programs.

6. Evaluate the outcome variables used in selected studies reported in the literature.

There are several ways to approach evaluation, and these often incorporate both qualitative and quantitative measures of the change process. In addition, cost containment concerns in health care may require programs to be evaluated in terms of cost-effectiveness. Some nurses approach evaluation using a model of structure, process, and outcome factors. Others use a formative and summative evaluation model or a goals-and-systems model, among others (Tinkham, Voorhies, & McCarthy, 1984).

EVALUATION AND THE ENERGY THEORY

Evaluation, the final step in the nursing process, is concerned about whether or not established goals are met. From an energy frame of reference, the question is whether or not the energy interventions were effective in establishing or reestablishing the energy balance for the particular concern in the community. One way to answer the question might be to evaluate changes in the "resulting-in" portion of the nursing diagnosis. For example, using the high infant mortality diagnosis presented in Chapter 7, the resulting-in portion of the diagnosis identified the effects of the community energy deficit and included factors such as a higher infant mortality rate than the state and nation, a higher rate than the *Healthy People 2000* (U.S. Department of Health and Human Services, 1991) goal, and that 75% of mothers delivering were unaware of health promotion and preventive activities during pregnancy. Did the energy interventions directed toward the "due-to" portion of the diagnosis cause a change in the energy deficit so that it is more balanced as identified by the rate's being closer to the state and national rates and the *Healthy People 2000* objectives, and do more women know about health promotion and prevention during pregnancy? If community balance has been achieved in this area, the health concern may be removed from consideration at this time. If not, there should be a reassessment of the problem.

DEFINITIONS AND CONCEPTS

PROGRAM EVALUATION

According to Patton (1986), program evaluation is the "systematic collection of information about the activities, characteristics, and outcomes of programs for use by specific people to reduce uncertainties, improve effectiveness, and make decisions with regard to what the programs are doing and effecting" (p. 14). Veney and Kaluzny (1991) say that the major purposes of program evaluation are to determine the program's relevance, progress, efficiency, effectiveness, and impact on clients. According to Posavac and Carey (1989), evaluation includes the methods that determine whether a service or program is needed and likely to be used, whether it is carried out as planned, and whether it actually helped the people it was intended to help.

STRUCTURE, PROCESS, AND OUTCOME

According to Donabedian (1966, pp. 169-170), structure standards are those that assess the environment in which care is provided and include assessment of factors such as the organizational framework, availability of resources, qualifications of staff members, and adherence to legal mandates. Process standards identify how care should be delivered and focus on reviewing health care provider activities (Donabedian, 1966, p. 183). Standards such as the American Nursing Association community health nursing standards determine if the health care provided was appropriate for the group. Outcome standards evaluate the end result of the care provided. These measure the behavioral changes in clients and evaluate what clients learned, what they did, or the effect of the interventions on aggregate statistics. Many of the *Healthy People 2000* objectives are outcome measures for aggregates.

FORMATIVE AND SUMMATIVE EVALUATION

FORMATIVE EVALUATION

A formative evaluation analyzes the daily ongoing activities and functions of the program and focuses on short-term data collection to improve the program. For example, a nursing clinic might be scheduled at a homeless shelter between 10 a.m. and 2 p.m. If few clients attend, an assessment of the situation may determine that they are all at school learning a job skill or working during those hours. As a result, the clinic may be rescheduled for evening hours when the clients are in the shelter and able to attend.

SUMMATIVE EVALUATION

A summative evaluation analyzes activities associated with the long-term effects of the program to answer questions regarding a change in health knowledge, attitudes, and practices of the participants. For example, following classes on nutrition, the presenter might determine whether clients scored higher than before or were able to select appropriate foods for a 24-hour period. This is similar to the outcome evaluation discussed earlier.

PROGRAM FOR EVALUATION

Posavac and Carey (1989) identify six steps useful for an ongoing program evaluation. First, one should identify relevant people to include in the evaluation process, such as program personnel, clients, sponsors, and community leaders. Next, a meeting should be arranged to discuss whether an evaluation is appropriate and desired or not. If an evaluation is desired, the type and frequency of evaluation and resources for carrying it out should be determined. These discussions lead to the third step, which involves the final decision about whether or not the evaluation will be carried out and which may be an administrative decision based on resource availability or an identified community need. The fourth step involves a review of relevant literature to determine the appropriate methods and techniques. During the fifth step, the methodology for evaluation is decided; the sixth step involves writing the plan for the evaluation.

EVALUATION QUESTIONS DURING STAGES OF THE NURSING PROCESS

Certain evaluative questions should be asked during the planning and implementation steps in the nursing process.

QUESTIONS ABOUT PLANNING

An important question during planning involves the need for the program and whether or not it should be developed. What are the needs of the population, and will the program meet the identified needs? Another question involves the appropriateness of any materials to be used. If pamphlets are to be distributed or if television or radio programs are presented, the material should be appropriate for the intended audience. Issues of appropriateness include accuracy of materials; appropriateness of language and reading level, if printed; attractiveness; whether symbols can be interpreted by the intended audience; and the general appeal of the material. These issues fall under formative evaluation, defined above.

Methods for evaluating the appropriateness of materials include expert panels or in-depth interviews. Expert panels may comment on the accuracy of materials and individuals from the target group may read the materials for comprehension.

QUESTIONS ABOUT IMPLEMENTATION

PROGRAM METHODS

Some questions regarding evaluation occur during the implementation stage. One question involves whether or not the program is being implemented as planned. Because all aspects of implementation would be impossible to evaluate, those aspects to be examined must be identified. This evaluation is important so that others who wish to replicate the program will know exactly what was implemented and how. This monitoring of the program's implementation may include record reviews or may involve creating new types of records for recording the data. Data about programs may also be obtained from interviews with clients or from direct observation of client-staff interactions.

Another evaluation question involves whether or not the program is reaching the audience for whom it was intended. If not, who does it fail to reach? For programs presented at specific locations, sign-up attendance data might be useful to answer the first question. Mass media or other types of programs may require surveys to answer the question. If the resource person knows segments of the population that might have been expected to participate in a program, surveys of these groups might answer the question. Data collected from those who failed to participate might answer questions about their awareness of program, the appeal and timing of program, and their perceived need for the program.

Another evaluation question relates to client satisfaction with the program. Although these data are usually biased toward positive answers (Stipak, 1982), satisfaction will influence outcomes. However, results should be evaluated cautiously.

Another question relates to the compliance of clients to the program requirements. For example, are they attending classes or reading the materials distributed? If not, changes may need to be made in the methods used. Other questions related to different aspects of the program may need to be included depending on the specific program. The above is a sampling of relevant questions about program implementation methods.

PROGRAM OUTCOMES

An important area of evaluation involves the program's outcomes or whether or not it is having the effect it was supposed to have. Outcome variables may be difficult to identify because of the varying effects of the planned interventions. For example, a smoking cessation program for pregnant women may influence maternal knowledge, maternal smoking patterns, infant birth weight, or infant mortality, and the program's outcomes could include any of these variables. Various questions regarding the soundness of the scientific evidence generated, the needs of the program agency for the data, or the cost involved in using one outcome variable over another must be answered. Other aspects of program outcomes and some variables that may be used to measure outcomes are discussed next.

OUTCOME VARIABLES FOR MEASURING COMMUNITY CHANGE

Many of the interventions proposed for the advanced practice nurse involve changes for significant portions of the community when using a multilevel approach. Thus, measuring community change and the variables for looking at community outcome are important. Some of these are addressed below.

MULTILEVEL INTERVENTION EVALUATION

Thompson and Kinne (1990) propose the following areas for evaluation: (a) individual changes, (b) community subsystem changes, (c) community interrelationship changes, and (d) total community changes, such as changes in norm and values.

Individual changes can be evaluated through surveys to determine how much individuals were influenced by the interventions. These changes can be evaluated in terms of awareness of, knowledge about, and participation in the program, as well as any change (cognitive, psychomotor) in behavior noted.

Organizations and groups are useful subunits of the community for measuring outcome variables of change. Areas of change for evaluation include (a) policy changes related to the program, (b) organizational or group support for the program, (c) program participation, and (d) other activities showing involvement with the program.

Measuring changes in the interrelationships between community subsystems can be identified by the extent of change in community organizations' involvement with each other or their social connectedness. Areas of change include (a) coalition development, (b) participation in community boards and task forces by subsystems, and (c) involvement in communitywide activities by subsystems.

Whole-system outcomes can be assessed by changes in norms or values of the community. Areas of evaluation include (a) changes in community policies related to the program (e.g., smoking), (b) enforcement procedures in the community, (c) shifts in norms as perceived by the public from both an individual and a subsystem level, and (d) external changes, such as new state and national laws.

COMPONENTS OF EVALUATION

Components of evaluation include (a) relevance, or need for the program; (b) progress, or the evaluation of activities to meet the established objectives; (c) efficiency, or the outcomes of the program in relation to its cost; (d) effectiveness, or the program's ability to meet established objectives—the results of the program; and (e) impact, or the long-range changes seen in the program population (Kaluzny & Veney, 1991).

Relevance includes questions about the need for the program or activities. It is often more important to look at relevance of existing rather than of new programs. For example, often, a program such as a lead poison screening program is established as a result of an identified community need. Then, it may continue for years without evaluating its relevance. Thus, periodic evaluation of the need for the program or relevance is necessary. New programs may then be hampered because of staff or budgetary constraints. In such instances, resources from a program that is no longer relevant might be redirected to meet the new identified need. Some of these issues were discussed in the case study on economics in Chapter 3.

Progress involves the monitoring of program activities, such as the hours of service, numbers of providers used, the numbers of referrals made, or the expected numbers of clients participating in the program. This ongoing formative evaluation allows assessment of and appropriate changes in the day-to-day operation of the program.

Efficiency refers to the costs and benefits of the program. It determines if the program's benefits warrant the cost involved for staff, materials, and so forth. An important question related to efficiency is whether or not the program could have been provided as well for less cost involved.

Effectiveness refers to how well the program objectives were met and the degree of client and provider satisfaction. It answers questions about the satisfaction of clients with the program and provider satisfaction with client involvement and with the activities implemented. It is concerned about immediate, short-term, or formative evaluation. The reader is referred to the next section on outcome evaluation for additional information.

Impact evaluation is concerned with the long-term outcomes of the program. It looks at changes in behavior, changes in morbidity and mortality, and other changes resulting from the program.

OUTCOME EVALUATION

In addition to outcome variables just mentioned, several others are of importance. Two references on outcome evaluation that may be useful to the reader are Lorig et al. (1996) and Schalock (1995).

KNOWLEDGE

An important outcome variable is knowledge. Information alone may not change behavior, but it increases the possibility of change. For example, without a knowledge of nutrition, weight loss might not be possible. However, knowledge plus motivation and other factors may make weight loss possible. Often, before offering a health education program for a community population or aggregate, a pretest may be given to use as baseline data. Following the program or programs, a posttest can be compared with the pretest results.

BEHAVIORAL CHANGE OR SKILLS ACQUISITION

One outcome of health interventions is behavioral changes or skill acquisition. Many of the multilevel interventions discussed in Chapter 8 would be directed toward behavior changes. In these instances, the resource person is interested in the proportion of the population that changed its behavior as a result of the interventions provided. Answers can be obtained by surveys (questionnaires or interviews), although the data may not be completely accurate because of human error. Observations following surveys are costly and time consuming and therefore are not always practical.

When one performs actions consistent with current knowledge, the actions are considered to be skilled. One learns to prepare formula for the newborn, give injections to the diabetic, or prepare a diabetic diet. These skills may be taught in groups and may be evaluated by observation of return demonstrations.

ATTITUDES

Another outcome measure is a change in attitudes. Attitudes are opinions and preferences about ideas, people, and things. Attitudes may predispose individuals to choose one action over another and are thus of importance to nurses. For example, community attitudes that health promotion activities reduce the community's costs for sick care may influence the economic subsystem on behalf of prevention.

Attitudes about health and health behavior can be changed by planned experiences. Measuring these attitudes before and after a community intervention will determine the effectiveness of the program. Such attitudinal changes may be instrumental in bringing about behavior changes that influence a higher level of health.

HEALTH STATUS

A change in health status of the population is the goal of many interventions. Programs often attempt to influence the rates of premature deaths, disabilities, injuries, morbidity, or mortality. Some emphasis has been on positive health using measures such as the percentage of the population that practices safe sex, abstains from smoking, or exercises regularly. Several of the outcome measures in *Healthy People 2000* focus on such positive factors.

SELECTED METHODS FOR EVALUATING PROGRAMS

CASE STUDY

Case studies are one approach for evaluating the adequacy of the program. A case study can be started at any point in the implementation process. It focuses on program activities data obtained by observation, reviewing reports, interviewing personnel or clients using a structured or unstructured format, or using questionnaires.

This method is useful for answering questions of relevance. For example, by obtaining data from clients and providers, the evaluator can determine the degree to which the program is meeting a community need. It also addresses progress by observing program activities being offered and comparing them with those being planned. Cost-effectiveness is more difficult to evaluate with the case method approach.

SURVEYS

Surveys include self-administered questionnaires and personal interviews and are useful in describing (descriptive surveys) or analyzing relationships (analytic surveys). They may describe the need for the program, the program's activities, characteristics of attendees, or the outcome of the program (descriptive). Descriptive data can be used for analysis also. For example, descriptive data of age, race, and sex may be analyzed in relation to hypertension control.

Surveys are useful to answer questions about the need for the program or its relevance when perceptions of clients, providers, and managers are solicited. Progress can also be evaluated, but efficiency, effectiveness, and impact are more difficult to determine with surveys.

PROGRAM EVALUATION MONITORING

Several methods have been developed to monitor the progress of program activities or to determine how well the program sequence is following the established plan. Monitoring usually follows objectives arranged in a sequence with time specified for each activity to be completed. Examples of monitoring methods include the program evaluation review technique (PERT), discussed in Chapter 8. Other methods include the Gantt chart and critical path method.

Monitoring charts are especially useful for evaluating a program's progress because they identify whether or not the activities are on schedule and within an established budget. This method may also be used to measure efficiency of the program by establishing the cost of resources per client. The impact of the program or the relevance cannot be evaluated with this method.

EXPERIMENTAL EVALUATION STUDY

An experimental design may determine the impact of the program by determining whether or not it made a difference. This method determines the outcome of the program in terms of changes in health behavior, attitudes, morbidity and mortality, and so forth. Although there are problems in implementing an experimental design (randomization, control, and study groups) it is the best way to measure the impact or to obtain summative data. It is also a good method for evaluating the effectiveness of the program. It is not useful for evaluating progress or efficiency.

COST-EFFECTIVENESS ANALYSIS

With rising health care costs and efforts at all levels of government at cost containment, the cost-effectiveness of programs has become very important. Two of the common methods for determining costs and benefits of a program are cost-benefit analysis and cost-effectiveness analysis. Both methods identify all costs (direct and indirect) and the consequences (negative and positive) of a program. These methods differ in the value placed on the consequences of the program. In the cost-benefit analysis, the benefits of the program are valued in terms of dollars, which makes it possible to compare one project against another. This allows an evaluation of whether or not the benefits in dollars exceed the costs in dollars.

The costs and benefits in the cost-effectiveness analysis are not measured in dollars, making it more difficult to compare one program with another or to evaluate the benefits over the costs. Variables measured as outcomes, such as suicides or other morbidity and mortality conditions prevented, are not always amenable to dollar amounts. However, this method may be used satisfactorily to compare one program with another when goals and objectives are similar. For example, two programs for increasing exercise among adolescents may have the same outcome and only the cost of the programs may vary. This makes the cost-effectiveness analysis an appropriate way to evaluate the two programs. However, neither approach will evaluate relevance, progress, effectiveness, or impact of the program.

The choice between these approaches to cost-effectiveness depends on the programs being considered. Sources of additional information include Drummond (1980); Weinstein and Fineberg (1980); Yassi, Tate, and Cooper (1995); Oldenburg, Owen, and Parle (1995); and Farnham (1994). Yassi et al. (1995) ask questions about both the costs (input) and consequences (outcomes) of the intervention and evaluate the effectiveness of a 2-year pilot project of early interventions for back-injured nurses at a large tertiary hospital in Canada. Effectiveness was measured in terms of days lost from work. Oldenburg et al. (1995) discusses a comparison of two or more options of activities and compares the economics of four worksite cardiovascular risk factor interventions using health risk factor assessment, risk factor education, behavioral counseling, and behavioral counseling plus incentives. The study found that behavioral counseling created the most benefits at the least cost. Hui (1995) discusses cost minimization analysis, which is appropriate when the outcomes of alternatives are the same. In this method, the multiple options are compared at the same time and the least costly one is selected. For example, when considering the outcomes of elderly stroke patients placed in day hospitalization versus traditional medical management, cost factors may be compared. He found the day hospital to be less expensive and the outcomes of each option similar.

Cost-effectiveness can be calculated after program outcomes and costs are determined. For example, you carry out two weight loss programs, and in Program A the cost was $120,000 for 1,200 pounds lost, whereas Program B cost $150,000 for 1,300 pounds lost. Weight loss per pound in Program A equals $100 per pound lost, and in Program B, $115 per pound. Program A is less expensive per pound lost. The additional weight loss of 100 pounds for all participants in Program B costs $300 per pound (program costs $30,000 more than

Program A for 100 pounds more lost or $300 per pound over the initial 100 pounds lost).

OUTCOME VARIABLES USED IN SELECTED STUDIES

In an article on a school nurse prenatal counseling program, Chen, Fitzgerald, DeStefano, and Chen (1991) evaluated the adequacy of the program by counting the prenatal care visits that pregnant women made to physicians and the birth weight of their infants compared with a matched group. Adequacy of prenatal care was measured by number of prenatal visits to a physician adjusted for the trimester of the first visit and the gestational age at delivery and placed into categories of adequate, intermediate, or inadequate. Birth weight was measured as weight at birth as recorded on the birth certificate. It was found that a significantly higher percentage of women receiving prenatal counseling also received adequate prenatal care. This study shows outcome measures for an aggregate of prenatal women.

Cohen, Stunkard, Michael, and Felix (1986), in a study regarding community change in disease prevention and health promotion, used a community resource inventory to measure changes in community health activities. This was completed by all organizations within a geographical area prior to the intervention and 3 years after. Data were compared with a matched control group. More than 300 organizations were used. The emphasis was on mobilizing organizations for risk factor reductions.

The community resource inventory included five risk factors for cardiovascular disease, including smoking, hypertension, physical inactivity, elevated levels of low-density lipoprotein cholesterol, and being overweight. Interventions were carried out by mass media initially and later in worksites, in the health sector, voluntary organizations, and schools.

Surveys included five types of data about health promotion activities:

1. Background data about population served, members in the organization, frequency of meetings, formal communication lines, and the presence or absence of a special person for health matters in the organization
2. The type of risk reduction activities over the past year for each of the five factors (programs such as films, literature distribution, speakers, seminars, newsletters, screenings, exercise classes)
3. Characteristics of the activities, such as frequency of activities and number of employees attending or reached
4. Interest in and future plans regarding risk reduction activities
5. Involvement in health promotion networks and the names of organizations included in the planning of risk reduction activities for next year.

Results showed an increase in health promotion activities in the organizations in the experimental county. The authors concluded that the community resource inventory is a good method for measuring community change when there is a long time between program initiation and outcome measurement.

Livingood, Woodhouse, and Natale (1991) report on a substance abuse prevention and intervention project (ALERT) by a coalition of funding agencies and service providers. Their objectives were stated in terms of numbers and types of projected services, and the outcomes were the number of programs conducted or numbers of participants in the programs compared with the projected number. For example, they predicted 8 to 10 professional workshops for professionals, and that was obtained. They predicted 36 courses for children with 288 children attending, and that was not attained. Other projections and their outcome were identified.

They also used qualitative data (summative and formative) to evaluate progress from in-depth interviews, monthly reports, and meeting minutes. They looked at the accomplishments of ALERT within the stated purposes and found that all had worked toward the mission of awareness and coordination to increase community understanding about substance abuse and to expand efforts to prevent and reduce substance abuse in the area.

Poland, Giblin, Waller, and Hankin (1992) report on the effect of a home visiting program on prenatal care and birth weight. They matched a sample of pregnant women visited by trained paraprofessionals with a sample who were not visited at home. Their evaluation criteria were the number of prenatal visits and the infant birth weights in the two groups. Women followed by the paraprofessionals had significantly more prenatal appointments and infants with average higher birth weights than those who were not visited.

Pearson and Theis (1991) present a comprehensive evaluation model used in a community-based respite care program. The plan considered three aspects, including the context of the program, the process used to meet the objectives, and the program outcomes. A model from Holzemer (1976) was used in which input evaluation involved the context into which the program was placed and looked at areas such as the existing philosophies of the organizations, the type of community in which the program was carried out, and the program objectives. Process evaluation included program activities, such as the time frame of the program and the clients to be seen (variety, number, services used, and staff-client interactions). Program outcomes were the goals of the program and included satisfaction of caregivers with the respite care and the impact of care on the caregivers' burden and quality of life.

REFERENCES

Chen, S., Fitzgerald, M., DeStefano, L., & Chen, E. (1991). Effects of a school nurse prenatal counseling program. *Public Health Nursing, 8*(4), 212-218.

Cohen, R. Y., Stunkard, A., Michael, R., & Felix, B. (1986). Measuring community change in disease prevention and health promotion. *Preventive Medicine, 15,* 411-421.

Donabedian, A. (1966). Evaluating the quality of medical care. *Milbank Quarterly, 44,* 166-206.

Drummond, M. F. (1980). *Methods for the economic evaluation of health care programmes.* New York: Oxford Medical.

Farnham, P. G. (1994). Defining and measuring the costs of the HIV epidemic to business firms. *Public Health Reports, 109,* 311-318.

Holzemer, W. (1976). A protocal for program evaluation. *Journal of Medical Education, 51*(2), 101-108.

Hui, J. (1995). Outcomes of elderly stroke patients: Day hospital versus conventional medical management. *Stroke, 26,* 1616-1619.

Kaluzny, A., & Veney, J. (1991). Evaluating health care programs and services. In S. Williams & P. Torrens (Eds.), *Introduction to health services.* New York: John Wiley.

Livingood, W. C., Woodhouse, L. D., & Natale, J. (1991). The ALERT partnership evaluation: Enhancing health program evaluation with qualitative techniques. *Family and Community Health, 14*(1), 28-35.

Lorig, K., Stewart, A., Ritter, P., Gonzalez, V., Laurent, D., & Lynch, J. (1996). *Outcome measures for health education and other health care interventions.* Thousand Oaks, CA: Sage.

Oldenburg, B., Owen, N., & Parle, M. (1995). An economic evaluation of four worksite based cardiovascular risk factor interventions. *Health Education Quarterly, 22,* 9-19.

Patton, M. Q. (1986). *Utilization-focused evaluation* (2nd ed.). Beverly Hills, CA: Sage.

Pearson, M., & Theis, S. (1991). Program evaluation application of a comprehensive model for a community-based respite program. *Journal of Community Health, 8*(1), 25-31.

Poland, M., Giblin, P., Waller, J., & Hankin, J. (1992). Effect of a home visiting program on prenatal care and birthweight: A case comparison study. *Journal of Community Health, 17*(4), 221-229.

Posavac, E. J., & Carey, R. G. (1989). *Program evaluation: Methods and case studies.* Englewood Cliffs, NJ: Prentice Hall.

Schalock, R. L. (1995). *Outcome-based evaluation.* New York: Plenum.

Stipak, B. (1982). Using clients to evaluate programs. In E. R. House (Ed.), *Evaluation studies review annual* (pp. 585-602). Beverly Hills, CA: Sage.

Thompson, B., & Kinne, S. (1990). Social change theory: Applications to community health. In N. Bracht (Ed.), *Health promotion at the community level.* Newbury Park, CA: Sage.

Tinkham, C. W., Voorhies, E. F., & McCarthy, N. C. (1984). *Community health nursing: Evolution and process* (3rd ed.). New York: Appleton-Century-Crofts.

U.S. Department of Health and Human Services. (1991). *Healthy people 2000: The surgeon general's report on health promotion and disease prevention* (DHHS Publication No. 91-50212). Washington, DC: U.S. Public Health Service.

Veney, J., & Kaluzny, A. (1991). *Evaluation and decision making for health service programs.* Englewood Cliffs, NJ: Prentice Hall.

Weinstein, M., & Fineberg, H. (1980). *Clinical decision analysis.* Philadelphia: W. B. Saunders.

Yassi, A., Tate, R., & Cooper, J. E. (1995). Early intervention for back-injured nurses at a large Canadian tertiary care hospital: An evaluation of the effectiveness and cost-benefits of a two-year pilot project. *Occupational Medicine, 45,* 209-214.

A P P E N D I X

COMMUNITY ASSESSMENT TOOL

ECONOMIC SUBSYSTEM

EMPLOYMENT DISTRIBUTION

	Number in Community	Percentage of Population
Employed persons		
Manufacturing		
White-collar		
Wholesale and retail		
Local government		
Federal government		
Unemployed persons		

LEADING INDUSTRIES

Name _____   Address _____

Number of employees _____   Manager _____

FAMILY INCOME

	Median income	Community	State	Nation
	Under $3,000			
Percentage of population	$3,000 to $5,999			
	$6,000-$9,999			
	$10,000+			

GOVERNMENTAL BUDGET

	Community Total in Dollars	Percentage of Total
Education	_____	_____
Transportation	_____	_____
Welfare	_____	_____
Health	_____	_____
Police	_____	_____
Fire	_____	_____

EDUCATIONAL SUBSYSTEM

NUMBER OF EDUCATIONAL FACILITIES

	Public	Private
Total	_____	_____
Elementary	_____	_____
Junior high	_____	_____
Senior high	_____	_____
Junior college	_____	_____
Colleges	_____	_____
Special schools	_____	_____

HEALTH COVERAGE

Adequate _____   Inadequate _____

Discuss _____

_____

EDUCATION LEVEL OF POPULATION

	Community	State	Nation
Less than 5 years	_____	_____	_____
High school graduate	_____	_____	_____
Some college	_____	_____	_____
College graduate	_____	_____	_____
Median school completed	_____	_____	_____
Currently	_____	_____	_____

HEALTH MANPOWER FACILITIES

	Number	Number Graduated Yearly
Total	_____	_____
Medical schools	_____	_____
Nursing schools	_____	_____
Dental schools	_____	_____
Physical therapy	_____	_____
Social workers	_____	_____

COMMUNICATIONS SUBSYSTEM

NEWSPAPERS

Name	Frequency	Circulation
_____	_____	_____
_____	_____	_____
_____	_____	_____

RADIO STATIONS

Name	Address	Audiences (number, kind— young/old, black/white, social class)
_____	_____	_____
_____	_____	_____
_____	_____	_____

TELEVISION STATIONS

Name	Address	Audiences
_____	_____	_____
_____	_____	_____
_____	_____	_____
_____	_____	_____

KEY COMMUNITY LEADERS/DECISION MAKERS INFLUENCING SUBSYSTEM

Name	Affiliation
_____	_____
_____	_____
_____	_____

If inadequate, list media as follows with deficits.

Name   *Deficits*

_____   _____

_____   _____

_____   _____

QUALITY

Good _____   Poor _____

If poor, list media below with deficits.

Name   *Deficits*

_____   _____

_____   _____

_____   _____

Is there a speakers bureau for health subjects?

Yes _____   No _____

List community organizations that have active health programs for the public.

Agency	*Type of Program*	*Qualified Personnel*	
		Yes	*No*
_____	_____	_____	_____
_____	_____	_____	_____
_____	_____	_____	_____

HEALTH MATERIALS IN SCHOOLS

Is health integrated into the school curriculum at all grades?

Yes _____   No _____

If no, discuss deficits. _____

_____

_____

Discuss areas of health covered by grade levels. _____

_____

_____

Is the information adequately covered?

Yes _____   No _____

POLITICAL SUBSYSTEM

POLITICAL PARTIES AND LEADERSHIP

Major party _____

Key leaders _____

Minor party _____

Key leaders _____

MAJOR ISSUES OVER LAST 5 YEARS THAT INFLUENCE HEALTH

	Yes	No	Party Favoring	Implemented
Housing	_____	_____	_____	_____
Transportation	_____	_____	_____	_____
Health facilities	_____	_____	_____	_____
Water, sewage	_____	_____	_____	_____
Immunizations	_____	_____	_____	_____
Fluoridation	_____	_____	_____	_____
Communications	_____	_____	_____	_____

RECREATION SUBSYSTEM

NUMBER AND LOCATION

	Total Number	Public	Private
Central	_____	_____	_____
North	_____	_____	_____
East	_____	_____	_____
South	_____	_____	_____
West	_____	_____	_____

LEADERSHIP AVAILABLE DURING RECREATION

	Area	Type of Leadership
1.	_____	_____
2.	_____	_____
3.	_____	_____
4.	_____	_____

HAZARDOUS SITUATIONS

Yes _____   No _____

Describe _____

_____

RELIGIOUS SUBSYSTEM

RELIGIOUS DISTRIBUTION

	Community Total Number	*Percentage of Total*
Protestant	_____	_____
Catholic	_____	_____
Jewish	_____	_____
Other	_____	_____

KEY LEADERS IN RELIGION (LIST)

Names	*Phone Number or Address*
_____	_____
_____	_____
_____	_____

TRANSPORTATION SUBSYSTEM

ROUTES AND SERVICES

Describe major transportation routes. _____

_____

Services available on these routes (buses, trains) _____

FUTURE PLANS

_____

_____

Transportation and health services _____

_____

Are transportation routes adequate for population getting to health facilities?   Yes _____   No _____

If no, discuss specific deficits. _____

_____

WELFARE SUBSYSTEM

AGENCIES

List agencies, location, area served, and service.

.

_____

_____

_____

Are these services adequate to meet population needs?

Adequate _____   Inadequate _____

If inadequate, discuss agency and inadequacies.

_____

_____

_____

POPULATION SUBSYSTEM

POPULATION CHARACTERISTICS

Population at last census _____

Population density _____

Population changes over 10-year period _____

Age distribution _____

_____

Age Group	Community _Current Percentage of Population_		State _Percentage of National Population_	
	Total	_10 Years Ago_	_Total Pop._	_% of Total %_
1-4	_____	_____	_____	_____
5-14	_____	_____	_____	_____
15-24	_____	_____	_____	_____
25-34	_____	_____	_____	_____
35-44	_____	_____	_____	_____
45-54	_____	_____	_____	_____
55-64	_____	_____	_____	_____
65+	_____	_____	_____	_____

SEX AND RACE DISTRIBUTION

Category		Community		State	Nation
Race	Sex	Current No./%	10 Years Ago No./%	Current No./%	Current No./%
White	Male	_____	_____	_____	_____
	Female	_____	_____	_____	_____
Nonwhite	Male	_____	_____	_____	_____
	Female	_____	_____	_____	_____

VITAL STATISTICS

Category	Community Current No./Rate	State 10 Years Ago No./Rate	Nation No./Rate
Live birth	_____	_____	_____
Neonatal death	_____	_____	_____
Infant death	_____	_____	_____
Maternal death	_____	_____	_____
General death	_____	_____	_____

SOCIAL PROBLEMS

Problem	Number	Percentage of Total
Illegitimate births	_____	_____
Venereal diseases	_____	_____
Syphilis	_____	_____
Gonorrhea	_____	_____
Narcotic users	_____	_____
Suicide	_____	_____
Alcoholism	_____	_____
Health problems	_____	_____

COMMUNICABLE DISEASE INCIDENCE

Disease	Current Year	5 Years Ago
Diphtheria	_____	_____
Encephalitis	_____	_____

Infectious hepatitis   _____   _____

Influenza   _____   _____

Measles   _____   _____

Tetanus   _____   _____

Tuberculosis   _____   _____

Typhoid   _____   _____

Other   _____   _____

Immunization level for acute communicable disease

	Percentage Immunized by Age			
Disease	Under 1	1-5	6-15	Over 15
Diphtheria				
Poliomyelitis				
Smallpox				
Tetanus				
Measles				
Whooping cough				

LEADING CAUSES OF DEATH

	Community		State		Nation	
Cause of Death	Number	Rate	Number	Rate	Number	Rate
1.						
2.						
3.						
4.						
5.						
6.						
7.						
8.						
9.						
10.						

HEALTH SUBSYSTEM

Hospital Services	Bed Capacity	Adequate	Inadequate
Medical	_____	_____	_____
Surgical	_____	_____	_____
Maternity	_____	_____	_____
Psychiatric	_____	_____	_____
Communicable disease	_____	_____	_____
Pediatric	_____	_____	_____
Rehabilitation	_____	_____	_____
Chronic disease	_____	_____	_____
Nursing home services:		Adequate _____	Inadequate _____
Ambulatory services:		Adequate _____	Inadequate _____
Occupational health services:		Adequate _____	Inadequate _____
School health services:		Adequate _____	Inadequate _____
Health Department services:		Adequate _____	Inadequate _____

Discuss any inadequacies _____

_____

_____

HEALTH PERSONNEL

Category	Budgeted Positions	Percentage Unfilled
Physicians	_____	_____
Nurses	_____	_____
Social workers	_____	_____
Psychologists	_____	_____
Aides	_____	_____
Sanitarians	_____	_____
Physical therapists	_____	_____
Other	_____	_____

	Community Health Nursing Agencies	Community Health Nursing Services
Name	_____	_____
Address	_____	_____
Purpose	_____	_____
Accredited	Yes _____ No _____	

SERVICES PROVIDED

Total number of clients seen in home _____

Percentage of these for home care _____

Types of services in home

Category	Number of Cases	Number of Visits	Percentage of Total
Cancer	_____	_____	_____
Heart disease	_____	_____	_____
Diabetes	_____	_____	_____
Tuberculosis	_____	_____	_____
Venereal disease	_____	_____	_____
Other diseases	_____	_____	_____
Maternity	_____	_____	_____
Infant	_____	_____	_____
Preschool	_____	_____	_____
School age	_____	_____	_____
Adult	_____	_____	_____

Clinic services

Type	Monthly Attendance	Purpose
_____	_____	_____
_____	_____	_____
_____	_____	_____

School services

Type	Monthly Visits to Nurse	Purpose
_____	_____	_____
_____	_____	_____
_____	_____	_____

PROTECTION

Fire protection: Adequate _____   Inadequate _____

    If inadequate, describe: _____

Police protection: Adequate _____   Inadequate _____

    If inadequate, describe: _____

Health services: Adequate _____   Inadequate _____

    If inadequate, describe: _____

Environmental services: Adequate _____   Inadequate _____

    If inadequate, describe: _____

Transportation services: Adequate _____   Inadequate _____

    If inadequate, describe: _____

Hospital services: Adequate _____   Inadequate _____

    If inadequate, describe: _____

Disaster services: Adequate _____   Inadequate _____

    If inadequate, describe: _____

Educational services: Adequate _____   Inadequate _____

    If inadequate, describe: _____

Exchanges With Nonhuman Environment

HOUSING CONDITION

Type of Dwelling	Good		Fair		Poor*	
	Number	Percentage	Number	Percentage	Number	Percentage
_____	____	____	____	____	____	____
_____	____	____	____	____	____	____
_____	____	____	____	____	____	____
_____	____	____	____	____	____	____

*Substandard Housing

HOUSING COMPLAINTS (NUMBERS)

Problem	Current Year	5 Years Ago
Heating	_____	_____
Lighting	_____	_____

Ventilation	_____	_____
Nuisances	_____	_____
Other	_____	_____

SANITATION

AIR CONTAMINANTS THAT ARE SOURCE OF COMPLAINTS

Smoke	Yes _____	No _____	Specify: _____
Gases	Yes _____	No _____	Specify: _____
Odors	Yes _____	No _____	Specify: _____
Vapors	Yes _____	No _____	Specify: _____
Pollens	Yes _____	No _____	Specify: _____
Others	Yes _____	No _____	Specify: _____

Sources of air contaminants

Industry	Yes _____	No _____
Vehicles	Yes _____	No _____
Homes	Yes _____	No _____
Incinerators	Yes _____	No _____
Other (Specify)	Yes _____	No _____

WATER SUPPLY

Source	Number	Percentage	Percentage With Adequate Treatment
Public	_____	_____	_____
Private	_____	_____	_____

SEWAGE DISPOSAL

Source	Number	Percentage	Percentage With Adequate Treatment
Public	_____	_____	_____
Private	_____	_____	_____

SOLID WASTE DISPOSAL

Adequate _____   Inadequate _____

VECTOR CONTROL PROGRAM

Program	Adequate	Inadequate
Mosquitoes	_____	_____
Insects	_____	_____
Rodents	_____	_____
Other (Specify)	_____	_____

Food and milk

Food source	Adequate	Inadequate
Restaurants	_____	_____
Stores	_____	_____

Exchanges Beyond the Community

HEALTH THREATS

Present _____ Absent _____

If present, describe. _____

_____

Programs to reduce threat _____

_____

HEALTH RESOURCES

List available sources.

Personnel _____

_____

Money _____

_____

SOURCE: *Community Health Nursing: Theory and Practice* by Carl O. Helvie. Copyright 1991, by Springer Publishing Co. Used by permission.

Index

Ganz, B., 378
Gariota, M., 380
Gelles, R., 115
Gender differences:
    in homeless population, 147, 150-153
    in rural health practice roles, 410-411, 416
    in STDs, 384
Gibbons, W., 89
Giblin, P., 433
Giger, J., 137
Ginsburg, E., 66
Glick, D. F., 394
Goeppinger, J., 275, 380, 417
Golden, K., 381
Goldfarb, R., 143, 144
Goldstein, M., 96, 154
Gonzalez, V., 428
Goode, W., 139
Goodman, R., 268, 269, 270
Goodwin, J. M., 246
Goodwin, J. S., 246
Goodwin, R. M., 275
Gordon, M. S., 169, 170, 225
Gordon, W., 128
Gottlieb, N., 263, 264
Grady, D., 115
Graubarth, R. P., 410
Gravely, E., 65
Greenberg, G., 58, 59, 62, 63, 64
Greene County School Health Cottage (Virginia),
    399-402
Greenfield, L. J., 149
Green, L., 139
Green, L. W., 247, 263, 264
Greenspan, B., 381
Grimm, R., 248, 249
Gruder, C., 304
Guerra, F., 71, 379, 381
Guided mastery strategy, innovation adoption
    facilitation through, 265
Gunning's Fog Index, 299
Gustafson, D. H., 247

Haan, M., 132, 143
Hacker, K., 389
Hale, J., 291
Hale, P. J., 394
Haley, N., 261, 262
Halfon, N., 139
Hall, J., 114
Hamburg, J., 148
Hamlin, R. H., 175
Hammond, J., 131
Hammond, K., 295
Hanchett, E., 169, 173
Handler, A. O., 131
Hankin, J., 433

Hanley, C. E., 131
Hanlon, J., 240, 255
Hanlon's model, of community intervention planning,
    240
Hanmer, M., 114
Hanson, C., 408, 411, 412, 413
Hardin, E., 381
Hardy, M. A., 376
Harlan, C., 143, 144
Harris, L., 137
Harrison, M. J., 224
Hartnagle, W., 392
Harton, M., 225
Harton, M. K., 169
Haskell, W., 303
Hate crimes, 114
Havelock, R., 263
Hayes, C., 384
Head Start, 145
Health belief model, of health education, 290
Health care costs. *See* Assessment of community,
    economic forces influencing
Health care reform. *See* Assessment of community,
    economic forces influencing
Health, Culture and Community (Paul), 132
Health education:
    in care provider role, 10, 16
    case study in, 313-318
    community assessment and, 33, 75
    effectiveness guidelines for, 299-301
    health belief model used in, 290
    mass media sources used in, 301-302, 313-318
    media advocacy and, 303
    multiple vs. single approaches to, 302-303
    planning process of, 298-399
    of professionals, 350
    by school nurse, 389
Health Information Center, 142
Health insurance purchasing cooperatives (HIPCs), 68
Health Maintenance Organizations (HMOs), 62, 64-65
Health patterns model, of community assessment,
    169-170
Health process:
    assistance needs and, 44
    homeless population and, 151-153
    preventive intervention model and, 17-18, 48, 49
Health promotion activities, 17
Health of Regionville (Koos), 141
Health subsystem, 127
    case examples of, 34-35, 203-204
    checks and balances to, 35, 46
    external energy exchanges of, 34-35, 37, 38
    information exchange and, 34-35
    internal energy exchanges of, 31-32
    population exchange and, 32, 33
    Rudyville community example of, 192-193, 220,
        221, 231
    secondary data sources on, 164

ABOUT THE AUTHOR

Carl O. Helvie is Professor of Nursing at Old Dominion University in Norfolk, Virginia, where he teaches community health nursing at the undergraduate and graduate levels. He also teaches an elective course on the homeless that is televised throughout Virginia. He began his nursing career more than 45 years ago in upstate New York at St. Lawrence State Hospital, School of Nursing. Later, he received a BS degree in nursing from New York University and an MS and post-master's degree in public health nursing from the University of California, San Francisco. After teaching at the University of California, he returned to school and obtained an MPH and DrPH with a major in mental health from Johns Hopkins University, School of Public Health. He has published numerous articles in nursing and health journals and has presented research papers nationally and internationally. Previous publications include two undergraduate community health nursing texts and a review book. He is currently under contract to coauthor a book on the homeless with his colleague Wilfried Kunstmann in Germany. He is also an associate editor for *Alternative Health Practitioner* and a manuscript reviewer for *Public Health Nursing*. He has been very active in professional organizations and has held numerous positions at local and state levels of the Virginia Nurses Association. He was also vice president of the Virginia League for Nursing and is currently Chair of Awards for Public Health Nursing of the American Public Health Association (APHA) and co-caucus representative to APHA from the Homeless Caucus.

ABOUT THE CONTRIBUTORS

Jacqueline Agnew, PhD, is Associate Professor of Environmental Health Sciences and Director of the Occupational Health Nursing Program at the Johns Hopkins School of Hygiene and Public Health in Baltimore, Maryland. She is Deputy Director of the Johns Hopkins Educational Resource Center, funded by the National Institute for Occupational Safety and Health (NIOSH) to prepare occupational health professionals. Her research focuses on occupational stress, ergonomic factors in the workplace, and the interactive effects of work exposures and age on the health of older workers. She is a member of the NIOSH Board of Scientific Counselors and also serves on the Workers' Family Protection Task Force.

Janie Canty-Mitchell earned a diploma in nursing from Lincoln Hospital School of Nursing, Durham, North Carolina, a BSN degree from Florida State University, and MSN and PhD degrees from the University of Miami. She was awarded a 2-year postdoctoral research fellowship at Indiana University School of Nursing in 1994. Her work in community health nursing spans 17 years, including work as a public health nurse, supervisor of public health nursing, assistant community health nursing director, and community health nursing university professor. Her nursing research has centered on stress, caring, and hope in inner-city adolescents. She was awarded a grant from the Agency for Health Care Policy and Research to conduct her dissertation research. She is a member of Sigma Theta Tau Nursing Sorority, the American Public Health Association, and the Midwest Nursing Research Society. She has numerous experiences working with youth and voluntary agencies in inner cities.

Barrie Carveth, RN, MSN, FNP, is former Instructor of Nursing at the University of Virginia and is case manager, Westhaven Nursing Clinic, Charlottesville, Virginia.

Jeri W. Dunkin received her PhD in nursing at the University of Texas, Austin, in 1988. She spent several years with the University of North Dakota, where she was director of the graduate Rural Health Nursing Specialization in the College of Nursing. At the same time, she served as chair of the Nursing Research Division at the University of North Dakota Rural Health Research Center. She is currently the Coordinator for the Center of Nursing Research, Medical College of Georgia School Nursing.

Christine Elnitsky is a doctoral student in urban health services at Old Dominion University in Norfolk, Virginia. She holds an MSN (community health nurse specialist) and a BSN from Old Dominion University. Her nursing education began with a vocational nursing program at Harris Hospital School of Nursing in Fort Worth, Texas. Her 20 years of nursing experience in community health and hospital nursing includes clinical, administration, teaching, and research activities. She participates in research and is published in the areas of health care delivery systems, outcomes, chronic illness, health policy, and older adults.

Sandra L. Ferketich, PhD, RN, FAAN, currently Professor at the University of Arizona College of Nursing, received a BSN from the University of New Mexico, an MS from Indiana University, and a PhD from the University of Arizona. She recently completed a year of analyzing health policy as a Fellow with the Institute of Medicine. Her publications and research have been on research methods, instrumentation, maternal role attainment, family functioning, childbearing, and nursing interventions with homeless persons on preventive therapy for tuberculosis and rural communities in partnership with community health nurses and lay health workers.

Sharon Garrett earned a BSN degree from the University of Wisconsin—Madison and is currently an MSN candidate at Indiana University School of Nursing—Indianapolis. She has been involved in diverse communities in a professional and volunteer capacity for more than 25 years. Her professional experience includes work as a staff nurse and head nurse at a major hospital, home health nurse, health services coordinator for a Head Start program, an instructor for a continuing education program, and a research and teaching assistant. Her accomplishments include developing a health curriculum for a Head Start program, coordinating a community bloodmobile, and cochairing a community television telethon that focused on alcohol and drug abuse. She received a good citizen award from a Wisconsin city for her community contributions. She has worked extensively with young adolescents and parents.

Laurel S. Garzon, PhD, is Associate Professor in the Advanced Perinatal/Neonatal Graduate Program at Old Dominion University School of Nursing in Norfolk, Virginia. She has participated in community empowerment projects involving women's health and adolescent parents. She is a graduate of the University of North Carolina at Chapel Hill, the University of Virginia, and the Catholic University of America.

Doris Glick, RN, PhD, is Associate Professor of Nursing and Director, Primary Care Nursing Center, the University of Virginia.

Bethany Hall-Long, PhD, RNC, is Assistant Professor in the College of Nursing at the University of Delaware. Her areas of undergraduate and graduate didactic and clinical teaching are community health nursing, health policy, and nursing theory. She has worked as a nurse educator, manager, recruiter, and clinician in a variety of acute care and public health settings. Her areas of scholarship and clinical expertise are community health nursing, community development, health policy, and multicultural women's health. She is a member of numerous professional and civic organizations.

Clare Houseman, PhD, RN, CS, is the Health Services Concentration Area Director for the PhD in Urban Services Program at Old Dominion University. She is also a Certified Clinical Nurse Specialist in Adult Psychiatric and Mental Health Nursing and maintains a part-time psychotherapy practice. She was a member of the HB1024 task force and at one point chaired the group. She also served as a consultant to the Virginia State Board of Nursing regarding the credentialing of clinical nurse specialists in the state. She is editor and author of a text titled *Psychiatric Certification Review Guide for the Generalist and Clinical Specialist in Adult, Child, and Adolescent Mental Health Nursing* (1994).

Kathleen M. May, DNSc, RN, currently Associate Professor at the University of Arizona College of Nursing, received a BSN from Saint John College of Cleveland, an MS from the University of Colorado, and a DNSc from the University of California, San Francisco. She has practiced nursing in hospital settings, home health, and public health. Her publications and research have been on community health nursing and nursing interventions with homeless persons on preventive therapy for tuberculosis, older rural elderly receiving health peer teaching on health promotion, and rural communities in partnership with community health nurses and lay health workers.

Sonda Riedesel Oppewal, PhD, is Associate Professor in the College of Nursing at East Tennessee State University in Johnson City, Tennessee. She teaches community health nursing and is Project Director of a federally funded school-based health center located in a rural high school. Her current research interests include adolescent health, rural health, and the diffusion of innovations.

Anna L. Pratt, RN, MSN, is currently Nursing Supervisor with the Virginia Beach Department of Public Health. A graduate of Hartwick College (1970, BSN) and the University of Rhode Island (1978, MSNEd), she has practiced community health nursing for 26 years. Her experience includes traditional home-based nursing care as well as various services provided in a public health clinic setting. Currently, she supervises a self-directed team of public health nurses and health educators whose focus is to provide health promotion and risk reduction education to residents in a wide variety of community settings. She also has adjunct faculty status with Old Dominion University's School of Nursing and is an active volunteer with the American Cancer Society in Virginia Beach, serving on its executive board of directors.

Angela B. Savage, RN, BSN, is currently Nurse Manager with the Virginia Beach Department of Public Health. A graduate of the University of Virginia (1969, BSN), she has 27 years of experience in community health nursing. She has provided home-based nursing care as well as maternal and child health and communicable disease services in public health clinics. Her career in middle- and upper-level management in public health spans more than 20 years. She is on the board of directors of a private, community-based clinic that provides free primary care to indigent residents of the city.

Sherry Weinstein, MN, CPNP, is former Instructor of Nursing at the University of Virginia and school nurse practitioner, Greene County (Virginia) School Health Cottage.

Cynthia Westley, RN, MSN, ANP, is Instructor of Nursing at the University of Virginia and care manager, Crescent Hall Nursing Clinic, Charlottesville, Virgina.